Pain in Childbearing and its Control

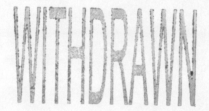

Pain in Childbearing and its Control

Rosemary Mander

MSc, PhD, RGN, SCM, MTD
Senior Lecturer
Department of Nursing Studies
University of Edinburgh

**Blackwell
Science**

© 1998 by
Blackwell Science Ltd
Editorial Offices:
Osney Mead, Oxford OX2 0EL
25 John Street, London WC1N 2BL
23 Ainslie Place, Edinburgh EH3 6AJ
350 Main Street, Malden
    MA 02148 5018, USA
54 University Street, Carlton
    Victoria 3053, Australia
10, rue Casimir Delavigne
    75006 Paris, France

Other Editorial Offices:

Blackwell Wissenschafts-Verlag GmbH
Kurfürstendamm 57
10707 Berlin, Germany

Zehetnergasse 6
1140 Wien, Austria

Blackwell Science KK
MG Kodenmacho Building
7–10 Kodenmacho Nihombashi
Chuo-ku, Tokyo 104, Japan

The right of the Author to be identified as the
Author of this Work has been asserted in
accordance with the Copyright, Designs and
Patents Act 1988.

First published 1998

Set in 10/12pt Souvenir Light
by DP Photosetting, Aylesbury, Bucks
Printed and bound in Great Britain by
MPG Books Ltd, Bodmin, Cornwall

The Blackwell Science logo is a trade mark of
Blackwell Science Ltd, registered at the United
Kingdom Trade Marks Registry

DISTRIBUTORS

Marston Book Services Ltd
PO Box 269
Abingdon
Oxon OX14 4YN
(*Orders:* Tel: 01235 465500
        Fax: 01235 465555)

USA
Blackwell Science, Inc.
Commerce Place
350 Main Street
Malden, MA 02148 5018
(*Orders:* Tel: 800 759 6102
                781 388 8250
        Fax: 781 388 8255)

Canada
Login Brothers Book Company
324 Saulteaux Crescent
Winnipeg, Manitoba R3J 3T2
(*Orders:* Tel: 204 224-4068)

Australia
Blackwell Science Pty Ltd
54 University Street
Carlton, Victoria 3053
(*Orders:* Tel: 03 9347 0300
        Fax: 03 9347 5001)

A catalogue record for this title
is available from the British Library

ISBN 0-632-04097-1

Library of Congress
Cataloging-in-Publication Data is available

Contents

Foreword

This book is distinguished from the burgeoning mass of publications on pain management. The very word 'management' grates in my ears and those of Dr Mander because it implies a distinct authoritarian manager who fixes the patients' problems willy-nilly from the manager's superior position of experience and knowledge.

From the beginning Dr Mander distinguishes between private suffering and public display. We all know what that difference is when we are ourselves in pain and yet it is peculiarly difficult to separate in other people. Grantly Dick-Read starts his seminal book *Natural Childbirth* in 1933 with an account of his witnessing calm unworried childbirth by women in Northern Kenya. He concludes that this is true natural childbirth which anyone could achieve free of fear, anxiety and tension. Fifty years later, a woman anthropologist who was familiar with the Tulkarm and could speak their language witnessed childbirth of the stoical variety described by Dick-Read. After the delivery, she asked the mother if she had been in pain. The mother replied that the pain had been intense. The anthropologist then asked why she had not complained and received the reply that it was not the custom of her people. It is apparent that the very concept of an idealised 'natural childbirth' had its origin in the mind of a white colonial doctor distanced from the world of the indigenous folk he managed.

It is evidently hugely difficult to penetrate the private world of individuals embedded in the powerful culture of their surround, especially when the observer is necessarily separated by experience, culture and learning and by the fact that the observer is 'in charge'. Patient and carer each have their expectations and they rarely match. Even answering a questionnaire intended to reveal private suffering is itself a form of public display by the one who suffers and attempts to satisfy the expectations of the expert. Mrs Eleanor Roosevelt wrote in her autobiography 'I was brought up in the type of household where one did not have a headache when guests were expected'. It is not possible to unravel from this sentence whether she did or did not have headaches. While at any one instant it might be possible to define separately the private and public components of pain, they undoubtedly feed back on each other and change with time. The mother during a contraction, between contractions, and her memory of both make up three different people, each equally important and a challenge to those who care for her.

Many years ago as a guest in China, the most important sentence I heard was 'We recruit the patients to be members of their own treatment team'. It was true. They did just that in an atmosphere far removed from the hurly-burly of what we are pleased to call modern medicine. Patients were admitted days and weeks before their operations. Apart from their widely spaced tests, they fed post-operative patients their meals, changed the beds, swept the floors and became familiar members of a task-oriented community. One saw them on the morning of their operation as fully qualified patients chatting with the staff with realistic expectations and familiarity.

Idealistic as this situation may seem, I do not believe that it is necessarily the optimum we should seek. I witnessed the easy confidence of some patients collapse when the unexpected event overwhelmed them. To treat the patient as an equal is surely a good start point, but the therapist's own greater experience, and consequent convictions about fact or fiction, cannot be ignored. Furthermore we are all familiar with the patient who refuses to become 'a member of their own treatment team' and insists on authoritative direction. The wonderful quotation from Willian Smellie that 'the mother should consult her own ease' is not possible for some mothers in our culture.

All therapists differ from almost all of their patients by virtue of their training and experience, they are thereby duty bound to question if their opinions are based on fact or fiction. I found the best part of this excellent book to be the insistence on questioning. The author exposes the fact that the great majority of procedures are untested and have simply crept in as common practice. Thoughtful questioning is crucial if authority is to be justified. I understand and regret the all too common attitude that research is for others and is generally a waste of time and no substitute for intuition acquired by experience. Furthermore I understand the threat of research done by others who intrude on the morale of understaffed harassed groups who are just getting on with their job. It is not enough to transfer decision-making to the patient, even as a participating member of the treatment team, if the therapist is not clear about the justification for the decision. For this reason every patient is the source of questions which can only be answered by planned research investigations.

Patrick D. Wall, FRS, DM, FRCP
Professor Emeritus of Physiology
St Thomas' Hospital

Preface

'Why ever do you want to write a book about pain?' she asked. 'You've never had a baby. What on earth do you know about it?' It may be that not having experienced childbearing puts me in an unusually strong position to write about it, because I can believe what the woman and the research tell me about pain. I have had many opportunities to believe women, mostly as a midwife privileged to be with childbearing women. My mind goes first to the women who have allowed me to be with them during labour, and who have permitted me to share with them, as far as is possible, their experience. This has taught me something of the variety of the pain of labour, as well as the frustration of unfulfilled expectations or of an unwelcome complicated birth. Inevitably, with women in labour, I have also shared the exhilaration of the woman becoming confident in the ability of her own body.

The pain of labour may be exacerbated by uncertainty, guilt and grief. I have been able to share these feelings when caring for the woman who decides that she must undergo a termination of pregnancy because her baby has a life-threatening disability. Similarly, my caring for the woman whose newborn baby has died has taught me the pain of her grief, superimposed as it is on the other pains of new motherhood. While I seek to help her to fathom the meaning of her loss, she begins to make sense of it and she eventually manages to resolve her grief and to learn from her experience.

Many women I have met during pregnancy have experienced a wide range of pains which, in the past, have been dismissed as 'discomforts'. This denigration may have served to aggravate the woman's anxiety, and hence her pain, and to make her fearful for her baby's well-being and possibly her own. We should remember too the feelings of the new mother who sees her newborn baby undergoing a series of invasive investigations and questions why the baby cries so much in response? Has this mother been 'reassured' that the neonate is incapable of feeling pain? If so, on what have these paltry crumbs of comfort been based?

These examples serve to remind us that it is not only the contractions of labour that cause pain during childbearing. Niven and Gijsbers have introduced the term 'perinatal pain' to illustrate the continuum of pain around the time of the birth (1996a). These researchers have further extended our understanding of childbearing pain, by linking it to the more humdrum kind of reproductive pain which a woman not infrequently encounters at other times throughout her life. Thus, pain may not be a new experience for the childbearing woman, and we are advised that we should not underestimate the contribution of the range of coping strategies which she may have learned previously (Niven & Gijsbers, 1996a).

These researchers discuss women's differing attitudes to labour pain, describing it as 'not often experienced as intensely aversive' (Niven & Gijsbers, 1996a). This observation may contrast with the more general impression of pain as totally negative. This impression is dominated by the masculine, medical and confrontational analogies of fighting and battle, seeking to convince us that pain needs to be defeated, by whatever means are available. Hence, the library catalogue presents me with titles such as: *Defeating Pain*, *The Challenge of Pain*, *The Conquest of Pain* and *Victory Over Pain*.

Such warlike images share little in common with the views of women who write about childbirth. O'Brien focuses on a woman going 'positively' to 'ride the great waves of pain with strength' (1986: 59). Langford (1997) refers to the pain, familiarly, as 'purposeful'. This constructive view of childbearing pain is reminiscent of Kitzinger's approach, when she writes: '. . . so a woman has less pain when she is calm, happy and self-confident, when she feels that she has the ability to handle whatever pain she experiences' (Kitzinger, S., 1989: 90).

It may be that women's experiences vary between these two extreme representations of pain. What both interpretations do have in common, though, is the recognition that the current situation needs changing. Unfortunately consensus is lacking as to the nature of the necessary change. The limited research into the woman's experience of childbearing pain and the methods used to control it is an example of a reluctance to view pain as a part of the complete childbearing experience (Howell & Chalmers, 1992). Our previous narrow focus on, for example, the techniques used to relieve or remove the woman's pain has inhibited a complete or 'holistic' understanding of the woman's experience of childbearing. Such inhibition has been facilitated by the 'inexpressibility' of physical pain and the way in which pain splits the sufferer from those close by (Scarry, 1985). Scarry goes on to remind us that this split is partly due to the unshareability of pain, which is aggravated by the limitations imposed by language, especially English; as Virginia Woolf observed in this context, 'language at once runs dry' (1925). These phenomena have contributed to doubts as to the existence of childbearing pain, discussed in Chapters 5 ('The history of childbirth education') and 6, which are compounded by professional reluctance to believe the accuracy of the sufferer's narrative. For these reasons, and perhaps in self-defence against reality shock, the woman sufferer may be overlooked, further weakening her already excruciatingly vulnerable position.

Thus, the political nature of pain emerges. Scarry's focus on the balance of power in the relationship between the sufferer and the attendant may be less than relevant in the context of childbearing. Or is it? To what extent are the 'caring professions' in a position to assist the childbearing woman to reduce or control her experience of pain? I intend that this book should illuminate a wide range of aspects of this situation in order to help the reader to answer this question.

Because the woman's experience is central to this book, I use for its theoretical framework one which emerged from a research project focusing on women's perceptions of their experience of childbirth (Halldorsdottir & Karlsdottir, 1996). Part I, 'Before the Journey's Commencement', establishes the context for childbearing and the pain experience; this includes historical, cultural, theoretical and research related issues. Part II concentrates on 'Beginning the Journey', which comprises childbirth education, including the extent to which it prepares the woman for her complete childbearing experience, and pain in pregnancy. Part III, 'The Journey', focuses on labour. Despite the increasingly tenuous link between labour and pain as interventive pain control becomes more effective, I include in Part III the issues and the interventions which may be used to control many types of pain. These topics fit together because the experience of labour and the desire to control pain are probably equally universal. In Part IV, I consider the period after the birth for the woman and child as 'The Journey's End'. The conclusion is included in Part IV and draws together the emerging themes.

Acknowledgements

I would like to recognise the help which I have received from a number of sources in the preparation of this book. First of all, I thank the Committee of the Nursing Studies Association of the University of Edinburgh and its then Convenor, Professor Alison Tierney, who presented me with the opportunity to realise that pain control includes crucial political dimensions which affect a range of actors in the maternity setting. I am grateful to all of the women and staff of the maternity unit in which I am privileged to hold an honorary appointment to practise as a midwife. This enables me to learn from them about their attitudes and behaviour. I would like to thank my colleagues in the Department of Nursing Studies in the University of Edinburgh, especially Tonks Fawcett, and the students for their forbearance, listening skills and support. My profound gratitude goes also to Iain Abbot for his assistance with the artwork and for help above and beyond. . .

PART I
Before the Journey's Commencement

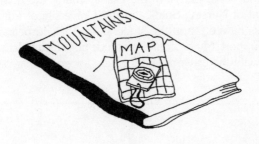

Chapter 1
The Past and the Peoples

The context in which the woman experiences childbearing pain is likely to affect her perception of it. In this chapter the focus is on the context of that pain.

History – attitudes and interventions

History is relevant to our knowledge of pain control because of the need to know where we've come from in order to understand our present situation (Beinart, 1990). I endeavour here to put pain, its control and the application of both to childbearing into an historical context; thereby facilitating our understanding of current developments. In the course of understanding this context, questions emerge about widespread assumptions relating to women's input into the use of pain remedies in childbearing.

Development of attitudes to and interpretation of pain

Ideas regarding pain develop as society changes and even relatively recent ideas soon become outdated. However, ancient ideas about pain in general, and pain as intense as labour pain in particular, may be deeply held and manifest themselves under the stress of childbirth.

In his account of the secularisation of pain, Caton (1985) traces the gradual change from regarding pain as a divine to a natural phenomenon; simultaneously it was transformed from being regarded as generally beneficial to a potentially destructive process. Caton discusses pre-Christian Greeks' and Jews' perceptions of pain having a dual role. First, pain operated as divine punishment for transgressors; thus Greeks, such as Homer, attributed pain to arrows released by the gods. Such external attribution was widespread and applied also to disease processes (Merskey, 1980a). Second and simultaneously, however, pain was regarded positively as an opportunity for healing through cleansing to achieve redemption from sin.

Similar ideas persisted from the fifth century AD through to the enlightenment; under Judaeo–Christian influence, pain continued to be

3

4   *Pain in Childbearing and its Control*

interpreted as divine retribution for wrong-doing. Through this powerful link spiritual leaders emerged as comforters and healers. Thus began the long-standing connection between the church and public health. Fundamental to these ideas was the church's dependence on the dogma of original sin, which materialised in woman's inherently evil nature (Achterberg, 1990). Inevitably self-inflicted pain was eventually substituted for spontaneous pain in a form of 'pre-emptive strike' to prevent disease by appeasing or propitiating the deity. Thus, an element of magical thinking developed. During the Spanish Inquisition this concept was extended to inflict pain on others to achieve their purification. Therefore, pain's dual role as both punishment and redemption emerges. These combined magical and mystical ideas became expanded by logic and observation, such as of substances to ease pain. These observations led to suspicions that human-controlled phenomena were involved and not just superhuman agencies. Such observations included public health measures, like isolation, which occasionally limited the spread of bubonic plague.

From about 1600 the age of faith made way for the age of reason. A link became established between the study of nature and the understanding of divine laws. Thus, the scientific approach to knowledge emerged. Divine laws became relatively less significant, to the extent that the contribution of the deity was eventually questioned by the influential thinkers of the enlightenment. Up to this time changing attitudes had resulted in only minimal changes in treatment, because the methods available were so limited.

In turn, the age of revolution led to the progress in many spheres which heralded the Victorian age. Influential philosophers facilitated the widespread development of new ideas in various arenas, and pain theory was no exception. One of the earlier philosophers, John Locke (1632–1704), clung to established ideas of pain as a divine gift to preserve life. Later, Jeremy Bentham (1748–1832) modified these ideas to interpret laws of nature as punitive interventions initiated by a deity and, thus, pain was 'inherently evil'. Later still, John Stuart Mill (1806–1873) denied any divine contribution and attributed pain to natural processes:

'Even when [nature] does not intend to kill she inflicts the same tortures in apparent wantonness. . . . No human being ever comes into the world but another human being is literally stretched out on the rack for hours or days, not unfrequently issuing in death' (Mill in Cohen, 1961).

Clearly, as ideas changed from the mystical to the secular, a focus on the present-time developed; simultaneously the orientation to reincarnation waned. These changes permitted interventions to ameliorate pain, which were made more effective by increased scientific knowledge.

During the nineteenth century humanitarian ideals manifested themselves in many different ideas; thus, various forms of physical and other pain aroused societal concern. Perhaps one outcome of such concern was the development of anaesthesia.

More recently moral or religious interpretations of pain have become obsolete in the developed world. As in other aspects of life, personal responsibility for individual welfare has become prevalent; in the context of pain, Caton (1985) suggests that personal responsibility has manifested itself in increasing use of psychological pain control methods.

Attitudes to childbearing pain

Historical accounts of childbearing pain invariably begin with a biblical quotation: 'In sorrow shalt thou bring forth . . .' (Genesis 3: 16) (Savage, 1987; Beinart, 1990). Although this 'curse of Eve' may have influenced attitudes to childbirth pain and its control, it contributes little to our understanding of these phenomena. The transition from regarding pain as a divine punishment to a natural process, mentioned above, applied to childbearing pain as much as any other (Arney & Neill, 1982).

Historically, common attitudes to labour pain have been shared among the major religions, but those of the more accessible Judaeo–Christian churches are more widely recognised (Gélis, 1991). Motherhood and pain are usually regarded as inseparable. The Christian churches regarded labour pain as evidence of original sin. So women were persuaded that childbirth pain served as redemption for woman for having caused the fall of man in the Garden of Eden; they were taught to accept labour pains as 'Never can they be as harsh as I deserve' (Gélis, 1991). This Judaeo–Christian concept is comparable with the ancient Greek attitude, which equated the rigours of childbirth for women with those of battle for men (King, 1988). The common factor was divine ordination to ensure life's continuity, thus removing any need for pain remedies and incriminating any woman who offered them as a witch (Achterberg, 1990).

In seventeenth and eighteenth century France, Gélis (1991) describes how labour pain was ignored. This was partly for religious reasons and partly because pain was not a priority; more important was the survival of the mother and, if possible, the child. Arney (1982) reiterates this attitude to childbirth pain and reports that early obstetricians regarded pain as little more than a potential distraction which might possibly impede their work.

As accoucheurs and obstetricians established their practice by disparaging the rival midwife, labour pain became differently significant. Pain was used to discredit the midwife, who was blamed for causing it, as quick labours were preferred, due to shorter duration of pain, and only obstetricians were thought able to shorten labour. Excessive pain was attributed to unnatural labour (Gélis, 1991), such as that associated with rachitic (rickety) pelvis. The woman's first labour was expected to be the most painful, as this baby would 'make the way' by opening up previously untried passages for subsequent, easier labours.

Gélis notes that fear, for example of death, was thought to weaken the woman's endurance and reduce her pain tolerance. Fear was banished by experienced and supportive companions, and simultaneously the woman's confidence in surviving was enhanced. From medieval times to the present century, 'sisters in God' or 'God-Sibs' supported the labouring woman. Because of female 'bonding' and male exclusion from these events, men turned the name of these women into 'gossips', replete with negative connotations (Kitzinger, 1996). Gélis (1991) reports that different societies regard differently the expression of labour pain. His French sources viewed crying out as permissible, even admirable. Like Cheung (1994), he observes that other societies regard crying out as dishonourable.

The dual dimension of childbirth was well-recognised in terms of physiological and psychological components; early obstetricians, however, ensured that the 'psychological' side of women did not interfere with their work (Arney, 1982). A major achievement of Dick-Read in the early twentieth century was his correction of this by 'retrieving the mind' (1933). By the 1950s the original, largely physiological sensation of pain and the woman's psychic reaction to it was differentiated. In this way, Arney argues (1982) that pain and satisfaction with birth were defined, and the significance and meaning of labour pain came to reflect the woman's internal and interpersonal relationships. Through childbirth education, attempts were made to change the woman's relationship with, for example, her body and thus to change her perception of pain. Perhaps unfortunately, this education inevitably carried with it the potential for changing the woman–physician relationship, hence medical opposition to childbirth education (Bonica, 1975). Arney and Neill detail the implications for women and obstetricians which 'natural childbirth' brought (1982). They identify how women's desire for control over their experience of pain challenged the dependency on which obstetricians had traditionally based their practice.

Thus it is clear that, in the same way as long-standing attitudes to pain in general were successfully challenged, established attitudes to childbirth pain have also been questioned.

Development of pain control in childbearing

While pain control in general may be traced back to the Babylonians (Astley, 1990), its place in childbearing is rarely considered to precede the work of Simpson (Savage, 1987). Examining pain control methods in ancient history, King (1988) describes physical as well as chemical remedies. In addition to the obvious herbal remedies, Fairley (1978) describes early opium-taking, the first recorded use of which was 5500 years ago. While admitting the difficulty of assessing the pharmacological effects of the interventions which she describes, King emphasises the crucial role of the interpersonal interaction which underpinned their administration. To the scriptural rationales for the historically limited use of pain control in childbearing mentioned already, King adds a familiar reason. She argues that, were the administration of a substance to be linked with a woman's deterioration or death, then the physician would be blamed. Clearly, defensive obstetrics is no modern phenomenon.

It is apparent that attitudes to the control of labour pain did not begin to change until attitudes to pain generally did. Despite this, attempts were made to alleviate the pain of childbearing, such as attempts by Agnes Simpson which resulted in her being burned as a witch in 1591 (Carter & Duriez, 1986). Acceptable interventions included the use of amulets and semi-precious stones, as well as manuscripts, magic girdles and the Christian liturgy. Perhaps surprisingly, all these interventions were sanctioned by the church, an example being St Hildegard of Bingen's eleventh century advocacy of jasper (Carter & Duriez, 1986).

The use of psychological methods was advocated in seventeenth and eighteenth century France in the form of 'charitable attitude', 'reassurance of progress' and 'distraction' (Gélis, 1991: 152). French midwives also used 'fungi, herbs or roots', so we may assume that such practices were fairly widespread. Surgeons in southern Europe had used soporific sponges since the Middle Ages (Gélis, 1991). The sponges were dipped into fluid containing henbane, hemlock, mandragora or ground ivy and applied to the woman's airways to produce insensibility.

Against this background in both the USA and UK inhalational analgesics/anaesthetics were introduced in the 1840s (Wertz & Wertz, 1979). The events in 1847 in the Simpson family's Edinburgh dining room, which supposedly ushered in 'chloroform à la reine', are well-known (Claye, 1954). As Beinart (1990) records, chloroform anaesthesia and the 'twilight sleep' which soon afterwards arrived from Germany were available only to a minority of women; that is, those who were affluent enough to employ a medical practitioner for the labour and birth. Although the demand for effective analgesia is said to have emanated from women (Bonica, 1994), we must question to what extent this is the case, or whether another agenda is operating? The demand for effective analgesia was a middle class phenomenon in the UK and USA in the early twentieth century (Beinart, 1990). Lewis endorses this view (1990), but maintains that in 1915 working class women were more concerned with a much-needed maternity allowance and health care than pain control. For this group of women pain was not an issue because it was 'natural'.

During the interwar years the vast majority of births happened in the woman's home with a midwife attending. Because midwives were forbidden to administer chloroform unsupervised, no analgesic medication was available to working class women. There is no evidence, though, that this was perceived as a problem. Beinart summarises such women's hierarchy of needs as, first, professional help for the birth, second, some form of pain control and, third, access to a hospital bed if needed. In 1936 the Minnitt apparatus for administering nitrous oxide and air was approved by the Central Midwives Board for midwives to use under well-defined circumstances. Contrary to the expected heavy demand for this form of pain control, local authorities showed no enthusiasm to train midwives in its use (Beinart, 1990).

One result of the wartime blockade of Germany was its production of the synthetic opioid which became known in the UK as pethidine. This drug was used by 68.9% of labouring women by 1970 (Savage, 1987), but has gradually been superseded by other agents.

Summary

History shows the various contributions to attitudes to pain in general and childbearing pain in particular, but women's inputs are notable by their absence.

Theoretical background

By thinking about the history of attitudes to its causation, I have shown how our understanding of pain has influenced its treatment. In the same way, our understanding of the physiological processes, sensations and emotions which together comprise the pain experience have developed as human knowledge has increased.

Development of pain theory

In order to discern the variety of theories which have been advanced to explain the universal human experience of pain, we need to remember that theories are just that. Their role is to facilitate our comprehension of the relationship between two or more variables; theories, like the understanding which they engender, are in no way immutable or fixed. Thus, our understanding of pain should be regarded as dynamic. In the same way as 'ropes' and 'bells' currently seem archaic (see 'Specificity theory'), in the future 'gates' (see 'Currently accepted pain theory') may also be viewed as anachronistic.

Specificity theory

Just as attitudes to the aetiology and treatment of pain changed with the advent of the age of reason in the seventeenth century (see 'Development of attitudes to and interpretation of pain'), so our understanding of the physiological mechanism of pain developed. Descartes (1596–1650) sought an anatomical and physiological explanation of the sensation of pain recognised by Aristotle; he employed the newly developing scientific method to find it. By dissection and by introspection Descartes came to regard the human body as no longer the temple of the soul but as a machine controlled by physical principles (Melzack, 1993). His dissections identified nerve fibres, on the basis of which he concluded that a specific system carries impulses from cutaneous pain receptors to a cerebral pain centre. This mechanism was analogous with 'pulling on one end of a rope makes a bell which hangs at the other end to strike at the same instant' (Wall & Jones, 1991). Cartesian ideas continued to determine knowledge and therapy until well into this century.

In the light of Bell's (1774–1842) recognition of the separate flow of sensory information through channels in the spinal cord, in 1842 Müller developed the doctrine of specific nerve energies. These energies were thought to comprise coded or symbolic messages which could be transmitted only by sensory nerves to the brain. A major flaw in this earth-shattering realisation was the belief that one single sense of touch encompasses all forms of pain.

Von Frey developed Müller's work and combined it with physiological observation and newly introduced staining techniques to identify four types of cutaneous receptor organs or 'modalities'. This theory persisted in affirming direct links to an appropriate cerebral centre and, on the basis of surgery, such pain 'pathways' were identified in the anterolateral or dorsal quadrant of the spinal cord.

The strength of these forms of specificity theory lies in their physiological specialisation. The multiplicity of weaknesses of specificity theory include the psychological assumption of straight-through transmission and the absence of any allowance for personal or temporal variation in pain perception.

Pattern theory

These weaknesses of specificity theory were clearly apparent to clinicians, so a search was begun to illuminate the complexity of transmission. The results comprise 'pattern theory'.

Following pathological observations, Goldscheider (in 1894) hypothesised that, together, central summation in the dorsal horn and stimulus intensity are the critical determinants of pain. Bonica (1990a) refers to this as 'Intensive (Summation) Theory', but the emphasis is clearly on the stimulation spatially or temporally of non-specific receptors (Fordham & Dunn, 1994). The earliest, or peripheral, pattern theory focused on intense peripheral stimulation being interpreted centrally as pain; physiological specialisation was effectively ignored.

The lack of any theory addressing phantom limb/body pain was recognised by Livingston, who in 1943 refined pattern theory to produce the central summation theory; a pattern of incremental and reverberatory circuits were thought to explain the otherwise inexplicable phantom pain experienced by amputees.

A still more complex hypothesis was advanced by Noordenbos in 1959 in the form of the sensory interaction theory, according to which a rapidly conducting fibre system inhibits synaptic transmission in a more slowly conducting pain-carrying system. This theory further proposed a multi-synaptic afferent system within the spinal cord. Thus the physiological stage was set for the gate-control theory (see 'Currently accepted pain theory').

Affect theory

Integrated into other pain theories is one which for centuries stood alone as the only explanation of pain. This is the 'affect theory' of pain, which defines pain as an emotion, rather than as a sensation (Melzack & Wall, 1991). Affect theory is closely linked with what Bonica (1990a) terms the 'Fourth' theory of pain, which differentiates the neurophysiological perception of pain from the cognitive aspects of the response to pain, as determined by a range of factors including culture and previous experience.

Psychological/behavioural theory

Psychological/behavioural theory is a disconcerting form of 'pain theory' proposed by Bonica, which is described as 'psychogenic', being 'found in patients with neurotic disorders, especially hysteria' (1990a: 11). Others have little time for such a 'theory' and dismiss it, writing: 'it is unreasonable to ascribe chronic pain to neurotic symptoms' (Melzack & Wall, 1991: 32).

Currently accepted pain theory

It is clear that, in the history of pain theory, the role of the central nervous system was insignificant, to the extent of the cerebral contribution being negligible. This imbalance was redressed by Melzack and Wall in the early 1960s, using new technology which permitted the electronic recording of individual nerve cells' activity. This work combined Melzack's study of the psychology of the somatic senses with Wall's interest in the physiology of the pain pathways to address certain paradoxes in our understanding of pain (Wall & Jones, 1991: 129):

- the variable relationship between injury and pain
- that innocuous stimuli may elicit pain
- the location of pain discrete from the site of damage

- pain in the absence of injury or after healing
- changes in the nature of pain over time
- intractable pain with/without obvious cause.

Melzack and Wall built on the already well-recognised phenomenon by which gentle stimulation inhibited pain sensation (Fordham & Dunn, 1994). The outcome of their research was the gate-control theory of pain (Melzack & Wall, 1965), which explains persuasively the psychological aspects of pain, the physiology of pain transmission and the modulating influences. The gate-control theory emphasises the body's in-built pain control mechanisms and provides a feasible explanation for the non-interventive or low-tech approaches to pain control, including psychological methods, back-rubbing and transcutaneous electrical nerve stimulation (TENS; Chapter 8). This theory may be summarised thus:

(1) The passage of nerve impulses from afferent fibres to spinal cord transmission cells and thence to local reflex circuits and the brain is modulated by a spinal gating mechanism in the dorsal horn. As with all CNS synapses this transmission is controlled by mechanisms which either facilitate or inhibit the passage of the impulse.
(2) The spinal gating mechanism is influenced by the relative amount of activity in large diameter (low threshold myelinated afferent) fibres and small diameter (high threshold myelinated A-delta and unmyelinated C) fibres: activity in large fibres tends to inhibit transmission (close the gate) while small-fibre activity tends to facilitate transmission (open the gate).
(3) The spinal cord gating mechanism, which is now thought to operate in a number of sites including lamina 2 of the substantia gelatinosa of the dorsal horn, is influenced by nerve impulses descending from the brain.
(4) A specialised system of large diameter, rapidly conducting fibres (the Central Control Trigger) activates selective cognitive processes that then influence, by way of descending fibres, the modulating properties of the spinal gating mechanism.
(5) When the firing rate or output of the spinal cord transmission cells exceeds a critical level, it activates the Action System – those neural areas that underlie the complex, sequential patterns of behaviour and experience characteristic of pain. The critical level is determined on an individual basis by the person's brain, and is dependent on a range of factors, such as previous experience (Melzack & Wall, 1991; Melzack, 1993).

The impact of the publication of the gate-control theory was 'astonishing' in terms of both its vigour and viciousness, although Melzack maintains that its greatest effect lay in its emphasis on the dynamic role of the CNS, especially the brain (Melzack, 1993). In the context of childbearing, this theory assists our understanding of how the emotions which childbearing women experience, such as fear or confidence, as well as cognitions, such as knowledge or meaning, affect the woman's pain experience.

Further hypotheses

The gate-control theory has impacted on the subsequent development of knowledge. One effect has been that simplistic theories are no longer appropriate, and that a holistic orientation to all aspects of pain is recognised as essential (Fordham & Dunn, 1994). Melzack and Wall have made progress separately in addressing the persisting paradoxes of pain listed above.

Phantom pain

Since 1965 Melzack has taken an increasing interest in the paradox presented by phantom (limb/body) pain (PL/BP). His understanding of this phenomenon derives from certain conclusions. He maintains that although the body is normally served by cerebral networks, in the case of PL/BPs the networks may continue to function without bodily inputs. To explain this we are reminded that all bodily 'qualities' (including pain) perceived in the brain are triggered, but not produced, by bodily stimuli. For each of us, our perception of 'self' is through identification centrally, that is through cerebral functioning. This cerebral activity is based on processes which are genetically determined. On the basis of these conclusions a theory of a 'neuromatrix' has evolved. This matrix comprises an anatomical substrate of the body-self and includes the thalamus, cortex and limbic system. The neuromatrix serves as a psychological template, which continues to function even after amputation or trauma to the spinal cord. This theory has the potential to help people with PL/BP (Melzack, 1993).

The concept of a matrix is advanced further by Kingham (1994), who suggests that referred pain and PL/BP may be explained by a continuous circuit of impulses between the periphery and the CNS. This theory describes a 'forwarding' of impulses, which is controlled in the spinal cord and in the thalamus, prior to onward passage for interpretation and action decisions. The comparison of current experience with previous experiences contributes to whether or not the impulse is forwarded.

Prolonged pain

In association with the gate-control, observations of small, unmyelinated afferent or C nerve fibres were observed to behave in an unusual way (Wall & Jones, 1991). Following an initial episode of acute and severe pain, those C fibres arising in deep visceral or joint tissues were found to show increasing activity, recognised as slowly increasing pain. These authors further suggest some cerebral control of this impulse-triggered prolonged pain. They give as an example the pain of a twisted ankle, which is initially sharp but is followed by a vague ache. It is also suggested that this mechanism may be relevant to surgery.

Alongside the gate-control and impulse-triggered prolonged pain mechanisms, Wall and Jones (1991) propose that damaged nerve fibres may engender prolonged pain due to local escape of chemicals normally transported only within the axon. This prolonged pain, termed trans-port-controlled prolonged pain, has been attributed to nerve growth factor. Again, C fibres appear to contribute crucially, perhaps by diagnosing a local problem, for which reason they have been labelled 'chemical pathologists'.

Summary

It is apparent from this discussion that our understanding of pain has developed hugely since Aristotle and that it is continuing to do so. In the same way as we now understand that pain is not a simplistic concept, we know that our understanding of it must also be multifaceted and multidisciplinary. It may be that, in historical terms, an understanding of the nature of pain has not been required to treat it; this situation has changed and our increasing understanding is facilitating more suitable methods of helping women to cope with pain.

Cultural aspects

It may be that childbearing and the associated pain are one of the few common experiences shared by the various component groups which comprise the current multicultural UK society. Although the experience is common, attitudes to it and their expression vary hugely and not invariably predictably. This chaotic situation is further complicated by the varying backgrounds, experiences and attitudes of those providing care during childbearing. In this section, I examine the cultural inputs into and perceptions of this conundrum of pain. I first consider the nature of culture and the factors which have been shown to influence it. I move next to the cultural factors that affect the sufferer's pain expression and carers' pain perception. Next are the cultural factors impinging on childbearing in general and the associated pain in particular. The themes emerging from this material are drawn together by considering the meaning of pain.

What is culture?

'Culture' is a term which carries many meanings; for this reason it is necessary to contemplate the sense in which I use it. Like so many abstract concepts, culture may exist at a variety of more or less abstruse levels. All too often, assumptions may be made about a person's culture from his or her physical appearance. This view is worryingly over-simplistic and verges on racial stereotyping and racism; in contrast Dobson (1991), who studied culture in nursing, emphasised culture's socially inherited nature and the extent to which it features shared ideals.

The complexity of culture is clearer in the unwritten and unstated assumptions and values which determine the behaviour of the members of the relevant group. These assumptions are 'powerfully influential' in controlling behaviour, and may be the only visible manifestation of group membership (Peacock, 1986). While culture describes complex abstractions, terms like 'ethnic/ity' are marginally clearer. These terms refer precisely to a person's racial origin or 'peoplehood' (Cohen, 1974); however, such straightforward terms become less comfortable when the word 'group' is added, as this introduces political nuances.

There are certain factors that have been shown to influence culture.

Geography

Critically reviewing the literature, Wolff and Langley (1977) maintain that it is usual to consider culture in terms of geographical origin. This is what Zborowski partially achieved in his seminal work on the cultural components of pain responses (1952). In a New York setting, he collected data on pain expression by patients of four ethnic backgrounds. The groups were selected following discussion with clinical staff, because staff found difficulty coping with the differing reactions to pain. The groups comprised Italians, Jews, Irish and a group long settled in the USA but of northern European extraction, entitled 'Old Americans'. The data were collected qualitatively by open-ended interviews with patients, observations of them while in pain and interviews with staff caring for them. Healthy members of the same ethno-cultural groups were also interviewed.

Thus, Zborowski made partial use of geographical origin as a proxy for culture; however, Davitz *et al.* (1976) were more discriminating in their interpretation of geographically based culture. These researchers focused on nurses from six different ethnic groups who were working in their country of origin; four of these are oriental countries (Japan, Thailand, Korea and Taiwan) and two are American (the USA and Puerto Rico).

Religion

These two examples (Zborowski, 1952; Davitz et al., 1976) show the extent to which culture is associated with geographical origin. This association is supported by an observation made prior to an attempt to measure the link between pain and culture, which identified 29 cultural groups whose pain responses had been researched (Lipton & Marbach, 1984). Religion and skin colour as well as geography featured as determining characteristics in five groups. Geographical origin and religious persuasion may be thought to be synonymous, but these authors state that such groups are few. The major religions influence culture by, for example, advocating pain acceptance, adopting either prospective or retrospective approaches; examples are the Muslim 'kismet' (destiny), Hindu 'karma' (reincarnated burden) or the Christian atonement (Illich, 1976).

The significant relationship between religious persuasion and geographical origin has emerged in pain studies such as Sternbach and Tursky (1965), who found that religion was closely linked with geographical origin. In their study 'Yankees' were Protestant, Italians and Irish were Roman Catholic, while Jews tended to be of Eastern European extraction. In contrast, Lambert et al. (1960) ignored geographical factors and explicitly recruited Protestant/Christian and Jewish female students in their attempt to probe the link between religious affiliation and pain tolerance. On the basis of their data, these researchers drew conclusions about the culture of minority groups in terms of their desire to emulate the dominant group. Thus, religious persuasion and geographical origin may be so similar in their determination of culture that they are interchangeable. This point was brought home forcefully to me when a woman of North African extraction was criticising the NHS staff's limited understanding. Her comments were unsurprising until she asserted 'You Christians...'. I was taken aback as I certainly do not regard my religious orientation as a prominent characteristic. For her, though, Western European was clearly synonymous with Christian, supporting my argument that culture is inextricably and equally linked, at least in observers' minds, with religion and geographical origin.

Education

With hindsight, I realise that the North African woman was applying a cultural stereotype to me, which I considered inappropriate. Thus, the usual stereotyping found in maternity care was reversed. Green and colleagues (1990) support this contention that stereotyping is invariably unidirectional. The stereotyping on which they focused was the woman's education relative to her involvement in childbearing decision-making. While their data supported the positive aspects of the stereotypical 'educated' woman, this study refuted the negative stereotypes of the less-educated woman.

Socio-economic class

This authoritative study persuaded Green and colleagues that education is inextricably linked to a person's cultural orientation. These researchers further considered whether social class is associated with education and culture, discussing stereotypes of 'uneducated working class women' (1990: 127). They dismiss social class (determined by the male partner's occupation) as not 'a very good indicator of women's attitudes' (1990: 128).

While Green *et al.* have debunked the myth of the stereotypical 'working class woman', McIntosh's research (1989) found that she is alive and, if not well, at least residing in Glasgow. McIntosh argues that women in lower socio-economic groups have their own shared perspectives of and attitudes to childbearing which are culture-bound. In his sample of 80 women, half belonged to social class IIIb and the remainder to social classes IV and V. He claims to have identified the stereotypical working class woman who is 'less opposed to medical intervention and control and less likely to espouse the cause of natural childbirth'.

The culture of social class was explored prior to a study of women's reproductive lives (Martin, 1989). She believes the crucial difference to be the reliance of middle class families on paid outside help and support; whereas 'working class' families are more likely to be able, or need, to pool their own resources.

The comments by Green, the argument by McIntosh and observations by Martin combine to demonstrate that socio-economic class carries a range of features contributing to a unique culture.

Other determinants

While warning against the pitfalls inherent in adopting a 'checklist' of cultures, Brodwin and Kleinman (1987) add gender and age to the factors influencing cultural orientation. Helman (1984) focuses on whether the expectations of society lead to cultural acceptance or non-acceptance of pain. His examples include, first, the groups who live in war zones and who accept battle-wounds and their pain as not merely inevitable, but actually admirable. Helman then suggests that cultures who are able to control pain effectively, such as the USA, tend to find pain unacceptable and analgesia is 'frequently demanded'.

Clearly, the range of factors determining culture do little to clarify its meaning. Such lack of conceptual clarity may be aggravated by its breadth, the response to which is narrowing of the interpretation of culture (Marteau, 1995). She maintains that this narrowing has led to its neglect by certain health disciplines, such as psychology. Marteau's criticism is supported as 'an unfortunate degree of ethnocentrism' by Cartwright (1979: 92). While considering culture as determined by certain characteristics, it is difficult to decide whether this relationship is unidirectional or whether a two-way effect exists.

Pain and culture

Even prior to the early studies mentioned above, the links between pain responses and culture were well-recognised, as reflected in the widely used though limited definition of pain, which allows for cultural variations in pain perception:

'Pain is an unpleasant sensory and emotional experience associated with actual or potential tissue damage or described in terms of such damage'. (International Association for the Study of Pain, 1979)

The cultural variations of pain perception have been demonstrated through a series of research projects undertaken by various disciplines adopting different perspectives. I now review some research findings relating to the client's expression and the carer's perception.

The person in pain

Focusing on the difficulty of making cultural comparisons of pain expression, Helman (1984) sought to distinguish public from private pain. Public pain involves some form of articulation, whereas private pain does not. Exemplifying the latter, he cites the 'stiff upper lip' so admired by 'Anglo-Saxon' peoples and the anecdotal absence of pain behaviour among warriors. Alternatively, this distinction reflects either the lack of sensitivity of the observer or a physiological shock reaction, rather than non-verbal/verbal behaviour in the sufferer. Even so, Helman concedes that 'an absence of pain behaviour does not necessarily mean the absence of private pain'.

The first 'observations' of the cultural implications of pain were made by 'missionaries, travelers and other laymen (and even some medically trained persons)' (Wolff & Langley, 1977: 313). These observations comprised merely assumptions that so-called primitive peoples are less sensitive to pain than their 'civilised' counterparts. Reflecting the thinking then prevalent, genetic inheritance was held responsible. The missionaries and their fellow travellers probably had in mind gruesome initiation rites and other rituals (Melzack & Wall, 1991). In these ceremonies, apparently painful behaviours typically produce no recognisable pain response in the 'celebrant'. As distinct from more humdrum everyday pains, these mystical ceremonies demonstrate the significance of culture; thus, the meaning of the situation, event and other unique factors are crucial in the perception, interpretation and expression of pain.

Despite the tendency to draw conclusions about the cultural factors associated with a person's perception and expression of pain, some anthropologists remain healthily sceptical about the validity of research findings (Wolff & Langley, 1977). Exemplifying Zborowski's study

(1952), these critics bemoan the continuing lack of experimental data supporting a cultural component of pain. They regret the lack of sound anthropological research on pain responses, blaming this on existing experimental studies being anthropologically naïve, and completed anthropological studies lacking the experimental rigour to permit valid conclusions.

As mentioned in 'Geography' above, an unprecedented study focusing on pain and culture sought the differing perceptions, interpretations and expressions of pain by patients and staff (Zborowski, 1952). Zborowski sought to illuminate the acceptability or otherwise of pain behaviour as viewed by staff and patients of differing cultural backgrounds. The immediate spur to this study was the seemingly infinite potential for conflict associated with differing attitudes to pain. Zborowski focused on four 'ethno-cultural' groups of patients. The sample comprised: Jews (n=31), Italians (n=24), Irish (n=11) and 'Old Americans' (n=26). Additionally, there were 11 patients of unstated ethnic origin. A qualitative research design involved interviews with the patients, staff and 16 healthy respondents, which were recorded on 'wire' and transcribed. There is no indication of how the observational data were organised.

The Italian and Jewish patients had been perceived as demonstrating similar emotional responses to pain, and were thought to have a 'lower threshold of pain' than other groups. Zborowski found that the situation was more complex than that. Although the responses to pain appeared similar, the underlying attitudes were diametrically opposed. The meaning and implications of the pain were the prime concern of the Jew, whereas it was the immediate experience that concerned the Italian. Thus, analgesia solved the Italian's problems, but the Jew perceived analgesia not just as no solution, but actually causing more problems by masking threatening symptoms. The Italian and Jewish patients were perceived by the American/ised staff as vocalising pain excessively to attract attention. The staff responded to this over-emotional reaction by minimising their assessment of the these patients' pain; thus, histrionics were counterproductive in gaining sympathy and treatment. Pain expression in these groups further differed according to whether the pain occurred at home or in hospital. The differences were determined by the tendency of the Italian to adopt a more macho and the Jew a more manipulative orientation. Thus, although these two groups exhibited similar pain behaviour, it derived from different attitudes to pain, served differing functions, and sought to achieve different ends. The 'Old American' patients were perceived by staff as being compliant and demonstrating the 'stiff upper lip' approach to pain. This group thought it pointless to fuss about their pain and believed it necessary to behave like a 'good American'. This group considered emotional displays counterproductive.

These attitudes suggest a future orientation in the Jew, compared with a present-time orientation in the Italian co-patient. Each group of patients expressed confidence in the staff, investigations and hospitalisation; while this was greatest in the Old American, the Jew tended to be more sceptical and pessimistic.

Not surprisingly, Zborowski (1952) identified individual differences between members of each of the four groups and sought the reasons for within-group variation. Some individual differences were attributed to the patient's degree of Americanisation, which correlated with the duration of time since the patient, or their forebears, had migrated. Zborowski considered that attitudes to pain and pain behaviour change more slowly than other behaviours. He noted that the pain behaviour of the Jew and the Italian may be similar to the Old American if the patient is third generation but, although behaviours may adapt, underlying attitudes persist. Also recognising the individuality of adherence to 'the old ways', Brodwin and Kleinman (1987) distinguish between ideological and behavioural ethnicity. The latter is the everyday version, whereas the former emerges for 'religious holidays and political rallies'. The extent to which these forms of ethnicity are amplified by migration is open to conjecture.

The gradual change in the behaviour of ethnic groups and the even slower change in underlying attitudes led Zborowski to explore how cultural attitudes to pain are transmitted. He concluded that early influences within the family are crucial. He suggests that 'appropriate' childhood behaviours are rewarded and, hence, reinforced. In contrast, other 'inappropriate' behaviours are disregarded, or even punished, to obliterate them from the child's repertoire. In the context of encouraging appropriate pain behaviour, Brodwin and Kleinman (1987) focus on the family contribution. These authors refer to pain behaviour as having been learned within the family of birth as a coping mechanism. 'Secondary gains' act as reinforcers, from which the sufferer benefits; examples include controlling situations, justifying dependency, punishing others and avoiding sex.

Zborowski may be guilty of racial stereotyping when describing certain groups of women as overprotective and rewarding of more dependent behaviour (Kleinman *et al.*, 1992). Zborowski's creation of 'cardboard characters', serving to dehumanise the subjects and their experience of pain, is also criticised. Despite these limitations, Kleinman *et al.* recognise this study's contribution to founding the study of culture and pain expression, in itself no mean feat.

Recently, aspects of Zborowski's much-criticised study have been supported by English researchers (McAllister & Farquhar, 1992), who also found that people of different cultures adopted differing attitudes to their health problems. Asian women (n=23) were compared with 'white indigenous' women (n=14) regarding their perceptions of health/illness causation. The relevant differences, attributed to culture, were that Asian women were less concerned about the causes of illness, and this was associated with greater confidence in medical and other health advisors. The Asian women attributed their health problems to psychological factors, such as stress, and to the British climate. The 'white indigenous' women, however, were more likely to blame lifestyle, including smoking and employment. These attributions reflect a weakness in this study recognised by the researchers; this is the way that the 'white indigenous' women's views related to health promotion material to which they were exposed, and which could not be read by many of the Asian women. Despite this, the cultural differences in attitudes to health, identified by Zborowski (1952), appear to be supported.

A contrary rationale for cultural differences in pain behaviour (Craig & Wyckoff, 1987) depends less on the individual and what they have learned from family than on their experience. These writers argue that the sufferer decides consciously whether to articulate their distress and seek help. This decision is based on their estimation, using previous experience, of what best advances their own interests. This interpretation of pain behaviour is reminiscent of the learning-free, forward-looking expectancy theory (Lewin, 1935), in which the individual scrutinises all aspects of the situation, including cultural, to calculate how to achieve the most desired outcome. Thus, a decision emerges about whether the pain is publicised or kept private. Regardless of the decision, the sufferer conforms to culturally determined rules governing emotional displays, rather than allowing any reflex pain behaviour.

Having indicated an alternative to the solely cultural interpretation of variations in pain behaviour, Craig and Wyckoff (1987) focus on the dangers of cultural stereotyping in pain assessment. While Zborowski identified major differences in attitudes to health and pain behaviour between cultural groups, he also noted differences within cultural groups. These inter- and intra-group variations are of a similar magnitude, but Craig and Wyckoff warn that stereotyping reduces their significance and renders care and treatment less relevant to the individual. A phenomenon which may aggravate stereotyping is the preparedness of minority groups to withhold information from the dominant group for fear of being labelled as 'weak' or 'mad'. These researchers maintain that this applies in therapeutic as well as research settings.

The carer's perception

As mentioned already (see 'What is culture?'), concern about the potential for conflict served as the spur to the original study of pain expression (Zborowski, 1952). That the attitudes of staff continue to arouse anxiety is demonstrated by continuing research in this area. A significant example is the multi-centre study by Davitz et al. (1976), which examined whether nurses' beliefs about patients' pain result from nurses' cultural backgrounds. The research instrument was a questionnaire comprising vignettes of patients in pain incorporating categories covering disease (5), age (3), severity (2) and both sexes. Davitz and colleagues found that Japanese and Korean nurses thought that patients suffered a great deal of physical pain, in contrast to their American and Puerto Rican sisters who believed the patients' level of pain was lower. This more empathetic attitude among Japanese and Korean nurses seems surprising in view of the western stereotype of oriental people as inscrutable. The researchers, however, found that the relationship between the assessment of physical pain and psychological distress was not straightforward. The Korean and Japanese nurses assessed the physical pain and the psychological distress as equally high. The American nurses were similarly consistently low in their estimation of both forms of suffering. The Puerto Rican nurses, however, linked low levels of physical pain with high levels of psychological distress. Limitations in the research design prevented conclusions being drawn about the reasons for this inversion.

In spite of these discrepancies, all the nurses agreed on their estimation of children's psychological distress as being less than adults. Similarly, they agreed that female patients experienced more pain than males. Whether this finding is associated with the totally female sample is difficult to assess. This research by Davitz *et al.* (1976) focused solely on the culture as determined by the geographical origins of the nurses. As mentioned already, culture has been shown to include a number of facets, but these researchers took no account of any of them. Particularly significant is their non-recognition of an occupational culture. It may be that nursing education has some influence on a person's interpretation of another's pain which acts independently of their geographically determined culture.

The findings by Davitz *et al.* (1976) are, however, endorsed by McCaffery (1983) in her observation that the carer's cultural background may inhibit his or her acceptance of the patient's pain expression. Her example is a man, whose culture encourages him to vocalise his pain, being cared for by a nurse who cannot accept such behaviour. McCaffery contemplates the implications should the nurse follow her culture and retreat from this patient's presence. Another example of culturally unacceptable behaviour was identified in childbearing (Bowler, 1993). Referring to the phenomenon as 'making a fuss about nothing' and contradicting Vangen *et al.*'s (1996) data, she found that midwives, who were invariably Northern European in origin, thought that Asian women made 'too much noise' and constantly grumbled about minor symptoms.

A later account of Davitz and Davitz's (1985) research built on the conclusions mentioned already and refers to another study which focused on the patient's ethnic and religious orientation. The influence of background factors on nurses' expectations of patients' physical pain and psychological distress was shown to be profound. Despite these generalised beliefs, which verge on stereotyping, the researchers found that care was well-individualised.

Admitting that their research was not concerned with the development of nurses' attitudes, Davitz and Davitz (1985) speculate that these nurses' views reflect more widespread 'American culture'. Superimposed on this, though, are the views, attitudes, even prejudices, which are passed from one generation of nurses to the next. These authors refer to such inter-generational effects as 'professional socialisation', and include in it both formal educational experiences as well as informal and unplanned interactions with experienced nurses. These observations answer my criticism (above) that their work ignores an occupational culture; they argue that this is how 'professional' belief systems become established.

Although the cultural background of caring staff in terms of their geographical and ethnic origin has been studied, the staff culture as such has not attracted much research attention. This contrasts with the culture of the work group, in general, which has been studied assiduously in more manual occupations (Argyle, 1989). A notable exception to this lack of research is found in the ethnographic study of a labour ward (Hunt & Symonds, 1995). These researchers reflect on how the culture of hospitals has moved on from the deprivation of the Victorian era, and has been superseded by an open, public and idealised, yet sanitised, atmosphere.

Culture and childbearing

Having considered the cultural significance of pain to the patient and to the staff, and before focusing on the cultural implications of pain in childbearing, we examine the cultural importance of childbearing itself. I suggest that the cultural aspects of childbirth have become significant for two reasons. The first relates to the intrinsic importance of birth to all human societies, which may be summarised as the anthropological argument. The second reason relates to a phenomenon currently emerging in the UK, if not in other societies; this is the political connotations of health in general and childbearing in particular among ethnic minority groups. These issues are becoming widely recognised and may be linked with accusations of racism.

Anthropology

Preceding her ethnographic study of birth in four cultures, Jordan (1978) discusses culture's contribution to the experience of childbirth. She, first, differentiates the almost inextricable pathophysiological and social components of childbirth. The differing practices and customs surrounding childbirth support her argument that it is the critical nature of childbirth, represented by risks of trauma or death, which lends this event its significance. Thus, unchallengeable packages of childbirth practices become culturally established. The cultural mores which evolve control a diversity of childbirth practices, such as who may be present (Jordan, 1978) or what the woman eats or drinks (Jeffery, 1989).

Jordan also focuses on how knowledge of others' childbirth practices may change or even improve practices prevalent in the West. She argues that experimentation with changing practices, such as medication or birth position, may expose the researcher/practitioner to accusations of unethical practice and perhaps to litigation. She suggests that understanding other cultures' practices may facilitate the 'unavoidable change of contemporary ways of doing birth' (1978: 4).

Emphasising the significance of childbirth, Jordan regrets the absence of suitable data. She blames this deficiency on the low status and female-oriented nature of birth. Perhaps as more female researchers become involved in this area, easier access and more data will emerge. Currently available data are of poor quality, she maintains, due to researchers' tendency to assume a medical orientation.

Politics of culture

Analysing maternity care provision for 'black' women, Phoenix (1990) reminds us that the majority of UK maternity carers are white. Hence, discriminatory attitudes develop and become institutionalised (Ahmad, 1993). Such discrimination has been shown to focus on those perceived to be less suitable to bear children, such as the unmarried, the very young and those with children already. Phoenix argues that black women have been stereotyped, particularly as belonging to the latter category, resulting, she argues, in discrimination in the form of institutionalised policies. One example (Phoenix, 1990) is the automatic categorisation of black women as 'at risk' on the grounds that certain groups have higher perinatal mortality rates (Ahmad, 1993). Such categorisation inevitably affects the woman's care. Parsons et al. (1993) suggest that this categorisation is due to Asian women's reluctance to accept care which they consider culturally inappropriate. Further examples of institutionalised discriminatory policies include the non-recognition of the need for interpreters, resulting in the husband or son translating the woman's intimate health history. Another example is staff's difficulty with non-British names, resulting in confusion and danger (Parsons et al., 1993).

Pain, culture and childbearing

Having related culture to both pain and childbearing, I attempt now to integrate these strands by focusing on cultural aspects of pain in childbearing, about which there is little research (Vangen *et al.*, 1996). This neglect is largely the responsibility of Western clinicians, whose child-bearing practices are regarded as a 'gold standard' by other 'less advanced' societies (Jordan, 1978: 35). Thus, childbearing has devel-oped into a medically dominated condition and the woman has been transformed into a patient. Jordan further identifies that the medical attitude to disease, as another problem to be resolved by intervention, has been applied to pain. The relevance of such an approach is uncertain and is seriously questioned by Jordan.

To support her argument, Jordan compares childbearing women in the USA, Holland, Sweden and Yucatan. Because the American woman must convince her carers that she needs medication to control her pain, she must display her need, leading to high levels of 'noise and hysteria in American obstetric wards'. Mayan women in Yucatan accept that pain is part of the childbirth experience. The woman prepares herself for pain, which is regarded as usual, healthy and finite. Jordan found similar attitudes in Holland. Dutch women, she states, accept childbirth pain and believe that nature will take its course. Hence, analgesia is 'neither expected or required' (Tasharrofi, 1993). Van Teijlingen (1994) links British women's attitude to pain in labour to their adherence to a medical model of health, reminiscent of the American woman's (Jordan, 1978). To explore this comparison, Senden and colleagues (1988) compared the expectations and experiences of labour pain in women in Iowa (the USA) and Nijmegen (Holland). In a sample of 256 women, a large majority of Dutch women (79.2%) did not use analgesia; this applied to only 37.6% of American women. The pro-portion in each group showing satisfaction with their pain control and the fulfilment of their expectations showed no significant difference. These authors, like Jordan (1978), attribute their findings to the con-fidence of Dutch women in the successful functioning of their bodies.

In contrast to the observations by Jordan, Bonica (1990a and 1994) reports his unpublished observational data of 'eight thousand women in the USA and almost three thousand in other countries'. On the basis of these data he refutes the contention that the expression of pain varies between women in different cultures. The method used to collect these data is not described, so the rigour of Bonica's approach is uncertain, as is the significance of his findings.

In the same way as other researchers have demonstrated the dynamic nature of culture in terms of the response to pain, Hunt and Symonds (1995) recount the changing cultural attitudes to childbirth pain in the UK. In the course of their study of the culture of a labour ward these researchers identified how, in the mid 1930s, the status of birth as 'natural' was rejected; simultaneously the pain of birth became less acceptable to women. Thus, attitudes that still prevail in Holland and Yucatan virtually disappeared in the UK.

The attitude of women in India appears to have much in common with those in Holland and Yucatan (Jeffery, 1989). The absence of pain control methods is not a problem but an irrelevance. In her ethnographic study, Jeffery found that 'intense' pain is regarded as beneficial, through the all-too-obvious connection with a speedy birth. The articulation of pain is also culturally controlled, through excessive vocalisation being thought to reflect 'shamelessness'; thus, the women she interviewed had been encouraged to 'accept the pains, calling on God's name'.

Examining pain behaviour, Schott and Henley (1996) discuss the extent to which racial stereotypes may cease to apply, due to the intensity of childbearing pain or to local influences. They comment on the UK tendency to value quiet, which has been elevated to institutional policy (Chapter 12), but which reduces the possibility of a woman using sound as a coping mechanism.

Recent research endorses Jeffery's observation. In a study of 137 labouring women, significant differences appeared in analgesia use between Pakistani (Punjabi-born) and Norwegian-born women (Vangen *et al.*, 1996). Of the 67 Pakistani women, 30% received no analgesia, compared with only 9% of the 70 Norwegian women. There is no suggestion that the Pakistani women's labours were any less painful. The researchers emphasise the communication difficulty between the Norwegian midwives and the Pakistani women, a large majority (82%) of whom spoke little or no Norwegian. Socio-economic backgrounds also differed markedly. The Pakistani women tended to receive analgesia, if any, which required minimal communication or instruction, such as intramuscular pethidine rather than nitrous oxide and oxygen or epidural analgesia. The Pakistani women were also more likely to undergo general anaesthesia, though not significantly. This research suggests that Western stereotypes of Asian women may not be accurate; however these researchers do not show whether language or culture or a combination of the two are responsible for the differing analgesia use.

Despite the shortage of research-based material on this topic, that which exists shows the considerable variation in and implications of the expression of childbirth pain between and within cultural groups over time.

Meanings

Throughout this chapter, the importance of the meaning of pain has become apparent. This concept emerged in the grisly initiation rituals, the celebrant's interpretation of which constrained his perception and expression of pain (Melzack & Wall, 1991). Zborowski (1952) found that certain ethnic groups were more concerned with the meaning and implications of the pain than its treatment; however, for others the immediate experience was the major concern. It may be that ascribing a meaning to pain constitutes a coping mechanism, which may apply no less to childbearing pain than to the more long-term forms on which the literature tends to focus.

The multiplicity of the meanings of pain are addressed in a phenomenological contemplation of pain (Leder, 1986). First defined are pain's meanings in terms of the very incarnation of 'the unhappy, the bad, the wrong' (p. 259). Leder then looks more closely at this 'immediate negativity', initially linking it with pathological processes and death, which have been associated with punishment, atonement and redemption, as by the early churches (Caton, 1985). This negativity is then contrasted with the potential benefits. The association with death imposes a realisation of our 'ownmost limitations and possibilities', by requiring a retrospective contemplation of our lives. Leder recognises that the pain of childbirth may additionally deliver both physical and emotional achievement, which he compares with an athlete passing through the pain barrier. While demonstrating the many meanings ascribed to pain, Leder (1986) reminds us of pain's potential to obliterate the meaning of those phenomena which help us to make sense of our lives. Although he fails to make a connection which may be apposite in childbearing, it may be that this obliteration of pre-existing common sense provides the opportunity to identify new understandings in our lives. Leder summarises the inevitable and enduring effects of pain in Bloy's words: 'Suffering passes but the fact of having suffered never passes'.

Pain may be meaningful to the sufferer in one or more of three ways (Fordham & Dunn, 1994). The philosophical/religious meaning of pain serves to provoke the sufferer perhaps into remedial action, or into contemplation. The sufferer may reflect generally on 'Why me?', but more appropriately in the present context, metaphysical questions of human experience, such as life and death, come to mind. The biological meaning of pain serves as a warning signal, a concept reminiscent of Bonica's (1990a) explanation of labour pain (Chapter 7). Fordham and Dunn's third meaning focuses on the psychosocial consequences, which are more appropriate for long-term pain.

Summary

This section on culture has emphasised culture's importance as a source of group values, which may be helpful to group members and to others. Superimposed on the group activity, though, must be the meaning of the experience to the individual, which serves as an additional means of coping with an experience such as childbearing pain. As individuals caring for individual women, it is crucial to identify our own beliefs about pain (McCaffery, 1983), including cultural assumptions and values and, perhaps, prejudices. While McCaffery stated this in personal terms it may apply equally to organisational culture.

Chapter 2
Experiences and Observations

This chapter seeks to address both the experience of pain and its observation by carers and researchers.

Emotional aspects of pain

It is apparent from our scrutiny of its history (Chapter 1) that pain had traditionally been envisaged as an emotion associated with previous sin. René Descartes' ideas at the beginning of the enlightenment introduced the distinction between bodily and other forms of pain, including guilt, tribulation and similar mental pain (Caton, 1985). The acceptance of Descartes' scientific ideas about a mind–body split was gradual. This is evidenced by its absence from philosopher John Locke's writing (1632–1704), which did not distinguish between pain which 'is physical and that which is mental'. A century later, though, Jeremy Bentham (1748–1832) had accepted the Cartesian distinction between physical suffering and mental anguish (Caton, 1985).

Defining pain

In order, in this section, to examine pain in broad terms, it is helpful to consider some of the recent attempts to define 'pain' before moving on to consider one aspect of this broad definition – emotional pain. The first example is found in a conventional medical text: 'Pain is that sensory experience evoked by stimuli that threaten to destroy tissue, defined . . . as that which hurts' (Mountcastle, 1980: 391). This definition's problems relate to the link between pain and tissue damage, which is too tenuous and too variable (Chapter 1) to be useful, while the obvious 'organic' emphasis in this definition limits the possibility of other forms of pain.

Merskey (1980b) prepared a more complete definition in an effort to encompass both 'organic' and 'psychogenic' pain, which was subsequently adopted by the International Association for the Study of Pain (IASP) (Bonica, 1990a: 18): 'an unpleasant experience which we primarily associate with tissue damage or described in terms of tissue damage, or both'. While some women might regard 'unpleasant' as an understatement of their experience of childbearing pain, this definition is sufficiently vague to encompass a range of pain perceptions.

The difficulty of devising an adequate and complete definition of pain has been attributed to its dubious homogeneity (Bendelow & Williams, 1995). This may be attributable to a deficiency in the English language, which has been contrasted with the multiplicity of terms for other important concepts. A well-known example is the great variety of Inuit words for the phenomenon which we know as 'snow' (Szasz, 1957: 10). Thus, the absence of applicable words means that 'pain' must be qualified by suitable adjectives to make its meaning more comprehensible (Szasz, 1957).

In a nursing context McCaffery (1979) coined a definition of pain which is useful both temporally and qualitatively: 'Whatever the experiencing person says it is, existing whenever he or she says it does'. While this definition does expand the experiences which are included in the concept of pain, the focus is still on physical pain. This problem is addressed by Melzack and Wall, who emphasise our limited understanding of pain, leading them to offer: 'a category of experiences, signifying a multitude of different, unique experiences having different causes, and characterised by different qualities varying along a number of sensory, affective and evaluative dimensions' (1991: 46).

Thus, I seek to consider pain in terms of Melzack and Wall's inclusive definition. In this section, however, I concentrate on those forms of pain that are thought to feature a significant emotional component and to a lesser extent, if any, physical aspects. The term 'suffering' is becoming appropriately used to describe such feelings (Spross, 1993; Rodgers & Cowles, 1997). Originally defined by Copp (1974) as 'the state of anguish of one who bears pain injury or loss', the spiritual effects of suffering have become included, thus: a 'state of severe distress associated with events that threaten the intactness of the person' (Cassell, 1982).

While non-physical pain may be ascribed to pathological or psychiatric processes (Merskey, 1980b), I avoid this assumption. Partly because it has been attributed to ignorance, I give no credence or further attention to the possibility of that pain which has been referred to as 'psychogenic' (Melzack & Wall, 1991: 32).

The mind/body split

Before focusing on emotional pain or suffering, we should consider the concept of mind/body dualism which has retarded our understanding of pain since it was first conceived by Descartes, and subsequently adopted by our medical colleagues (Bendelow & Williams, 1995). Concluding his philosophical investigation into pain and pleasure, Szasz (1957) pleads for a re-examination of Cartesian dualism. While Melzack and Wall's gate-control theory (1965) might have answered Szasz's plea by ending the Cartesian mind/body split, this is not the case, as evidenced by later major texts omitting material relating to affective aspects of pain (e.g. Bonica, 1990a). The persistent legacy is the scientific or, more precisely, medical understanding of pain as purely physical. This understanding, preferred as it is to all others, impedes acceptance or utilisation of a holistic interpretation of pain (Bendelow & Williams, 1995: 161–2). This mind/body split has been associated with the tendency noted already to ascribe the emotional component of pain to psychiatric conditions rather than regarding the pain experience as one complete entity. While making no apology for attributing the persistence of this concept to certain disciplines, we recall that the nature of pain itself aggravates the dichotomy by alienating our minds from our bodies, thus perpetuating this Cartesian dualism (Bendelow & Williams, 1995).

Suffering

When discussing pain, the assumption is ordinarily made that it is largely physical in origin, as shown in the definitions above (see 'Defining pain'). Recognition of the existence of emotional pain, though, is longstanding and featured in the last century in the work of Durkheim and Marx (Bendelow & Williams, 1995). The use of the term 'pain' in this context is further supported by the clear picture which it presents of both emotional turmoil and physical suffering in the well and less healthily functioning body and mind (Bendelow & Williams, 1995). In order to consider that pain which is predominantly emotional and which may be termed 'suffering' (Rodgers & Cowles, 1997), I examine first its healthy and pathological forms. I next move on to suffering which is more directly associated with bodily pain and, finally, I discuss how suffering may manifest itself during childbearing.

Healthy suffering

Under certain circumstances suffering may be an unpleasant but healthy response to the difficult or otherwise distressing situations which we meet occasionally throughout our lives. Nyatanga (1993) discusses suffering, referring to it as 'emotional pain', which he distinguishes from physical pain. Emotional pain, he maintains, is a response to the person's environment and the actors who inhabit it. A complex interplay of emotions becomes established with the other actors, together with the recollection of past bitter experiences; these include losses such as bereavement, loss of personal faculties or loss of affection or self-esteem. Emotional pain, Nyatanga argues, manifests itself in physical form in some sufferers. It may present as altered body language or as symptoms, examples being eneuresis or other regressive childhood behaviour. This healthy, if unwelcome, experience of suffering is regarded by Copp as an unavoidable fact of life, when she refers to it as 'life pain' (Copp, 1994: 222). She maintains that life pains increase as the sufferer ages, presumably because such pain is associated with loss. These losses may be through death or other forms of separation, by loss of income or employment, loss of relationships or loss of meaning for life.

While Copp does not mention it explicitly, Nyatanga like Bendelow and Williams (1995) refers to grief as a form of emotional pain. The fundamental link between attachment and loss engendering painful grieving is widely accepted (Bowlby, 1969; Mander, 1994b) and grief has appropriately been referred to as 'the cost of caring'. Grieving is essentially healthy and beneficial, and enables adjustment to the losses confronting us as we move through life (Marris, 1986). Grief facilitates progress, although not directly, from the initial feelings of distraught hopelessness, eventually achieving some degree of resolution which permits our usual functioning for a large part of our lives. Although grief may sometimes be viewed as apathetic passivity, it is better regarded as a time during which the person actively strives to complete the emotional tasks facing him or her; the phrase 'grief work' describes this active striving.

The stages of grief through which the person needs to work have been recounted in various ways, but Kübler-Ross's account is well-known and useful (1970). Individual variation combined with a 'one step forwards two steps back' progression inevitably affects grieving. The initial denial response of grief constitutes a defence mechanism which protects from the full impact of realisation. This helps to insulate from the unthinkable reality, allowing a 'breathing space' in which to marshal our emotional resources. As denial ceases to be effective, awareness of the reality of the loss dawns, simultaneously powerful emotional reactions and their physical manifestations materialise, featuring sorrow, guilt, dissatisfaction, compulsive searching and anger. Realisation dawns in waves as the bereaved person attempts various coping strategies to 'bargain' with him- or herself to delay accepting reality. The despair of full realisation of the loss eventually supervenes, bringing apathy, poor concentration and bodily changes. After eventual acceptance the loss is integrated into the person's life. This process is complex, involving slow progress and setbacks, described as 'oscillation and hesitation' (Stroebe & Stroebe, 1987). Although we never 'get over' the loss, we integrate it into our experience of life. This ultimate degree of 'resolution' is recognisable in the bereaved person's ability to think realistically and with equanimity about the strengths as well as the weaknesses of the lost relationship.

The healthy suffering of grieving matters mainly because it contributes to the balance or homeostasis in the life of the affected or bereaved person. Grief is crucial in helping us to recover from the painful effects of loss.

Pathological suffering

As with many arbitrary distinctions, the boundary between healthy and pathological suffering may be unclear. Grief, mentioned above, exemplifies how the physical manifestations of healthy suffering in the form of sorrow may be indistinguishable from true depression (Beutel *et al.*, 1995). Depression, a commonly experienced mental illness (Fishel, 1981), constitutes a good example of pathological suffering. While the suffering involved in depression takes a variety of forms in addition to the characteristic lowering of mood, the experience is often explained by the sufferer in terms of pain. Dominian (1981) gives verbatim accounts of this 'inner world of pain, anguish, misery, confusion' in his self-help guide:

> 'A kind of isolation sets in: a peculiar paralysis of mind and body in which you exist as a state of pure pain. . . . Pain is the proof that you are still alive if not kicking' (p. 16).
> 'Shape, colour and forms are experienced acutely with a corresponding increase in the pain felt. I can only think it is painful because the frustration which is continual leads to you becoming more aggressive' (p. 19).
> 'Time seems to be running out . . . [which] seems to be the most desirable thing in the world . . . the relief from the agony of despair; peace from all that threatens, or release from existing. And yet there is another side to it; for the feeling of being close to total disintegration is also part of the pain and darkness of being depressed' (p. 19/20).

These personal statements show clearly how, though in no way physical, the person suffering the pain perceives it as very real. These accounts are supported by research which focuses on the pathological anguish of depression associated with work-related stress experienced by one occupational group (Shurtz *et al.*, 1986). Similarly, anguish has also been identified in other psychiatric conditions (Rosenbaum *et al.*, 1994). The inclusion of mental illness as a form of pain is certainly justified by the symptoms that a depressed person is likely to encounter. Even if Merskey's narrow definition of pain is used, the symptoms fall well within the scope of an 'unpleasant experience' (Bonica, 1990a: 18). Pathological suffering in childbearing is discussed below .

Physical-related suffering

While considering the suffering that a person may face in the absence of physical pain, we should recall that mental suffering not uncommonly co-exists with physical and other pain. The concept of 'total pain' was introduced by Saunders to emphasise the complexity of the physical, emotional, social and spiritual components of the suffering inherent in advanced cancer (Baines, 1990). On the basis of this concept, she argued that effective pain control is not feasible until each aspect has been adequately addressed. The role of the recommended multi-disciplinary team comprising carers and family in this situation is to plan care, taking account of the wide range of factors that impinge on the person's pain experience (Baines, 1990).

Baines describes the emotional vicious circle which is likely to develop and escalate when the patient experiencing physical pain becomes anxious or depressed due to inadequate pain control. Such mental suffering, she maintains, lowers the patient's pain threshold, thus exacerbating the original problem. The 'conspiracy of silence' in which staff and family connive further aggravates the patient's anxiety relating to the disease or other matters. The pain is exacerbated by spiritual concerns which fill the mind of the person facing an experience like death (Baines, 1990). Memories of previous losses, unsatisfactory relationships, unfinished business, feelings of guilt and the meaning-lessness of life emerge, further reducing the patient's coping ability.

Emotional pain in childbearing

While childbirth is generally regarded as a happy event, we must bear in mind that some degree of emotional pain or suffering not uncommonly features. This suffering may take the very mild form of momentary regret which a mother may encounter on learning that her baby is not of the gender for which she was hoping (Mander, 1994b). The process of adaptation to motherhood has been explained in terms of suffering which interferes with the woman's other relationships and needs time for these to be renegotiated (Barclay *et al.*, 1997). These researchers warn, however, of the difficulty of differentiating maternal suffering or distress from emotional pain which is serious, that is depression (Barclay & Lloyd, 1996).

Healthy childbearing suffering

A mother experiences healthy suffering if there is some form of loss in association with her childbearing. Her loss might comprise miscarriage, stillbirth or the neonatal death of her baby (Mander, 1994b). Less likely to come to mind, but still engendering grief, are the losses associated with termination of pregnancy, the birth of a baby with a disability, relinquishment of a baby for adoption or diagnosis of infertility. Researching how women cope with the pain engendered by unexpected pregnancy, Marck (1994) discusses the women's coping strategies. Featuring prominently is the emotional pain of loss, which Mary felt following her dilatation and curettage, which Vanessa feels because someone else is mothering her son or which required Maggie to seek a blessing after her termination. Marck extends this emotional pain to include that which the mother invariably experiences as an inevitable component of loving, or even anticipating loving, her child (1994). These 'mothering pains' essentially only begin after the physical pains of childbirth are completed, but last indefinitely.

Pathological childbearing suffering

While postnatal depression (PND) is rarely said to feature pain, its distressing nature is widely recognised (Niven, 1992; Littlewood & McHugh, 1997). There is no reason to believe that it causes any less suffering than depression at other times in the life cycle. The term 'postnatal depression' is a source of considerable debate among mental health practitioners (Cooper *et al.*, 1995), but its value to those working with childbearing women is that it differentiates the relatively inconsequential mood changes, or 'blues', from the significant ones. Like the appropriateness of the name, the condition's incidence is uncertain. This is due to the problem of making a diagnosis, which is compounded by sufferers having difficulty seeking help due to feelings of guilt or fear of stigma. Although an incidence of around 10% is quoted, this may be an underestimate, as Leach suggests that 'up to 60% of new mothers experience some form of PND' (Welford, 1996).

A range of causes has been suggested, including genetic, psychodynamic, socio-cultural, obstetric and hormonal (Cox, 1986). It may be that knowledge of the causes is of limited value, when focusing interventions on vulnerable women has so little impact on the incidence and severity of PND (Stamp *et al.*, 1995). Despite the limited benefits of prophylactic interventions, the socio-familial causes and effects of PND attract attention, including that of feminists (Jebali, 1993). The male-determined societal expectations of motherhood are thought to engender in women unrealistically romantic views of childbearing. Similarly, Littlewood and McHugh (1997) regard the pain of PND as exemplifying the oppression of women. When women fail to achieve such romanticised expectations, a male-dominated medical system diagnoses the woman's disappointment as psychiatric pathology. Jebali concludes that more realistic views of motherhood are needed, rather than the pronatalism currently prevalent. It may be that midwives are ideally situated to facilitate such realism.

Total pain

Never having experienced labour, it is through being with women in childbirth that I have formed the impression that the transition phase of labour equates with total pain. UK textbooks rarely mention the stage of labour known as the 'transition phase' (Bennett & Brown, 1993), although North American texts include it (Bobak & Jensen, 1993). Kitzinger (1987a: 223) defines transition as 'the very end of the first stage of labour. .... It is often the most difficult part of labour, but may last for only a few contractions'. It is my observation that the woman begins to despair of her ability to complete her labour successfully at the time when her contractions are becoming more intense in preparation for the birth and when she feels there is little she can do to help herself. This psychological low point in combination with seemingly unproductive pain correlates with the mental and physical pain labelled 'total pain' by Saunders (Baines, 1990). Tucker lists the characteristics of the transition:

- 'You may suddenly lose your ability to keep things in perspective.
- You may no longer be able to keep on top of your contractions.
- You may shake uncontrollably.
- You may find yourself very confused mentally; you may want to go home, feel irritated with those around you, and find it difficult to cooperate' (1996: 154).

Vogler, however, describes the transition more objectively:

- 'Expresses sense of extreme pain
- Expresses sense of powerlessness
- Shows decreased ability to listen or concentrate on anything but giving birth' (1993a: 471).

At this time the skills of the midwife are challenged, if she is to maintain rapport, while supporting the woman through this supremely demanding phase.

Summary

In this section I have discussed the concept of emotional pain and have established its right to be considered alongside other, perhaps more easily recognisable, forms of pain. I have indicated situations in which a person is likely to experience emotional pain, which may be known as 'suffering', including those associated with childbearing. To conclude, words of comparison may be appropriate:

'Mental pain is less dramatic than physical pain, but it is more common and also more hard to bear. The frequent attempt to conceal mental pain increases the burden: it is easier to say "My tooth is aching" than to say "My heart is broken"' (Lewis, 1940: 144).

Assessing pain

The research which I mentioned in the sections on culture and pain theory in Chapter 1 has demonstrated the crucial yet challenging role of pain assessment. I now consider issues associated with the measurement and assessment of pain. I begin by examining the problem, meaning the widely recognised underestimation of pain by nurses (Allcock, 1996a; Price & Cheek, 1996), and evidence that a similar situation exists in maternity. I next look at the rationale for assessment and instruments to assess pain, emphasising acute pain. Finally, I contemplate the relevance of these instruments to maternity care.

Traditional observation

The difficulty which the nurse encounters in assessing and remedying the patient's pain is due to the innate fear of pain which lurks within us all (McCaffery, 1983). Such fear engenders denial of the patient's pain and is compounded by two other factors. First is medical underprescription of analgesia, both in terms of the dosage and the frequency of administration. The second compounding factor is the nurse's tendency to further reduce the patient's analgesia by administering the medication in smaller doses and less frequently than prescribed (McCaffery, 1983).

McCaffery's longstanding observation has been endorsed by research in England (Willson, 1992) and in a Scottish post-operative setting (Lloyd & McLauchlan, 1994). The complex interrelationship of patient and carer characteristics cannot be ignored (Allcock, 1996b). The nurse's tendency to underestimate the patient's pain was reiterated by the Scottish study, finding that over 70% of nurses 'accepted' that they did this. The nurse's reluctance to administer analgesia post-operatively emerged in the majority of nurses who agreed 'that it should be used for as short a time as possible'. As previously identified by McCaffery, almost one-quarter of these nurse respondents were concerned that the medication carried addiction risks.

McCaffery's hypothesis of nurses' denial of patients' pain as self-protection has been applied to midwives (Niven, 1992). Niven pursues her argument to contemplate the damage that the midwife's unsympathetic attitude causes to the mother–midwife relationship. For this reason or for fear of addiction, pain medication in labour has been demonstrated as providing inadequate analgesia. Rajan (1993) re-analysed Chamberlain *et al.*'s data (1993; see below) to ascertain the perceptions of women, midwives, obstetricians and anaesthetists about analgesic effectiveness. Rajan found that generally the staff assumed pain control to be satisfactory to the woman, whereas the women experienced it as inadequate. This applied, typically, when pethidine was used; however, the reverse held when nitrous oxide and oxygen (N_2O & O_2) was used and the women found it more effective than perceived by staff. Unlike the nurse administering inadequate medication due to denial (McCaffery, 1983), Rajan suggests that the midwife's different knowledge base is the reason. She maintains that the midwife compares the woman's observed pain with the extremely painful labours which she has attended, and provides analgesia proportionate to the appearance of pain. The woman, on the other hand, compares her pain with other pain she has experienced, which pales into insignificance by comparison, and expects pain medication proportionate to that. This mismatch of expectations, Rajan states, remains unarticulated and self-perpetuating, being exacerbated by social, cultural and linguistic differences. While regretting the discrepancy between women's and staff's perceptions, Rajan observes the greater congruency between the perceptions of individual staff members, which compounds the woman's frustration that her pain perception is accepted by none of her carers. Congruent perceptions of the effectiveness of pain control could serve as an indicator of empathy and as a quality assessment tool (Robinson, 1997).

Just as Rajan found that analgesia in labour was perceived by the mother as inadequate, Waldenström (1988) also identified the midwife's concern about using pain medication. In Sweden, however, Waldenström found that the midwife's concern related not to the possibility of addiction, but to the drug's effect on the woman's labour and baby. The Swedish midwives compensated for their reluctance to administer medication by their belief in the beneficial effect of their presence.

An omission in both of these important studies is the lack of any explanation of the midwife's assessment of the woman's pain or the drug's analgesic effect. No pain measuring instruments are mentioned, leading to the conclusion that none was used. Thus, it is necessary to examine the reasons for using such tools and their form before considering their place in maternity care.

The rationale for assessment of pain

There are various reasons for assessing the pain being experienced by someone in our care. The reasons are associated first with interventions to alleviate the pain. In clinical situations the nurse assesses pain to make a nursing diagnosis, on the basis of which pain control is implemented (Johnson, 1977). This involves the nurse facilitating the patient's own coping mechanisms, with or without the use of medication. The meaning of the pain to the individual is likely to affect, first, her ability to cope with it and, second, the support and other interventions which may help. In a study of the meaning that patients ascribed to pain, Copp (1974) found that over 25% of patients perceived some value in their pain experience. This may have been attributable to short-term severe pain, such as following cholecystectomy, or being able to end long-term pain, such as that due to biliary colic. After the interventions the nurse re-assesses the pain to evaluate their effectiveness and plan future therapy.

Adopting a multidisciplinary orientation, Melzack (1983) draws our attention to the number of different occupational groups involved in caring for a person with pain, particularly if it is long term; examples include physiotherapists, social workers and occupational therapists as well as nursing and medical personnel. Melzack emphasises the need for shared interdisciplinary understanding of the patient's pain experience, which is facilitated by using recognised assessment instruments. Although pain assessment instruments may be criticised for spurious objectivity, I have already established that subjective assessments tend to be particularly unreliable. Thus, pain assessment can only improve the carer's evaluation of this most personal, private and subjective of all human experiences (Sternbach, 1968).

In order to write about the various aspects of pain, I have separated the assessment of pain from the interventions that are used to either prevent or remedy it. Such a separation is totally artificial and clearly has no place in practice. Wright (1988) reports that in some clinical settings pain assessment is undertaken routinely, without affecting patient care, to the detriment of that care. Collecting information which is not utilised to facilitate care raises serious ethical problems.

Instruments for assessing pain

The science of pain measurement has been termed 'dolormetrics' (Rollman, 1983) and it incorporates a wide range of technical and simple approaches. The close relationship between research and practice in this area is illustrated in two ways: first, the assessment instruments in clinical use may also be used to measure pain in laboratory-based and other research (Stewart, 1977); the second example of these close links materialises in the use of some tools, originally experimental pain research instruments, which have become, rightly or wrongly, incorporated into clinical practice (Stewart, 1977). We should, however, question the clinical value of research jargon such as pain threshold, meaning the point at which pain is just perceived, and pain tolerance, meaning the point at which pain can no longer be tolerated. Such supposedly 'objective' measures are of questionable value clinically when biological stability or constancy are absent, even in one individual.

For reasons such as this the tools have changed towards self-assessment by the person in pain. Despite this change, it is sometimes necessary for the carer to make the first move to open up the topic of pain. Observation may lead the carer to suspect pain, even though the person has not verbalised his or her pain or may have, for various reasons, denied it (Fagerhaugh & Strauss, 1977).

In describing the many pain assessment instruments, it is necessary to bear in mind that these techniques are in no way exclusive. For this reason, after considering the main techniques, I examine those instruments that combine a number of techniques. The multiplicity of techniques reminds us that patients may encounter more than one pain at a time; then each pain must be assessed separately (Fordham & Dunn, 1994).

Physiological indicators
While physiological sequelae of pain, such as tachycardia, may be useful indicators of its intensity, they lack specificity. Many physiological, psychological and pathological phenomena alter the heart rate in addition to pain, rendering this observation of little value (Vogt *et al.*, 1973).

Verbal descriptors
The traditional forms of pain observation, mentioned already, tended to rely on verbal interaction. These have developed into systematic formats which are applied interactively or in writing. Verbal descriptors are usually used in combination with other approaches. These may combine verbal and numerical scales (Linton & Gotteskam, 1983); the best known is the McGill Pain Questionnaire (MPQ; see 'A combination of methods'; Melzack, 1975a). A long-recognised problem in using words to denote, particularly, the intensity of pain is their variability of meaning between individuals (Stewart, 1977); thus, what constitutes severe pain to me may only be moderate to you. In a therapeutic setting, though, this problem is less significant than in research, but our multicultural society requires us to take account of the patient's language skills.

Numerical scales
Descriptive words often have numerical values added in an effort to further clarify the relationship between the various levels of pain. This may result in a painometer (Wright, 1988), a pain thermometer (Hayward, 1975) or a pain rule (Bourbonnais, 1981). The importance of 'anchor words' to indicate the extremes of the pain experience cannot be overemphasised; examples are 'no pain' as the minimum and 'pain as bad as it could possibly be' as the maximum. Despite this, though, people in pain may still experience difficulty in ascribing numbers to an experience as human as pain. For research purposes, establishing the relationship between the intervals is necessary to permit mathematical calculations.

Visual Analogue Scales (VAS)
Whereas numerical scales are subdivided to indicate differing levels of pain, often with words attached to each level, a Visual Analogue Scale (VAS) provides only anchor words at each extreme. If words are used to indicate imprecise levels without numbers, the scale is known as a

'Graphic Rating Scale' (Stewart, 1977). The absence of numerical indicators increases the sensitivity of these scales, but the lack of fixed points may offer patients more freedom of choice than they can handle, resulting in difficulties.

Body outlines

Providing a gender-free outline of the front and back of the body permits the patient to indicate the location of the pain. These instruments do not require anatomical literacy or common language. They carry the disadvantage, however, of being two-dimensional and being unable to indicate the pain's superficiality/internality. Melzack (1975a) attempts to overcome this weakness by requesting that an 'E' (external), 'I' (internal) or 'EI' (both) be used to pinpoint the pain more precisely.

A combination of methods

The MPQ (Melzack, 1975a) combines verbal descriptors with numerical values attached and a pair of body outlines. This instrument evolved out of the recognition of the multidimensional nature of the pain experience and that instruments which focused solely on the intensity of pain were too limited in their approach (Melzack, 1983). The MPQ seeks to determine the intensity, the quality and the duration of the individual's pain and aids diagnosis, assists therapeutic decisions and evaluates interventions' effectiveness (Melzack & Katz, 1994).

In the MPQ information about the nature of the pain is sought through offering the patient 78 words describing the pain. These words originated from those frequently used by patients and medical personnel to describe pain. They are subdivided into 20 groups, which are based on statistically derived levels of agreement between respondents. From these words the patient chooses those that best describe her pain. The words cover sensory aspects of pain, such as 'tugging', affective aspects, such as 'fearful', evaluative aspects, such as 'unbearable', and miscellaneous aspects, such as 'wretched'.

Application of the MPQ provides quantitative information in the form of a series of scores which indicate the sensory, affective and evaluative dimensions of pain. These are the Present Pain Intensity (PPI), the Pain Rating Index (PRI) and the Number of Words Chosen (NWC). These scores are used to evaluate the effectiveness of pain interventions (Melzack, 1975a).

Its widespread use supports the claim that the MPQ is 'valid, reliable, consistent and, above all, useful' (Melzack & Katz, 1994). Inevitably, this instrument is not without its critics, such as Wilkie *et al.* (1990) whose criticisms derive from a meta-analysis of 51 studies that used the MPQ. Developed initially for researchers with the aim of facilitating common understanding and communication between them (Melzack, 1975a), the MPQ has subsequently been used increasingly in clinical settings.

The likelihood of common understanding, however, is jeopardised by the differing forms of the MPQ. Wilkie and colleagues observe that only the body outline and the presence of 78 words are common and consistent features, suggesting that limited comparability results. The instructions relating to the administration of this questionnaire are contained in the original journal paper (Melzack, 1975a). They are neither well-detailed, comprising a critique of patients' comprehension rather than precise instructions, nor easy to follow, as is crucial if being applied clinically. Wilkie and colleagues further note the skewed distribution of MPQ scores, rather than the normal distribution claimed by Melzack. As the bias appears to be to the left it is possible that this instrument may be underestimating pain as has traditionally happened. These writers recommend that when the MPQ is used for research, the description of the method must provide maximum information, including details of both version used and application.

Assessment of pain in childbearing

In this section I focus on the assessment of labour pain, because other childbearing pain is probably comparable with other experiences of pain, whereas the nature of labour pain is unique. Thus, the general discussion of the assessment of pain up to this point is relevant to other pain in childbearing; examples would include postoperative pain, postnatal pain and in certain pregnancy-related conditions. I deal with neonatal pain assessment separately in Chapter 11. Hence, it is necessary now to consider what progress has been made in the assessment of labour pain and whether this progress benefits either the labouring woman or those who care for her. Because more attention has been given to research into assessing labour pain, I examine this first.

The difficulties of using the MPQ in labour were demonstrated by a large study (n=141) by Melzack *et al.* (1981) evaluating prepared childbirth. The instrument was applied once when the woman was in established labour. There was some variation in the data due to the precise stage of each labour being unknowable. Although details of the application were provided, the version of the MPQ was not. Because the questionnaire could only be completed between contractions the possibility of recall biasing the data emerges and makes this application different from the usual assessment of current pain. There is no explanation of whether the woman was asked to assess her most recent contraction or her strongest contraction. However, because, the MPQ takes 5 minutes to administer (Heywood & Ho, 1990), the focus on one particular contraction becomes difficult when the woman has a 'rest' of under 1 minute between contractions. It is, thus, possible that she could experience at least five contractions between beginning and completing the MPQ.

Despite these difficulties the MPQ has been used in other research on labour pain. Niven and Gijsbers (1984a) undertook a smaller study in which each woman completed the MPQ once in established labour and again within 24–48 hours of the birth. This study suggests that women with experience of non-childbearing pain are likely to have lower scores, indicating that they perceive less pain; whereas inexperienced women reported more pain. The MPQ was read to the woman in active labour. These researchers appear to have experienced no problems with administration of the MPQ, reporting 'All subjects responded well ... showing little difficulty selecting words'. Refuting criticisms that the MPQ is 'cumbersome', they contend that their study shows it to be acceptable and valid and recommend its use in further studies.

In an attempt to develop a more user-friendly instrument Fridh *et al.* (1988) devised a tool comprising three elements:

(1) a set of Visual Analogue Scales of affective aspects of labour for prenatal administration
(2) a painometer including 11 affective and 12 sensory word descriptors differentiating intensity of pain by each carrying a pain intensity score. Examples of the words (scores) include 'torturing' (5), 'killing' (5), 'pricking' (1), 'sore' (1). The scores are totalled, as in the MPQ
(3) a VAS comprising a 10-cm line with verbal anchors only at the extremes. These were 'no pain' and 'pain as bad as it can be'.

Assessments of pain intensity were made at three points in the labour: at 2–4 cm cervical dilatation, at 5–7 cm and at 8–10 cm.

While admitting that the instrument had not yet been subjected to rigorous testing, Fridh *et al.* claim it presents a simple, multidimensional view of labour pain. After applying this instrument to 50 primigravidae and 88 parous women, the authors conclude that through better understanding of the woman's pain more appropriate pain relief measures may be implemented.

Attempting to produce a simpler tool involved the use of physiological indicators to develop a behavioural pain index (Bonnel & Boureau, 1985). This instrument observed various phenomena, such as respirations, grasping movements, agitation and tension. Because it requires continuous observation throughout labour by an obstetrician or midwife its value is limited.

On the basis of this examination of pain assessment tools in general and their use in labour, it is necessary to contemplate whether they have any clinical relevance in labour. Current methods of assessing and treating the woman's labour pain are clearly inadequate (Rajan, 1993), hence research into and the introduction of innovative assessment methods could only improve the care of labouring women. In view of the time-consuming nature of pain assessment, Heywood and Ho (1990) recommend that a brief scale, such as the PPI (Present Pain Intensity) scale of the MPQ, could appropriately be applied half hourly in labour. The obvious question, though, is the value of the data which would be collected and the use to which it would be put. Rajan has shown that women are dissatisfied with the pain control that is provided. Is it likely that an instrument to clarify this dissatisfaction would actually improve matters? As Rajan suggested, midwives use their occupational experience to make decisions about pain control, and it is hard to imagine that introducing a PPI scale would change this.

Researching pain

Origins

'The outstanding event in the history of pain relief in childbirth' was the first administration of ether to a woman in labour by Simpson in 1847 (Moir, 1973). The research basis of this development, like so many in obstetrics, was scanty, to say the least. The 'research' which subsequently led to the 'almost universal' use of chloroform in labour was undertaken in the not uncongenial surroundings of Simpson's dining room in Edinburgh's up-market New Town (Smith, 1979). Unfortunately for generations of women, those who participated in Simpson's research were in no condition to identify the hazards of this drug in childbearing. Chamberlain (1993) reports chloroform's then well-known side-effects, such as irregular heart beat, liver damage, respiratory depression and uterine atony. These hazards jeopardised the life of the woman, baby or both, but did nothing to impede chloroform's widespread administration well into the twentieth century. Thus underresearched, the medical control of childbearing pain, and perhaps childbearing itself, was established. In this section I consider whether the research basis of this aspect of maternity care has changed in 150 years.

The mid-Victorian preoccupation with pharmacological pain control inevitably produced a backlash, represented by Dick-Read's (1933) ideas. His precepts shared little in common with those who originally opposed what was then termed 'natural childbirth'; these opponents' views continue to be promulgated (Bonica, 1994: 615). A common factor, though, was both sides' dearth of any research foundation. Dick-Read's teaching emanated from his jingoistic, eugenic and religious convictions (Kitzinger, J., 1989), while his opponents claimed women's support (Lewis, 1990).

Physiological research

It had been realised during the Middle Ages that the brain, rather than the heart, is the centre of sensory, and therefore pain, perception.

Descartes (1596–1650) sought to advance knowledge by explaining the function of sensory nerves, utilising the new scientific method; his anatomical dissections and suppositions persuaded him that bodily functioning is analogous to any machine's operating. The role of the sensory, including pain, nerves was compared with the bell-rope in church towers; a person or stimulus at one end initiated the action which resulted in the bell at the other end ringing, or sensation in the brain. The connecting structures or nerves were thought to be tubes containing threads, linking stimulus and perception (Bonica, 1990a).

Descartes' theory led to the belief that specific nerve endings in the skin led, via the dorsal horn of the spinal cord and the anterolateral spinothalamic tract, to the pain centre in the brain (Fordham & Dunn, 1994). This belief resulted in nineteenth century anatomists' search for sensory structures at the distal nerve endings. Clinical neurologists' recognition of localised cerebral lesions being consistently associated with specific deficits supported this 'specificity theory' (Chapter 1). Such observations were further supported by technical advances, such as staining techniques and microscopy (Wall & Jones, 1991). The 'intensive' or 'pattern' theories emerged to contradict specificity theory, being promulgated by differing groups of physiologists and psychologists (Bonica, 1990a). Based largely on animal experiments, the gate-control theory seemed to resolve this contradiction (Melzack & Wall, 1965; Chapter 1, 'Currently accepted pain theory'), although Melzack (1993) maintains that testing this theory engendered 'an explosion' of physiological and pharmacological research.

Recent research into prolonged pain mechanisms (Wall & Jones, 1991) suggests that the initial bombardment of the CNS with pain impulses may have long-term repercussions; simultaneously there may be changes in the chemicals produced and transported within nerve fibres (p. 136). The implications of this research and its relevance to childbearing remain uncertain, but a promising line of research is the role of the naturally occurring analgesics, the endorphins (Eisenach *et al.*, 1990).

Psychological research

The gate-control theory suggested that various factors affect the individual's perception of pain intensity (Melzack, 1993) and some of these may be psychological, rather than physiological. In childbearing, social support is likely to be one of these moderating factors (Chapter 8) as endorsed by research into the role of the father and midwife during labour (Niven & Gijsbers, 1984b; Niven, 1985; 1994).

Early this century Dick-Read conceived the idea of fear engendering or at least aggravating labour pain (Chapter 5). The relationship between anxiety and pain remains unclear and, while the interaction between these factors may be researched in other areas (Hayward, 1975), the unpredictable nature of labour presents the researcher with greater challenges.

The surprise finding that women's satisfaction does not necessarily correlate with the most effective pain control emerged from a study investigating epidural analgesia (Morgan *et al.*, 1982). This distinction between effective pain control and a satisfactory birth experience dawned as a revelation and helped illuminate issues of control, which subsequently became more significant.

Pain intervention research

Unlike other aspects of childbearing pain research, there is no shortage of research into the interventions to control pain (Oakley, 1993), such as the UK-wide study funded by the National Birthday Trust (NBT; Chamberlain *et al.*, 1993). This was a descriptive prospective study involving mothers and partners as well as midwives and medical staff. The study aimed to demonstrate the methods used to control labour pain and the circumstances under which these methods are used. Comparisons were sought between the consumers' and the staff's evaluation of pain control. Side effects of pain control methods were investigated and there was also a 6-week follow-up (Wraight, 1992).

The researchers encountered difficulty in contacting the sample, as 9% of Directors of Midwifery Services declined to participate (Wraight, 1993). A further seven maternity units contributed no data due to poor staffing, other research demands, high workload and staff sickness. The result was that only 88% of maternity units were involved in the survey, compared with a range of 99–94% previously (Wraight, 1992). The reasons given certainly applied in 1990, but this poor response leaves a nagging concern that research is low priority in an understaffed area where organisational changes threaten morale.

Mothers' low response (66% compared with the range 98–99% previously) was because 'they have things to do in these busy days' (Chamberlain *et al.*, 1993: 115). The response rate reflects the salience of the topic to those approached and/or the quality of the research design (Atkinson, 1988), but happened despite the researchers' efforts to involve consumers (Wraight, 1993) and staff (Wraight, 1992) and piloting the instruments (Wraight, 1993). Thus, it is necessary to question whether the inclusion of some other, perhaps more consumer-friendly or qualitative, method of data collection would have achieved a better response (Barker, 1991).

Despite this inadequate sample, the researchers draw conclusions (Chamberlain *et al.*, 1993) which relate to the organisation of maternity services and reflect satisfaction among mothers with pain control. Additionally, the closure of small maternity units is recommended 'unless geographically necessary' (1993: 117), as is the encouragement of women to accept epidural analgesia for operative deliveries and also the availability of 'non-medical volunteers' to stay with women in labour. The research basis of such recommendations is unclear.

The epidural analgesia data detail its availability and also the anxiety engendered in women planning to use an epidural and finding it unavailable. In her secondary data analysis, Rajan (1993) observes the difficulty which midwives reported when unable to contact an anaesthetist because she or he was outwith the maternity unit or busy elsewhere. A woman describes her feelings after this happened:

> 'To be told that staff shortages meant that there was no one around to give my epidural upset and panicked me . . . it is wrong to hand out books promising pain relief options that are not available in practice.' (Wraight, 1992)

This woman correctly identifies the ethical problem of stating that a 24-hour epidural service exists when this may not be so. My personal observation, that in this situation labour progresses well in terms of duration and maternal achievement, compares adversely with the woman's disappointment and anger. This problem is currently thought to apply to up to 25% of the women who request epidural analgesia in labour (Audit Commission, 1997).

Literature provided for women states: 'An epidural can be requested by you and the service is available 24 hours a day' (Stewart & West, undated). Certainly material such as this correctly indicates that an anaesthetic service covers the labour/delivery area for the full 24-hours, but omits to mention that this service also covers the theatre suite, which is included in the labour/delivery area. Thus, this service is effectively unavailable while caesarean or other operations are in progress. While Morgan (1993a) recounts the number of maternity units per region providing 24-hour epidural services as between 34% and 100%, the question must be asked whether this applies to dedicated epidural services or to labour/delivery/theatre services. Perhaps, yet again, the woman is denied accurate information on which to base pain control decisions (Mander, 1992b).

Following up the NBT study, Oakley (1993) points up some of the problems of researching childbirth pain; her criticisms appear strangely reminiscent of the NBT study. She highlights, first, the lack of qualitative data on this topic. She then notes the lack of serious methodological and theoretical questions, relevant to this report, which omits a literature review and includes a totally descriptive 'Method' section. She finally discusses the limitations of the survey as a data collection tool in such a sensitive area; criticism is absent elsewhere in the NBT report.

The research basis of midwives' pain control interventions is further scrutinised in relation to 'the most frequently used obstetric analgesic drug' (Allbright *et al.*, 1986). Thomson and Hillier (1994) examine the quality of the plentiful research data on pethidine and conclude that evidence to support its use is lacking. This deficiency applies, first, to the effectiveness of this drug and, second, to the likelihood that it may actually prolong the labour and, hence, the unrelieved pain (Chapter 9).

Thus, the quality of research on pain control and the limited effect of existing research findings are apparent.

Woman-orientated research

In view of these problems with quality and utilisation of research, it is necessary to consider the use and misuse to which research findings may be put. As identified elsewhere medical research claiming to reflect women's views provides ammunition in the ongoing conflict between obstetric anaesthetists and the active birth movement (Mander, 1994a). Of doubtful quality, this medical research appears to be considered acceptable if it only examines the 'softer' aspects of care, such as women's experiences (Oakley, 1993), whereas strict requirements apply to technical research. This double standard emphasises the minimal significance attached to the human aspects of care (Robinson, 1996b). All too frequently consumers remain unconsulted or disregarded; thus, the consumer view is qualitatively and quantitatively under-researched (Oakley, 1993).

To correct this deficit, the vulnerability of the labouring woman has been the basis of a plea for more appropriate research protocols (Robinson, 1996c). Using examples of labour pain control research, Robinson raises a number of ethical issues, summarising them as 'Research should be done with women not on women'. To achieve this, research ethical committees (RECs) should recognise the woman's right to appropriately timed information (to keep) relating to funding of the study, withdrawing, stopping interventions, not answering all items, being informed of findings and contacting the REC. Further arguing that women be more than research subjects, Robinson asserts the need for women's involvement in planning research, such as through REC membership. She comments further on RECs' cursory scrutiny of 'social science research'. Like Robinson, I have found that RECs' ignorance of non-medical research is profound; however, my experience is that this results in greater scrutiny, not the reverse (Mander, 1992a).

In view of Robinson's concerns and proposals, research on the involvement of women in research projects assumes greater significance. Elbourne (1987) studied women's feelings about their participation in a randomised controlled trial (RCT) on women holding their own maternity records. The enthusiasm of the women for this and any future studies emerges clearly. Whereas other researchers report difficulty explaining the concept of randomisation, this sample was quite comfortable with it. While Elbourne's sample negates Robinson's concerns, in contrast Garcia (1987) reinforces the woman/subject's need for support. Garcia focused on staff views about providing women with information about a recently completed RCT on fetal monitoring. A large proportion of staff were unconvinced of the value of giving women this information, fearing 'overload' or concern that she would not understand the information, because of staff's difficulties. An even more disquieting rationale for not giving women the findings was the 'professional' argument that the staff 'knew best'. Not only did this view deny choice to the woman, but also the research cast doubt on whether the staff actually knew best.

Pain research issues

As mentioned above, some health care providers disregard research findings. In a nursing context, this strategy is advocated by Pulsford (1992) on the grounds that research neither informs nor improves practice. Additionally, in caring it is unlikely to 'prove' anything decisive, so it is a waste of resources. As well as being irrelevant, Pulsford argues that researchers may endanger their subjects by exposing them to dehumanising experiences, such as questionnaires and interviews. While it is tempting to condemn Pulsford's heretical ideas, there is a grain of truth, as shown by Harris' work (1992) which demonstrated the negligible impact of research on midwifery practice. By choosing the well-researched area of perineal pain, Harris showed research findings' infrequent and then appropriate use.

A study in which midwives evaluated research reports believing them to be by midwives or medical personnel further supports Pulsford's argument (Hicks, 1992). Midwives belittled and ignored research that they thought was by midwives. This study raises serious concerns about midwives' valuing of their own knowledge base and may explain midwives' reluctance to utilise midwifery research.

Further probing Pulsford's criticisms, an attempt was made to ascertain why an apparently effective research-based pain control intervention was underutilised (Allcock, 1996a). Sofaer had sought to improve nurses' post-operative pain control (1985), but difficulty emerged in finding a suitable research design. This was partly due to the large number of variables inherent in human situations and the problem of isolating one independent variable which is ethically manipulable experimentally. We should also question the appropriateness of the tendency towards hard-edged, that is experimental, methods in the caring professions. Allcock suggests that action research may supply some of the answers in such complex human research. Although Sofaer's research intervention achieved an improvement in care, it was unsustained. The transience of staff in the surgical area reduces their ability to maintain a change as does their status in the multidisciplinary hierarchy. It may be that these issues apply equally to midwives researching childbearing pain and that more woman-orientated research may provide the information from which midwives and those with whom they practise will benefit.

The criticisms articulated by Pulsford are answered authoritatively in the context of cancer nursing (Gaston-Johansson & Fall-Dickson, 1995). These authors argue that because these cancer nurses are the personnel who are with the person in pain and because it is they who 'deliver pain treatments directly' (p. 598–9), they inevitably carry a research responsibility. This argument applies at least equally to midwives. These authors identify that pain in certain groups is woefully under-researched, such as minority populations. Because of the tremendous cultural input into childbearing, midwives should consider whether they have made any better progress than their nursing cousins. Unlike Allcock's more human argument, these authors advance the need for more powerful and hard-edged research designs, meaning the increasing use of RCTs.

The ultimate answer to Pulsford's inanity is provided, however, by Chalmers (1993). He states unequivocally that, far from an irrelevant luxury, it is the obligation of midwives to provide women with research-based care. He goes on to require midwives to base their care on strong research evidence, thus challenging them to evaluate that which they contemplate applying. Like Oakley (1993), Chalmers reiterates the need for research on questions which are of not just interest, but also importance to women and midwives. Chalmers' example illustrating the serious implications of unresearched practice is the introduction of epidural analgesia three decades ago. As with many interventions, this form of pain control was introduced when inadequately researched. The result is that now such research is likely to be increasingly difficult, though 'certainly still feasible' (1993: 9). Although this 'high-tech' form of pain control constitutes a glaring example of the need for research, there are many relatively low-tech and midwifery interventions which would benefit from similar research attention.

Summary

To end this section on researching pain in childbearing, I answer my initial question of whether the research basis of our pain interventions has improved in the past 150 years. Unfortunately for those for whom we care, the conclusion must be that, despite a plethora of research, the increase in our knowledge of the woman-orientated implications of our interventions is barely, if at all, discernible.

Chapter 3
Medication: Constraints and Consequences

Although the midwife utilises many interventions in labour which are variably beneficial, it is her use of medicines that traditionally has been and still is most stringently controlled. Further, midwives in a range of educational settings find the consequences of disobedience to these controls being impressed on them. In this chapter we consider the constraints, especially the legislative framework within which the midwife practises and is able to prescribe and administer medicines to the woman for whom she cares. We look first at the reasons for the legislation and second at what it comprises. Third, we examine the operation of the legislation and, then, how the legislation relates to an area which is of increasing interest, that is, complementary medicines. An important constraint on the midwife's administration of medicines is their fetal and neonatal effects, which is examined next. Finally, there is some discussion of the consequences of non-adherence to the constraints.

The rationale for legislation

In general terms Bayliss (1980) reminds us of the benefits and hazards which are difficult to avoid in the use of drugs. He draws attention to the fact that drugs may be perceived as a double-edged sword, imparting both advantages and dangers. The aim of the legislation, he maintains, is to permit the benefits to accrue while limiting the dangers. While this arrangement sounds ideal, he fails to relate such altruism to the nature of the legislation, which is almost entirely reactive, rather than proactive. His example is the Medicines Act (1968) which reached the statute book as a reaction to the thalidomide debacle, and which sought to redress the lack of statutory controls on the safety of new drugs.

A further reason for the legal control of medicines is protection in an even wider sense. This reason is particularly relevant in the context of pain control in childbearing because of the risk of addiction to many of the drugs which midwives administer to control pain. Thus legislation is intended to reduce the likelihood of addiction in both recipients and health care personnel. While this aim is laudable, it is necessary to question why these substances are the subject of legislation, when many agents that are similarly dangerous are not. Equally, some drugs that are dangerous and probably addictive are subject to comparatively lax legislation, examples being alcohol and tobacco. Yet another rationale has been identified in the context of the currently developing role of the midwife as an increasingly independent practitioner (Simpson & Smith, 1995a). These authors emphasise the increasing importance of the midwife's understanding.

The regulations

The legislative framework which guides and controls the midwife's actions in relation to her prescription and administration of drugs derives from the Medicines Act (1968), the Misuse of Drugs Act (1971) together with subsequent amendments, the Medicines (Prescription Only) Order (1983), the *Guidelines for the Safe and Secure Handling of Medicines* or Duthie Report (1988), as well as the United Kingdom Central Council for Nursing, Midwifery and Health Visiting, *Midwives Rules* (UKCC, 1991b) and *Midwife's Code of Practice* (UKCC, 1991a). These documents cover the classification of drugs, and the supply, surrender, recording and destruction of drugs (Simpson & Smith, 1995b).

The confusion caused by standing orders drawn up to avoid retrospective or prospective prescribing has caused some highly publicised problems for our nursing colleagues (Simpson & Smith, 1995b), which have hopefully been resolved by the introduction of midwife and nurse prescribing. The introduction of self-administration of drugs in hospital (Chapter 10, 'Pharmacological methods') was addressed in UKCC guidelines (1992). Practices that may be regarded as the extended role of the midwife, such as topping up epidural analgesia, are also controlled by the *Midwives Rules* (Roch 1993).

The developing system

A recommendation for nurse prescribing featured in the Cumberlege report on neighbourhood nursing (1986). The Crown report (1989) sought to operationalise this recommendation by applying it to 'the supply of drugs, dressings, appliances and chemical reagents to patients'. The list of approved substances would be incorporated in a 'Nurse's Formulary'. Similar practice developments have been introduced into midwifery and 'Prescribing Guides for Midwives' have been drawn up. The Medicinal Products: Prescribing by Nurses, Midwives and Health Visitors Act (1992) authorises initial prescribing by these groups. In order to comply with this legislation, the midwife must address four issues; these are authority, ability, context of activity and competency.

Legislation relating to complementary medicines

Although some people may think that homeopathic and other complementary remedies are of so little effect that they must be harmless, this has by no means been established. For this reason, complementary remedies are subject to regulation in the same way as allopathic medicines. The regulations controlling the midwife's use of complementary remedies are also included in Section C of the *Midwives Rules* (UKCC, 1991b) and in Section 3.4 of the *Midwife's Code of Practice* (UKCC, 1991a). Additionally, the UKCC document entitled *Standards for the Administration of Medicines* (1992) spells out the regulations under the Medicines Act (1968) covering these remedies. The quality, safety and efficacy of all medicines are controlled at entry to and removal from the market by the Medicines Act (1968). Because most complementary medicines were already on the market when the Act came into operation in 1971 they are covered by special arrangements which applied to drugs already in existence. These drugs were granted Product Licences of Right which exempted them from additional scrutiny.

In terms of prescription and administration, the usual arrangement is for homeopathic substances to be prescribed by a recognised practitioner. Additionally or alternatively they may be self-administered by the woman, a practice endorsed in rules 34 and 35 of the *Midwife's Code of Practice* (Jones, 1994).

Fetal and neonatal constraints

As well as the written requirements, other important considerations that influence the midwife's administration of medicines are the fetal and neonatal effects. The fetal effects are due to the transplacental transfer of drugs by passive diffusion, which may be facilitated or inhibited by certain factors. These factors include the molecular weight of the drug which, when greater, slows diffusion. Similarly, ionisation, low concentration gradient, lipid insolubility and increasing pH slow that movement (Cupit & Rotmensch, 1992). The transfer of drugs via breast milk is by a similar process with similar inhibitors. This means that 'virtually all drugs cross into the breast milk' (Rubin, 1987). Of greater concern, though, is the effect of the drug. According to Rubin, the presence of many drugs is undetectable in the baby; this applies particularly to highly protein-bound drugs, such as warfarin. There is a larger group of drugs whose effect on the neonate is not significant. Another group is those that are likely to be transferred to the baby in sufficient quantity to cause harm. Of particular importance in this group are opioids, lithium, carbimazole, cytotoxics and immunosuppressants.

The consequences

It is a fact of life that medication errors happen, despite legislative and institutional precautions aiming to prevent them. As well as educational approaches (Carlisle, 1996), other recommendations have been made to reduce both the likelihood and the impact of medication errors. That such errors are not just a reflection of an individual's irresponsibility is recognised in the policy implications of these errors. As well as no-fault reporting, the system of 'failure mode analysis', developed from the aircraft industry on the assumption that if anything can go wrong it will, has been advocated. At the same time it is increasingly recognised that the dire punishment often resulting from medication errors serves to deter staff from admitting mistakes, thus compounding the risk to the patient.

The personal implications of medication errors were the subject of a qualitative study (Arndt, 1994). This researcher identified general enthusiasm for 'the procedure' of disciplining those who admit a medication error, although this enthusiasm was reduced among those who had been through it. Support following a medication error was earnestly sought and the need for it may serve to persuade a nurse to openly admit such an error. This support may be sought from a range of colleagues, but medical staff were found to be especially helpful, perhaps reflecting their contribution to such errors through, for example, illegible handwriting. On the basis of her study, Arndt recommends that the focus of the problem should be transferred away from the 'guilty' nurse and on to the situation which permitted the error to happen.

Summary

As with so much of the legislative framework within which the midwife practises, the purpose of the drugs regulations may be questioned. Perhaps in this area, legislation is more beneficial to the midwife than in other aspects of her practice. This is because it is clear that the legislation serves not only to protect the midwife and her client from medication errors and their consequences, but also to protect her from accusations of inappropriate practice.

Chapter 4
Scientific Background
Hally McCrea
BSc, MSc, DPhil, RN, RM, RMT, Former Lecturer,
School of Health Sciences, University of Ulster

Introduction

Pain is an integral part of labour and delivery (Melzack, 1984). It is not as was previously believed, a direct result of only social, cultural and emotional influences in civilised societies (Velvovsky, 1954; Dick-Read, 1962), but rather it is a culmination of both physiological and psychosocial factors. This chapter will focus mainly on the physiological basis of pain in labour although references will be made, where appropriate, to psychological influences. The chapter outlines the neuroanatomy/physiology of pain with specific reference to labour pain, the pain pathways involved, including ascending and descending pathways, bodily responses to pain and concludes with an examination of the methods used to block the physiological processes of pain.

Neuroanatomy of pain

The sensation of pain is produced by a complex network of nerve fibres that involves both the peripheral and central nervous systems. In labour pain, the autonomic nervous system and particularly the sympathetic component also plays a role in the sensation. Before proceeding to examine the more complex neurophysiology of these systems, a description of the basic structural unit of pain is considered.

Basic structural unit of pain

The nerve cell or neurone consists of a cell body and two sets of processes which are primarily responsible for the transmission of nerve impulses, including pain impulses (Fig. 4.1). Projecting from the cell body are short branched processes called dendrites which receive sensory stimuli from the outside environment of the cell and transmit them toward the cell body. These processes are called afferent (sensory) neurones or nerve fibres and are the receptors for all stimuli, including noxious (pain) impulses.

Each cell also possesses a single process called the axon which varies in

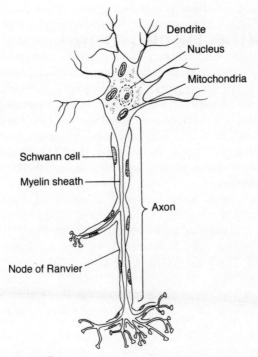

Fig. 4.1 Structures of the neurone.

length and along which nerve impulses are conducted away from the cell body of a neurone to the dendrite of another neuron or to efferent structures such as muscles or glands. These nerve fibres are called efferent (motor) neurones. Most of the axons are covered with two layers; a spiral sheath composed of specialised cells called Schwann cells, and a myelin sheath which is a liquid substance contained in the Schwann cells and which acts as an electrical insulator. It is arranged along the axon like a string of sausages separated by the nodes of Ranvier which allow electrical transmission of nerve impulses in myelinated nerve fibres.

It is now known that there are two specific types of peripheral nerve fibres which transmit and process pain sensations separately; A-delta and C-fibres (Perl, 1971; Hallin & Torebjork, 1974; Bonica & Albe-Fessard, 1976). A-delta are small, thinly myelinated fibres which innervate the skin and subcutaneous tissues as well as viscera, muscle and other deep structures. They transmit impulses quickly and pain associated is easy to localise and generally described as 'pricking and sharp'. C-fibres are also small but unmyelinated and make up two-thirds of the nerve fibres in the peripheral nervous system. They transmit information more slowly than A-delta fibres and are responsible for conducting slow, burning pain, generally described as 'deep, aching' and hard to localise.

Some of these nociceptive (pain) fibres are activated by strong mechanical stimulation and are called mechanical nociceptors. Some are stimulated by extreme cold or high temperature and are referred to as thermal nociceptors. A number are also activated by both mechanical and thermal stimuli and by pain-sensitive chemicals and are called polymodal nociceptors. Approximately a quarter of the A-delta fibres respond to very strong mechanical and thermal stimuli (Perl, 1971; Burgess, 1974; Bonica & Albe-Fessard, 1976) and these fibres innervate not only the skin and subcutaneous tissues but also viscera, including the uterus. Additionally, 10–20% of C-fibres supply mechanical nociceptors and approximately 30–40% supply polymodal nociceptors.

The role of these two nerve fibres in the transmission of noxious stimulation accounts for the concept of 'double pain'; the first, sharp pain is conducted by myelinated A-delta fibres, whereas the second, dull, aching pain is mediated by slow conducting C-fibres (Bonica, 1980). This brief outline is the basic neuroanatomy of pain associated with somatic and autonomic stimulation. There are, however, certain distinct features of the autonomic nervous system and in particular the sympathetic component which apply to visceral pain including labour pain.

The autonomic nervous system

The autonomic nervous system controls the activities of smooth muscles and viscera such as the uterus and may be known as the involuntary nervous system because these organs function without conscious control. There are two distinct components: the sympathetic and parasympathetic systems. These systems act synergistically where they innervate the same organ, but they also act alone, for example the sympathetic nerves supply the uterus and form an essential part of the neuroanatomy of labour pain.

Afferent neurones transmitting information from noxious stimulation from the autonomic to the central nervous system travel from the viscera mainly via sympathetic nerve fibres. These fibres have their cell bodies in the dorsal root ganglia from which central processes (dendrites and axons) travel into the spinal cord. In the dorsal horn region they synapse, a process which will be discussed later in the chapter (see 'Synapse'), with connector neurones. Both somatic and autonomic afferent neurones synapse in the dorsal horn region and it has been suggested that they may interact, resulting in a phenomenon called 'referred pain'. This is the predominant pain felt during labour and particularly during the first stage (Brownridge, 1995) and will be considered later in the chapter (see 'Referred pain').

Autonomic afferent neurones ascend through the spinal cord and brain stem alongside somatic afferent neurones, but whereas the majority of the fibres in the latter continue to the thalamus, many of the autonomic afferents travel to the hypothalamus before radiating to the thalamus and then finally to the cerebral cortex. Here noxious impulses and their emotional components are integrated and interpreted before a response is transmitted through descending pain pathways.

A further distinct feature of the autonomic nervous system is the fact that efferent neurones emerge from the central nervous system only through three regions:

(1) in the brain (3rd, 7th, 9th and 10th cranial nerves)
(2) in the thoracic region (T1 to T12, L1 and L2)
(3) second and third sacral segments of the spinal cord.

The thoracic region forms the outflow for the sympathetic nervous system which supplies visceral organs such as the uterus.

The majority of autonomic efferent neurones leave the central nervous system and synapse with excitatory neurones at peripheral sites where these cells collect to form 'ganglia'. The ganglion may lie some distance away from the organ which it supplies (in the case of the sympathetic component) or it may lie close to or within the organ (in the case of the parasympathetic component (Bond, 1981).

Prior to synapses, efferent neurones are referred to as pre-ganglionic neurones and in the sympathetic system they travel to a ganglion via white rami communicantes, so called because these neurones are covered with a myelin sheath. Following synapses they are termed post-ganglionic neurones and in the sympathetic system they leave the ganglion via grey rami communicantes because these neurones are unmyelinated. The neurones may take one of a number of different pathways before reaching their final destination. Unlike the neurones of the parasympathetic system which tend to be mostly pre-ganglionic and therefore have fewer synapses, efferent neurones of the sympathetic system have approximately eight synapses before reaching the organ(s) they innervate.

Peripheral pathways of labour pain

Experimental work on the autonomic nervous system indicates that both the sympathetic and parasympathetic components supply the majority of the abdominal and pelvic organs, including the uterus. Anatomically, the smooth muscle of the uterus is supplied mostly by unmyelinated C-fibres and some small myelinated A-delta fibres. Bonica's work during the 1950s and 1960s (exact dates are not given) provides some of the information on the peripheral pain pathways during labour. This was a long-term clinical study which utilised a sample

of 187 women (162 parturients, 25 gynaecological patients) to investigate the influence of neural block of different spinal cord segments on
labour pain. Neural blocks such as paravertebral somatic nerve block,
trans-sacral nerve block, segmental epidural block and lumbar sympathetic block were used to study their effects on pain produced by manual
stretch of the cervix, uterine contraction pain, perineal pain and other
pain associated with labour. Drawing on the results of this study, Bonica
(1980) provides a description of the pain pathways during labour (Fig.
4.2).

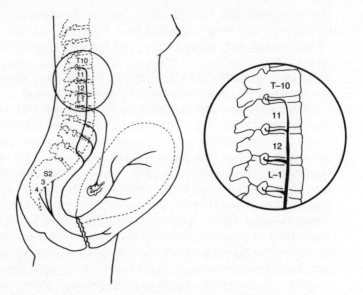

Fig. 4.2   Peripheral pathways of labour pain.

Nociceptive fibres in the uterus and cervix pass through the uterine
and cervical plexuses and then (in sequence) through the pelvic plexus,
the middle hypogastric nerve, the superior hypogastric nerve and then
to the lumbar sympathetic chain. From here, the nociceptive fibres pass
through the lower thoracic chain and then leave it by running through
the white rami communicantes linked with T10, T11, T12 and L1
spinal nerves. Finally they pass through these nerves and their posterior
roots to enter the spinal cord and link up with the dorsal horn neurones.
Nociceptive fibres from the perineum pass through the pudendal nerve
and into the spinal cord through the posterior roots of S2, S3 and S4.
Additionally, the lower lumbar and upper sacral segments supply nerves
to pelvic structures which are involved in labour pain.

During the first stage of labour, pain is due to dilatation of the cervix
and lower uterine segment and distension of the body of the uterus

(Bonica & Chadwick, 1989). The intensity of the pain during this stage is due to the strength of the contractions and the pressure thus generated. This assertion is based on the finding that an amniotic fluid pressure of over 15 mmHg above tonus is required to distend the lower uterine segment and the cervix and thus produce pain (Caldeyro-Barcia & Poseiro, 1960). In fact pressures of over 50 mmHg have been recorded as being the 'norm' during the first stage of labour (Caldeyro-Barcia & Poseiro, 1960). It is logical therefore to expect that with higher amniotic fluid pressure, distension will be greater, causing more severe pain. The pain is referred to dermatones supplied by the same spinal cord segments that receive nociceptive input from the uterus and cervix. Dermatones are body areas that are innervated by specific spinal nerves, for example dermatone 12 refers to the twelfth thoracic dermatone (T12). The pain is felt as an ache in early first stage and limited to the eleventh (T11) and twelfth (T12) thoracic dermatones. Later in the first stage of labour, pain in T11 and T12 dermatones becomes more severe, sharp and cramping, and spreads to T10 and L1 dermatones.

Descent of the fetal head into the pelvis in the late first stage causes distension of pelvic structures and pressure on the roots of the lumbosacral plexus, producing referred pain by way of segments L2 and below. Consequently pain is felt in the region of L2, low in the back and also in the thighs and legs.

In the second stage of labour, additional pain is caused by stretching and tearing of tissues such as the perineum and pressure on skeletal muscles of the perineum. Here the pain is due to stimulation of superficial somatic structures and is described as sharp and localised, mainly to areas supplied by the pudendal nerves. Some women may experience pain in their thighs and legs, described as aching, burning or crampy. This may be caused by stimulation of structures in the pelvis which are pain-sensitive and which results in mild pain referred to the lower lumbar and sacral segments.

Transmission of nociceptive impulses from the dorsal horn and spinal cord to ascending systems to the brain is said to follow the same pathways as other types of acute pain and is discussed in 'Pain pathways', (this chapter).

Referred pain

The phenomenon of referred pain has been mentioned on a number of occasions and requires an explanation. It describes the manner in which pain caused by tissue damage in one organ is experienced as though it were occurring at some distant organ. The classic example here is left shoulder pain associated with angina pectoris. A less obvious case is pain during the first stage of labour which is mediated by mechanical distension of the lower uterine segment and cervix (Bonica & Chadwick, 1989), but the pain is referred to the abdomen, lower back and rectum (Brownridge, 1995). There are a number of explanations for this phenomenon, but the most plausible is that nociceptive fibres from visceral organs enter the spinal cord at the same level as afferent fibres from the referred area of the body, so that nociceptive fibres from the uterus travel to the same spinal cord segments as somatic afferents from the abdomen, lower back and rectum.

Synapse

The transmission and processing of peripheral stimulation occurs through the process of synapse. Nociceptive impulses must be converted into electrochemical energy before they can travel from one neurone to the next. They are transmitted from one part of the nervous system to the other along a chain of neurones. There is no physical contact between them; rather, impulses (referred to as action potential) are transmitted from one to the other by chemical substances released as a result of electrical activity. These substances, called neurotransmitters, travel to receptor sites on the dendrites of nerves to which the transfer is being made. This causes depolarisation of the nerve membrane and increased electrical activity in the next neuron of the chain.

Depolarisation is a change in the electrical state of a nerve fibre caused by chemical, mechanical and/or thermal stimulation. This alters the distribution of ions within a cell so that sodium and chloride ions flow into the cell and potassium ions flow out (Bond, 1981). The space across which neurotransmitters cross is called the synapse (Fig. 4.3) and it is bordered by the membranes of the two nerves involved. The membrane of the transmitting nerve is referred to as the presynaptic and that of the receptor as the postsynaptic.

There are two types of synapse: excitatory and inhibitory. In the former, the neurotransmitter released causes depolarisation of the

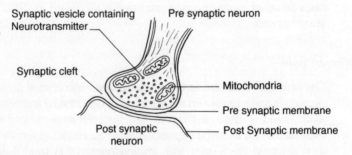

Fig. 4.3 Processes involved in a synapse.

nerve membrane which in turn generates depolarisation in the receptor nerve. In the latter case, the neurotransmitter released causes hyperpolarisation which inhibits an action potential emerging in the receptor neuron.

Experimental work on neurotransmitters provides some information on their physiology in producing pain sensation (Sicuteri, 1974; Taub, 1974). It has been established that pain can be caused by mechanical, chemical and thermal stimuli. These stimuli irritate and cause injury to tissues which then sets in motion a process at the cellular level that leads to pain perception. When pain impulses are received, they stimulate nerve endings which respond by releasing the appropriate neurotransmitter(s). These are the chemicals that cause depolarisation of nerve membranes and include potassium and hydrogen ions (Bond, 1981), histamine, serotonin, bradykinin, prostaglandins (E-type), substance P, acetylcholine and noradrenaline. The neurotransmitter in the autonomic nervous system is acetylcholine whereas noradrenaline is produced by excitatory neurones in the sympathetic component of the autonomic nervous system.

Neurotransmitters can produce pain directly. Experimental work has shown, for example, that when these substances are applied to the skin of humans, they can cause pain (Keele & Armstrong, 1964). They are also known to act in combination to effect pain. It has been demonstrated for instance that excitation of muscle nociceptors by bradykinin can be increased substantially if serotonin or prostaglandin E2 is also present (Zimmerman, 1981). Most midwives will be familiar with prostaglandins which are used for the induction of labour. What may not be so obvious is the fact that fluid and electrolyte imbalance which may coexist with labour pain can in fact increase pain sensation. This may be a particular problem for women who experience a difficult and/or long first stage of labour.

Since the human body cannot endure pain indefinitely, nature has a built-in mechanism for reducing and eliminating the sensation. This mechanism makes use of substances called neuromodulators which are produced by the body in response to stress and pain. They act by blocking the release of excitatory neurotransmitters (Snyder, 1977). A number of neuromodulators have been discovered and they are categorised into three main groups: beta-lipotrophin, enkephalin and dynorphin. Beta-endorphin is a sub-group of beta-lipotrophin and has been shown to inhibit the formation of prostaglandins and reduce their effects.

The endorphins are endogenous opiates which have a morphine-like action and are produced in varying concentrations in the brain, spinal cord and the gastrointestinal tract in response to stress and pain. Stimulation of beta-endorphins during labour is an important physiological pain block and will be considered in greater detail under 'Blocking the physiological processes' (this chapter).

Pain pathways

Nociceptive impulses are transmitted from the peripheral spinal nerves to the dorsal horn cells and then to the brain. Textbooks on neurophysiology provide varied definitions and descriptions of pain pathways to the brain, but there seems to be agreement that essentially there are three main ascending pain pathways to the brain that include the spinothalamic, spinoreticular (also known as the lemniscal tract) and spinocervical tracts. The dorsal horn forms an integral part of the pain pathways since it is the first synaptic link between the peripheral and central nervous systems. It is also recognised as an important structure in pain sensation.

Dorsal horn

The dorsal horn is a complex structure consisting of six layers called laminae. Lamina 1 cells receive information from A-delta and C-fibres and it is assumed therefore that they play a role in pain. Their axons project through the spinal cord and ascend as the spinothalamic tract (Kerr, 1975). Laminae 2 and 3 cells make up the substantia gelatinosa which lie on either side of the posterior horn of grey matter and are said to have a modulating effect on pain impulses (Wall, 1964). These cells project to the brain. Lamina 4 cells respond to gentle pressure and may not play a role in pain. These cells project to the dorsolateral pathway. In contrast, lamina 5 cells respond readily to noxious stimuli (Hillman & Wall, 1969) and especially from viscera such as the uterus (Pomeranz *et al.*, 1968). The majority of lamina 5 cells travel through the spinothalamic tract and then on to the brain.

One of the most significant roles of the dorsal horn in labour pain is the fact that all of lamina 5 cells respond to both visceral afferents and somatic afferents from skin innervated by the same spinal cord system. It has been suggested that somatic and visceral fibres converge with lamina 5 cells to produce the phenomenon of 'referred pain' which occurs during each uterine contraction (Bonica, 1980).

Ascending pain pathways

Information from the body is transmitted to the brain via the three main pain pathways: spinothalamic, spinoreticular and spinocervical tracts (Fig. 4.4). The most important spinal cord pathway for the transmission of noxious stimuli is said to be the spinothalamic tract (Albe-Fessard *et al.*, 1974). It is composed of lamina 5 cells, some of which link up with afferent visceral fibres and may be the basis for referred pain of labour (Wilson, 1974). It consists of two parts: the neospinothalamic and the paleospinothalamic systems. The neurones of the former travel directly

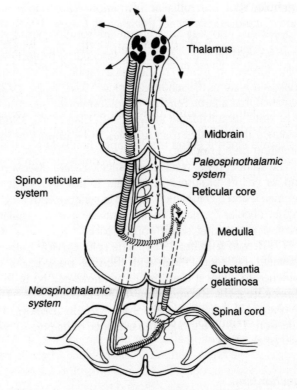

Fig. 4.4 The main ascending pain pathways.

to the thalamus whereas those of the latter system travel to the reticular formation, the medulla and midbrain and then end in the thalamus. The neospinothalamic system consists of long fibres, has fewer synapses and transmits impulses rapidly, which results in 'localised, sharp pain'. It is thought to be involved in the discrimination of spatial and temporal aspects of pain. In contrast, the paleospinothalamic system consists of short fibres, has frequent synapses and transmits impulses slowly. It is believed to be responsible for the less discriminative aspects of pain; the motivational-affective component which is concerned with aversive drive and responsive behaviours (Meinhart & McCaffery, 1983), for example preventing or avoiding painful stimuli. The spinoreticular tract begins with A-delta fibres which enter the dorsal column and then travel to the medulla, synapse with second order neurones and cross over before synapsing with third order neurones in the thalamus. The message is finally transmitted to the cerebral cortex.

This tract is also believed to be involved in the motivational-affective rather than the sensory-discriminative aspects of pain (Melzack & Casey, 1968; Price & Dubner, 1977). There is evidence to suggest, for example, that the reticular formation may trigger arousal and thus motivate individuals to act (Melzack & Casey, 1968; Price & Dubner, 1977). The role of the spinoreticular tract in pain sensation is strengthened by the finding that descending projections from the reticular formation inhibit nociceptive input and stimulate endogenous analgesia systems (Basbaum & Fields, 1978; Willis, 1982). There is also evidence that a large number of spinoreticular neurones are responsive to noxious stimuli (Haber *et al.*, 1982; Blair *et al.*, 1984). Based on the evidence thus far this tract appears to be important in modifying and inhibiting pain impulses.

The spinocervical tract is a relatively recent discovery (Morin, 1955) and as yet its precise role in pain is not known. It originates from laminae 4 and 5 cells which ascend to synapse with third order neurones in the reticular formation before travelling to the thalamus. The fibres are fast acting and some appear to be nociceptive (Cerveno *et al.*, 1977; Brown & Fyffe, 1981). The spinocervical pathway seems to be activated by mechanical and thermal nociceptors. There is also evidence to suggest that it may be stimulated by both A-delta and C-fibres (Gregor & Zimmerman, 1973; Brown *et al.*, 1975). It may be involved in behavioural responses to pain (Bishop, 1980; Ignelzi & Atkinson, 1980), although the evidence of its precise role in pain is not fully established.

Brain mechanisms

Traditionally it was believed that the centre of pain is located in the cerebral cortex, but recent evidence suggests that the thalamus, hypothalamus, reticular formation, limbic system and the cerebral cortex are all involved in pain sensation. Exactly how this complex system of neuronal networks functions is not clear, but it is believed that sensory as well as motivational-affective processes are involved. The reader is referred to Melzack's (1973) *The Puzzle of Pain* for further information on this aspect of pain.

Descending pain pathways

Wall (1970) provides some evidence to suggest that vibration can reduce the subsequent response of neurones in the posterior horn of the grey matter to nociceptive stimuli. These neurones can also be influenced by centrifugal impulses travelling down the spinal cord from the brain (Hagbarth & Kerr, 1954). It would appear therefore that nociceptive impulses can be modified once they reach the spinal cord by impulses from the cord itself and/or from the brain.

There is in fact evidence to suggest that ascending nociceptive afferent impulses can be modulated by descending inhibitory pathways

(Bishop, 1980). Findings from experiments using electrical stimulation (Terman *et al.*, 1984) and opiate mechanisms (Ignelzi & Atkinson, 1980; Zimmerman, 1981) imply that modulation can take place at any point where synapses occur. This may be at the first synaptic transmission in the substantia gelatinosa, in the brain stem, the thalamus or the cerebral cortex. Some researchers claim that the brainstem structures are primarily responsible for the descending control of pain information (Mayer & Price, 1976; Fields & Basbaum, 1989). Electrical stimulation of some neurones in the midbrain, for example, has been shown to produce analgesia which is comparable to very large doses of morphine (Bonica, 1980; Willis, 1982). Stimulation appears to activate an inhibitory neural system which blocks transmission of pain in the spinal cord and other parts of the nervous system.

One of the most important descending inhibitory systems is the opiate mechanism first described by Reynolds (1969). Since Reynolds' discovery, new evidence (Basbaum *et al.*, 1976) demonstrates that when endogenous opiates are released, they bind to opiate receptors and activate descending inhibitory neurones. These neurones release serotonin which acts as a neuromodulator to inhibit nociceptive information in the spinal cord.

Pain and stress are also known to activate descending inhibitory pathways, although the opioid and non-opioid pathways may respond to different types of stress (Terman *et al.*, 1984; Phillips & Cousins, 1986). As new evidence emerges, it is becoming clear that descending pathways have a crucial role to play in pain sensation, especially chemical mechanisms, which will be examined in greater detail in 'Blocking the Physiological Processes' (this chapter).

Labour pain and bodily responses

Pain associated with uterine contractions affects the physiological mechanisms of a number of body systems which invariably leads to generalised and widespread physiological stress response (Brownridge, 1995). Many of the involuntary responses are probably nature's way of preserving homeostasis, but severe and prolonged labour pain can affect ventilation, circulation, metabolism and uterine activity (Fig. 4.5).

Ventilation

Pain associated with uterine contraction causes hyperventilation, with respiration rates of 60–70 breaths per minute being recorded (Cole & Nainby-Luxmoore, 1962). Hyperventilation in turn can cause lowering of the $PaCO_2$ level (normal pregnant level is 32 mmHg, decreased level is 16–20 mmHg; Bonica, 1973) and a consequent increase in pH level. Similar findings have been reported by a number of researchers in the

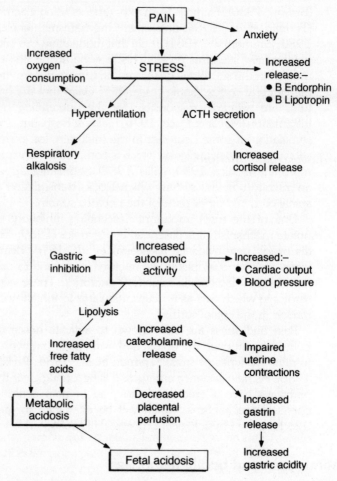

Fig. 4.5   Diagram illustrating the physiological changes associated with labour pain.

area of labour pain (Fisher & Prys-Roberts, 1968; Marx *et al.*, 1969; Huch *et al.*, 1977; Peabody, 1979). One of the dangers of a low maternal $PaCO_2$ level is lowering of the fetal $PaCO_2$ level resulting in late decelerations of the fetal heart.

Ventilation may increase markedly when women in labour use breathing exercises (Brownridge, 1995). This could affect the acid–base balance of the circulatory system, producing alkalosis with pH of 7.5 and above. The evident danger of alkalosis during labour is a decrease in oxygen transfer to the fetus. It could also induce vasoconstriction of the uterus (Motoyama *et al.*, 1966), prolonging labour and further exacerbating alkalosis. Thus a vicious cycle is set in motion.

Increased ventilation together with the energy expanded in pushing during the second stage of labour could raise maternal oxygen consumption and thus compromise fetal oxygenation. Evidence that these respiratory changes are pain-mediated has been demonstrated by the finding that effective pain relief, using regional analgesia, prevents their occurrence (Pearson & Davies, 1973; Hagerdal *et al.*, 1983). Pain relief, such as narcotics, does not seem to prevent hyperventilation and may in fact depress further ventilation and thus aggravate fetal hypoxia (Pearson & Davies, 1973).

Cardiovascular functions

Cardiac output increases progressively as labour advances mainly because of labour pain (Ueland & Hansen, 1969). The increase could be as much as 15–20% above that of pre-labour during the early first stage and as much as 45–50% during the second stage (Hendricks & Quilligan, 1956; Ueland & Hansen, 1969). It has been estimated that each uterine contraction increases cardiac output 20–30% over that when the uterus is relaxed (Hendricks & Quilligan, 1956; Adams & Alexander, 1958). The increase in cardiac output is due partly to the fact that with each contraction, approximately 250–300 ml of blood is squeezed from the uterus into the maternal circulation. It is also possible that increased sympathetic activity brought about by labour pain, anxiety and fear may be responsible for some of the rise in cardiac output as labour advances (Hendricks & Quilligan, 1956; Ueland & Hansen, 1969).

The pain from uterine contractions could also cause a rise in both systolic and diastolic blood pressure and may help to explain why some obstetricians advocate epidural analgesia for women who develop pre-eclampsia or have a history of hypertension. Increases in cardiac output and systolic blood pressure associated with labour pain generally do not pose any major danger to healthy women in labour. It could, however, increase the risks for women with cardiac diseases, pre-eclampsia or hypertension (Bonica & Ueland, 1969; Morishima *et al.*, 1980).

Metabolic effects

The increase in sympathetic activity caused by labour pain can lead to an increase in metabolism and oxygen consumption and decreased gastrointestinal and urinary bladder motility. The pain and anxiety associated with labour can cause further delay in gastric emptying (Nimmo *et al.*, 1975; 1977). Increased oxygen consumption, loss of sodium bicarbonate from the kidneys to compensate for the respiratory alkalosis caused by labour pain, and often reduced carbohydrate intake (due to restricted dietary policy during labour) all contribute to a state of metabolic acidosis which is then transferred to the fetus.

Endocrine effects

Stress caused by labour pain has been linked to an increase in maternal catecholamine release which in turn decreases uterine blood flow (Shnider *et al.*, 1979; Morishima *et al.*, 1980). Evidence of increased adrenaline/noradrenaline levels during labour has been reported by Lederman *et al.* (1977) whilst decreased levels postpartum have been noted by Shnider *et al.* (1983) and Abboud *et al.* (1985). One of the side effects of increased adrenaline level is decreased uterine activity which may lead to prolonged labour (Lederman *et al.*, 1978). In these cases, abnormal fetal heart rate patterns and lower Apgar scores at 1 and 5 minutes following birth have been recorded (Lederman *et al.*, 1981).

When maternal and/or respiratory diseases coexist or there is evidence of fetal distress, then endocrine and metabolic changes induced by labour pain may place the health of the mother or baby or both in danger. Epidural analgesia has been shown to reduce maternal catecholamine levels and through this speed up the process of labour. This form of pain relief could also increase intervillous blood flow in healthy and pre-eclamptic women (Hollman *et al.*, 1982; Jouppila *et al.*, 1982).

Other hormonal effects

Pain and other stress-related factors are known to influence the release of hormones such as beta-endorphin, beta-lipotrophin and adrenocorticotrophic hormone (ACTH). These hormones are also increased during painful labour. Abboud *et al.* (1983) for example, provide evidence to show that beta-endorphin levels decreased by about 50% in women who received epidural analgesia whereas there was no significant change in concentrations for women who received no pain relief. Similar findings have been reported by Gintzler (1980) and Thomas *et al.* (1982).

Uterine activity

Labour pain can affect uterine contractions through secretion of increased levels of catecholamine and cortisol and consequently influence the duration of labour. Noradrenaline, for example, has been shown to increase uterine activity whereas adrenaline and cortisol cause decreased activity (Lederman *et al.*, 1978) leading to prolonged labour. Pain can also cause incoordinate uterine activity leading to prolonged labour.

Pain and overt bodily responses

In addition to the physiological responses to pain outlined, labour pain is also associated with observable behavioural responses such as vocalisation, facial expressions, bodily movements and verbalisation. Vocalisation refers to the sounds produced in response to labour pain and may include moaning, groaning, and/or shouting and crying. Facial expressions on the other hand may be the only evidence that a woman is experiencing pain in labour. In fact it may be the first observable sign to midwives that a woman is in distress although it does not indicate that pain relief is needed or indeed necessary (McCrea, 1996). Facial expressions associated with labour pain include clenched teeth, tightly closed lips, tightly shut eyes and tightened muscles in the jaw. Body movements such as immobilisation, tensed muscle and restlessness are also behaviours related to or in response to labour pain. Some women may find that they have to walk about in order to cope with the pain whereas others may find lying in bed more tolerable. Some may hold themselves rigidly during a contraction whilst a few may 'roll' their pelvis in response to the pain during a contraction. These behaviours are evident depending on individual women's responses to labour pain. Verbal accounts of labour pain by women themselves were studied by Melzack and Wall (1965), which contributed to the development of the McGill Pain Questionnaire (MPQ). This research instrument measures the sensory, affective and qualitative components of pain as experienced by women in labour and is discussed in greater detail in Chapter 2.

It is evident that labour pain produces physiological and observable behavioural responses which are associated with the autonomic nervous system as well as learned behaviours that pain creates (Abu-Saed & Tesler, 1986). Learned behaviour is individual and generally represents coping strategies that women may have used in previous experience(s) to deal with pain. Thus complex perceptual and cognitive processes in the central nervous system influence nociceptive impulses so that they are interpreted with emotion, belief and expectations of the present situation. It is because of these processes that the meaning, quality and intensity of pain and the behavioural and psychological responses to it are determined in relation to people's personality, cultural background, past experiences and the psychological context in which the pain is being experienced (Chapman, 1985).

Blocking the physiological processes

The physiological processes that lead to pain sensation can be blocked by chemical, electrical and thermal blocks. However, the most researched is opioid-mediated (chemical) analgesia (Fields & Basbaum, 1989).

Chemical blocks

Reynolds (1969) first showed that electrical stimulation of the grey matter in the midbrain produced analgesia. Later, opiate receptors were identified in the brain, spinal cord and the gastrointestinal tract. The discovery of opiate receptors throughout the brain and neuroaxis revealed that concentration levels vary; the highest level is found in the thalamus, brain stem and the spinal cord, especially in the dorsal horn. In fact the dorsal horn grey matter has the highest concentration of opiate receptors (Bishop, 1980). From the evidence that has accumulated, it seems that opiate receptors are located on primary afferent fibres (LaMotte *et al.*, 1976).

These discoveries led to the search for substances that would bind with opiate receptors and thus far three main groups of endogenous substances with morphine-like properties have been discovered as natural constituents of the brain (Terenius & Wahlstrom, 1974). These include beta-lipotrophin, enkephalin and dynorphin (see 'Synapse' for discussion). The beta-endorphin of the beta-lipotrophin group is the most important in labour pain. It is known to be activated by stress and pain of labour and is produced by the pituitary gland. It binds firmly to opiate receptors and serves as a chemical messenger and acts as an analgesia. Although its exact role is not clearly established, it seems to block nociceptive impulses. It is known, for example, that when a noxious stimulus is received, it generates a pattern of change in the nerve. The stimulus is converted into the form of an impulse which is then transmitted from one end of a cell to the other. This process causes disturbance of sodium and potassium ions with consequent depolarisation of the nerve membrane. Opiates, including beta-endorphin, are said to prevent this depolarisation by inhibiting substance P, a nociceptive neurotransmitter, and thus block the impulse from being transmitted (Jessel & Iversen, 1977; Wall & Jones, 1991). Beta-endorphin also has an analgesic role and has been shown to have an analgesic effect lasting up to 2–3 hours.

Since the discovery of naturally produced opiates in the central nervous system, attempts have been made to produce synthetic opiate-like substances which can be used in the form of local anaesthetics to block pain. The basis for using chemical blocks is the interruption of specific nerves. In labour, blocking the sympathetic pathway at the level of the second lumbar vertebra is the main nerve block used for the relief of pain. Other chemical blocks used in obstetrics include pudendal nerve block and local infiltration as, for example, in suturing episiotomy.

Electrical blocks

Electrical stimulation of opiates in a number of central nervous system sites has been shown to produce analgesia, but the exact mechanism is still not clear. From the experiments conducted it appears that nociceptive fibres in the spinal cord dorsal horn are selectively inhibited by stimulation at analgesia-producing brain stem sites (Guilbaud *et al.*,

1973). There is also evidence to suggest that damage to specific sites of the spinal cord can block transmission of noxious stimulation (Basbaum *et al.*, 1976). The finding that electrical stimulation of large C-fibres inhibits the effects of noxious stimulation in the spinal cord led to the use of transcutaneous electrical nerve stimulation (TENS) as a method of pain relief. This form of blocking the physiological processes of pain is based on the gate-control theory (Melzack & Wall, 1965).

According to this theory, low level activity in small fibres which transmit nociceptive impulses can be blocked at the first synaptic junction by activity in large ascending fibres and by activity in fibres descending from higher centres in the brain. Melzack and Wall (1965) proposed that intense activity in small fibres triggered by painful stimulation opens the 'gate' at the first synapse whereas intense activity in large fibres closes the 'gate' to painful stimulation. Based on this theory, electrical stimulation of A-delta fibres using TENS (the application of gradual current) can therefore desensitise the affected area to noxious stimuli and thus block their transmission by closing the 'gate' to pain sensation. TENS also appears to stimulate the release of endorphins (Salar *et al.*, 1981) although its effects last for only 25 minutes. The rapid onset and short-lived effect of this method of pain relief may only be suitable for the early first stage of labour for some women.

Thermal blocks

Thermal blocks such as heat treatment, massage and manipulation have been used for many years as forms of pain relief (Haldeman, 1989) and are discussed in greater detail in Chapter 8.

Summary

The evidence presented in this chapter strongly indicates that the central nervous system is primarily responsible for the control of pain, including labour pain. However, as our understanding of the physiological processes increases, it is becoming clearer that psychological as well as physical factors play a role in pain sensation. The stress and fear of labour pain and the intensity and length of the pain experienced are all important in influencing pain sensation in labour. An understanding of its physiological basis and the psychological factors that influence it is therefore necessary for effective pain control during labour.

PART II
Beginning the Journey

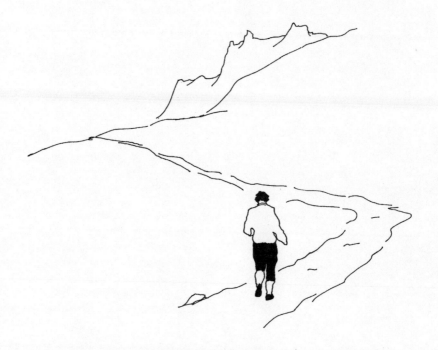

Chapter 5
Childbirth Education

The remit of childbirth education is wide and the timing is equally variable and so I am looking at it before pregnancy (Chapter 6). The 'classes', on the other hand, tend to be provided only during pregnancy and a large proportion of the material focuses on labour. For these reasons, I include this topic alongside the material on pain in pregnancy and before labour. In considering how childbirth education relates to pain, I discuss first its development. Approaches to teaching about pain changed during this development, and I look at these approaches next. Finally this chapter focuses on the effectiveness of childbirth education, particularly in relation to pain, as demonstrated through evaluative research.

History

Childbirth education has been happening through 'women's networks' for almost as long as women have been bearing children (Nolan, 1997). The tendency of experienced mothers to recount their experiences to new mothers-to-be carries benefits as well as risks for both; however, the account invariably features the experience of pain (Perkins, 1980). While Nolan (1997) argues that childbirth education was a self-help response among isolated middle class women, others relate its development to the increasingly 'scientific' nature of obstetrics (Simkin & Enkin, 1989). These authors' claim that the original goal of these programmes was 'the prevention of pain in childbirth' contradicts Nolan's emphasis on the programmes satisfying the need for preparation for motherhood.

An example of the pain prevention goal is found in Dick-Read's pioneering work. His first book (1933) introduced the concept of pain being culturally learned and leading to an escalating cycle of potentially counterproductive fear and tension. To break this cycle, he advocated education, relaxation and breathing exercises. His methods were easily accepted in the USA and dubbed 'natural childbirth' (Combes & Schonveld, 1992), but they encountered resistance in the UK. This may be associated with the societal, patriotic, medical and evangelical

Christian inputs into Dick-Read's approach to birth (Arney, 1982: 214; Kitzinger, J., 1989).

In contrast, psychoprophylaxis was easily accepted throughout the West, despite its Eastern European origins. These techniques were derived from the concepts developed by Pavlov on learning by conditioning (Velvovsky *et al.*, 1960). Because of their French advocate (Lamaze) and group sessions, this approach became known as 'Lamaze classes'. Hence, from early days, social support, as well as learning about 'preventing' pain, was crucial to childbirth education. Despite the acrimony between these two approaches' disciples (Kitzinger, J., 1989), they shared common features, such as their reluctance to admit the reality of labour pain. While I understand that some women experience pain-free childbirth, my personal observation suggests this is not the case for the majority of mothers. The early proponents of prepared childbirth, however, denied that uncomplicated labour is painful; to the extent that Lamaze claimed that his method provided 'complete absence of sensation' (1956). Dick-Read did eventually concede, though, that 'the last few contractions' are possibly painful (Jimenez, 1988). The persistence of belief that labour pain is mythological is evident (Langford, 1997), but such condescending approaches and their legacy, the euphemistic 'contraction', barely deserve consideration.

Pertinent to the discussion of Dick-Read's approach are questions of the relevance of the pervasive medical orientation of much client, including childbirth, education (Fleming, 1992). Similarly, it is necessary to question the role of men, such as Dick-Read, his Russian equivalents and more recently Odent (1994), in defining women's childbirth experience as painless. Fleming argues against the medical control of childbirth education by describing the ultimate desired outcome. This is not the health of the woman and baby, or even the mother's satisfaction with her birth experience, but (she argues) 'the rewarding of staff with "compliant patients"'. These thoughts are powerfully reminiscent of Kirkham's research-based observations (1989). Monto (1996) suggests that these medical/antimedical orientations are clearly apparent in different educational approaches and that a woman seeks the education that accords with her view. Although statistical significance is not claimed, in Monto's sample of 31 women the desired birth tended to be achieved.

Another recurring theme, which continues to appear in the literature of childbirth education on pain control, is the antagonism between medical and childbirth education lobbies. An early inconclusive evaluation provoked:

'... the acknowledged leaders of American obstetrics to voice their opinions. The concerns which they expressed indicate the degree of [medical] resistance at the time and which remains to some degree today' (Simkin & Enkin, 1989: 329).

This antagonism manifests itself explicitly in the epidural debate (Mander, 1994a), while appearing regularly in more general and, supposedly, authoritative material:

'Antenatal education no longer attracts only the highly motivated people who wish to avoid pain medication. . . . Vocal and assertive, this small minority exerts a disproportionately large influence on maternity care practices. They carefully investigate and select antenatal classes, read extensively, exercise their right to choose their caregivers and places for birth (changing in mid-pregnancy if they feel unsatisfied), and expect full participation in the decisions concerning their own and their baby's care' (Simkin & Enkin, 1989: 320).

Similarly, the original unjustifiable medical claims of 'painless childbirth' are still used to discredit childbirth education. Such a diatribe concludes: 'prepared childbirth training and epidural anaesthesia should be regarded as complementary, compatible procedures' (Melzack *et al.*, 1981: 357).

Teaching about labour pain

Before contemplating what is taught about childbearing pain, we must ask whether anything is taught about it? There exist textbooks on the topic which omit even to index 'pain' (Wilson, 1990; Priest & Schott, 1991); exceptionally, though, Robertson (1994) devotes a full chapter to teaching about pain. The rationale for these omissions may be approached in two ways.

Feasibility

First, it is necessary to question whether it is possible to teach a woman about what pain she should expect in labour? Drew (1992) admits the inability of educators to prepare women for 'the type and degree of pain involved in labour'. Additionally, Bergum (1989), on the basis of her qualitative research, attributes this inability to the 'horror' of the pain, combined with the limitations of the English language (Scarry, 1985; see Preface).

On the other hand, Crowe and von Bayer (1989) maintain that teaching the reality of birth is feasible. Their research suggests that a woman who is taught realistically about the anxiety of the birth has a less painful experience of birth. These authors consider that a woman with some grasp of what birth is like, and who has been taught how to control the pain, is more likely to have a positive childbirth experience.

Despite the findings of Crowe and von Bayer (1989), teaching the reality of birth tends to be avoided, probably for the reasons given by Bergum (1989). The result is that the focus of childbirth education tends to be on coping with or controlling or relieving the pain (Trenam, 1994).

The P-word

The second rationale involves a long-running argument, which followed the debate about the existence of labour pain, relating to the use of the word 'pain' itself. Williams and Booth (1985) argue that by discussing 'pain' the woman, who has been conditioned to expect that 'labour equals pain', may interpret any 'unusual sensation' as pain. These authors then suggest that the word should be used 'occasionally': 'it seems unnecessary to reinforce the conditioning which certainly does exist by describing every contraction as a pain' (p. 110).

Drew (1992) discusses this resistance to the word 'pain' in terms of 'a four letter word best avoided' which some fear may become a 'self fulfilling prophecy'. She maintains that the childbirth educator walks a tightrope in relation to emphasising pain. She concludes that childbirth involves a positive form of pain which, unlike most pain, does not constitute pathology; she reinforces Kitzinger's aphorism that labour comprises 'pain with a purpose' (1978). This view is endorsed by recent research by Hallgren and colleagues (1995), which used 'sense of coherence' (SOC), a form of confidence, as the theoretical framework. Decreased SOC was associated with increasing need for pharmacological pain control (p. 134).

This issue is confronted by some midwives (Leap, 1997), who discuss pain antenatally in preference to 'pain relief'. This orientation is thought responsible for these midwives' clients' limited use of pharmacological pain control (69% used none), although the clientele are self-selected.

Teaching approaches

The approaches to childbirth education (Perkins, 1980; Drew, 1992) are particularly relevant to teaching about pain, as shown by a major research project by Perkins (1980). Huge variations emerged in teaching about pain between classes and between teachers; attitude to pain was the defining feature in the three different approaches to childbirth education.

The first, entitled 'old wives' tales', comprises a range of traditional horror stories in which pain invariably predominates. The second approach, entitled 'new wives' tales', draws on up-to-date horror stories, usually involving medical technology, resulting iatrogenic pain and further medical interventions to resolve the pain. The last of Perkins' approaches is her 'free spirit's tales'. This 'everything in the garden is lovely' idealisation of childbirth seeks to help the woman to cope with pain by redefining it 'as a new, overpowering sensation'. The woman is taught techniques to help her to work with her pain, rather than against it. Despite her criticism of this approach, Perkins admits 'paradoxically, this romantic view of childbirth is the most practical one, in that the woman has something she can do to help fulfil her expectations' (p. 48). Although Hallgren and colleagues (1994) use different terms from Perkins, their research shows that variability in childbirth education approaches persists. They discuss the obstetric perspective, the parent-oriented perspective and the mixed perspective.

An innovative form of childbirth education (Fleming, 1992) advances Perkins' free spirit approach by drawing on the principles of critical social theory (Freire & Shor, 1987). It proposes that the traditional didactic and medically orientated format of childbirth education be replaced by a transformational, negotiated curriculum in which both woman and educator share their experiences and legitimate theoretical standpoints. The resulting joint search for the meaning of the birth experience fosters an educational opportunity which is likely to 'create a climate that is more favourable for personal growth' (Fleming, 1992: 162).

It is apparent that traditional antenatal teaching may not actually teach the woman about pain. More liberal approaches focusing on the education of the mother may prove more enlightening.

Research on the effectiveness of childbirth education

As I mentioned above (see 'History'), since its inception, a major, if not sole, goal of childbirth education has been the alleviation of labour pain. It is unsurprising, therefore, that much childbirth education research has focused on the extent to which it relieves pain. Despite the plethora of research projects, evidence supporting the effectiveness of childbirth education is still sparse (Nolan, 1997). Additionally, the shortcomings in terms of both methodology and applicability of much of the research inevitably mean that 'more research is needed'. Because of the commercial importance of childbirth education in the USA, much of the research has been undertaken there. This leads to the question of the relevance of research undertaken in relatively medicalised, interventionist settings to those countries where intervention is less institutionalised.

A study which was undertaken in the context of a health care system more comparable with the UK examined the influence of 'childbirth classes' on pain medication decision making (Handfield & Bell, 1995).

Using postal questionnaires, these researchers found that a majority of women (n=59) reported having changed their minds regarding their choice of pain medication. Equal proportions attributed their change of mind to the classes and to their experience of labour. Of the women who attributed their mind-change to the classes, those who became favourable to pain medication approximately equalled those who came to 'be wary' of its effects.

In evaluating childbirth education, methodological problems arise out of the mother's decreasing ability to employ her chosen technique as her labour progresses (Copstick *et al.*, 1985). The presence of a support person, be it partner, midwife or doula, has also been shown to affect the mother's ability to cope with labour; thus, these research design problems are further compounded. Methodologically, the Hawthorne effect is a major obstacle: 'reporting benefits from classes may have testified more to the enthusiasm of the proponents than to the effectiveness of the approaches' (Simkin & Enkin, 1989: 323).

In spite of this, certain well-organised RCTs have suggested the effectiveness of childbirth education in pain control. Using a three-group technique, it has been established that women who are prepared for their labour are likely to use less pharmacological analgesia and anaesthesia in labour than their unprepared and otherwise educated sisters (Enkin *et al.*, 1972; Timm, 1989). Admittedly, medication intake is an imprecise substitute for pain assessment, making the findings of the lower pain scores in prepared mothers all the more significant (Melzack *et al.*, 1981).

Summary

Teaching methods and evaluation of childbirth education attract considerable attention. Equally, pain is a variably taught topic and an unsatisfactory outcome measure. In the same way that effectiveness has been shown to need research attention (Nichols, 1995; Shearer, 1995), the extent to which the inputs meet women's needs also requires attention.

Chapter 6
Pain in Pregnancy

Healthy pregnancy

Although we are frequently reassured that pregnancy and childbearing are physiological events, perceptions to the contrary have arisen from a number of sources. Historically, our Victorian greatgrandparents were embarrassed by pregnancy's sexual connotations, and in their denial referred to it as 'an interesting state'. Culturally and for similar reasons, pregnancy is still a private matter among certain ethnic groups (Scott & Niven, 1996). A further factor that has contributed to the perception of childbearing as other than physiological is its medicalisation (Oakley, 1980). The extent of the perception of the non-physiological nature of pregnancy was demonstrated by research comparing the views of care providers (Schuman & Marteau, 1993). The obstetricians (n=15) regarded pregnancy as significantly more risky than their midwife colleagues (n=14), with the pregnant women (n=136) assuming a marginally more risk-free stance. Interestingly, of the three, the midwives were significantly more likely to view pregnancy as a 'normal' event. The researchers contemplated whether such differing perceptions adversely affect care.

Thus, the physiological nature of pregnancy is not as obvious as we sometimes assume, and referring to it as 'an altered state of health' may be more accurate. In this chapter I consider some alterations in the woman's health during pregnancy, focusing on those experienced as painful. These alterations vary hugely in their implications for maternal and fetal wellbeing. Some have traditionally been described as 'minor disorders' or 'discomforts' (Brucker, 1988; Jamieson, 1993:117). Such patronising terminology discounts the woman's experience and will be avoided here. Similarly, I avoid categorising the intensity of the pain associated with the various conditions.

To show the close relationship between perinatal pain and women's other pain (Niven & Gijsbers, 1996a), I address the painful conditions in order of their relationship with the pregnancy. Thus conditions associated with pregnancy are followed by those aggravated by it, then those unique to it or, finally, coincidental to it. Each condition is considered in terms of its pathophysiology, origins of pain and possible remedies. Limited attention is given to analgesia, except specific types, as pain remedies are discussed in Chapters 8 and 9.

Conditions associated with pregnancy

The physiological changes of pregnancy, which are largely hormonally determined, may cause painful conditions for which the woman may seek advice or even treatment.

The gastrointestinal tract

The activity of the gastrointestinal tract is reduced or reversed by rising progesterone levels (Olds *et al.*, 1996), and the woman's symptoms may be exacerbated by mechanical or positional changes (Brucker, 1988).

Heartburn

Its various names clearly indicate the nature and site of heartburn's pain; likewise, the North American term 'pyrosis' suggests the burning nature of this retrosternal pain. Technically, 'reflux oesophagitis' means that irritation due to regurgitation of acid stomach contents into the oesophagus is responsible. The pain has been defined as 'a burning sensation or discomfort behind the breastbone that often extends upwards to the throat' possibly accompanied by pharyngeal regurgitation or 'clear fluid reaching the mouth/throat and causing a bitter or acidic taste' (Marrero *et al.*, 1992: 731).

Atlay and colleagues' estimate that heartburn occurs in 66% of pregnant women (1973) was confirmed by a survey of 607 antenatal clinic attenders (Marrero *et al.*, 1992). The incidence increased to 72% in the third trimester when the expected relief associated with 'lightening' failed to materialise. These researchers also found that heartburn was significantly more likely to present in women affected by it prior to pregnancy and in multiparous women.

The cause is largely positional, being associated with stooping or lying down (Bracken *et al.*, 1989); clearly the effects of postural changes are exacerbated by the growing uterus (Feeney, 1982). Progesterone's relaxing effect on the cardiac sphincter is partly responsible, and this is likely to be aggravated by that hormone's reduction of gastrointestinal motility and delaying gastric emptying (Hytten, 1991).

The suggested remedies are intended to counteract the underlying postural causes or symptoms of heartburn. Non-pharmacological remedies include attention to posture, reduction in meal size and avoidance of fatty, spicy and very cold substances (Brucker, 1988). The recommendation of milky drinks is of uncertain value (APA & NPSP,

1982), as milk may irritate the gastric mucosa. Following their survey, Marrero *et al.* (1992) recommend that at risk groups should adopt preventive measures, such as raising the head of the bed, prior to symptoms appearing, to prevent oesophageal sensitisation.

The woman may need pharmacological remedies if simpler ones fail to resolve her pain. Antacid medications may be recommended, but there may be risks involved in taking any drug during pregnancy, the problem in this situation being the danger of sodium bicarbonate inducing sodium overload and systemic alkalosis (Bracken *et al.*, 1989). If long-term use is considered, the medications based on magnesium salts appear safer than those derived from aluminium salts (Brucker, 1988).

Acute appendicitis and other abdominal pain

When thinking about acute appendicitis and other abdominal pain in pregnancy we must remember the huge anatomical changes occurring in the abdomen at this time (Nathan & Huddleston, 1995). As well as predisposing to certain conditions, these changes impede the diagnosis and treatment of acute appendicitis and other abdominal pain. In this section I focus on the more significant conditions in terms of their frequency and implications, but, for completeness' sake, I indicate in Table 6.1 these conditions' relative frequency.

Table 6.1 Frequency of painful abdominal conditions in pregnancy (from Nathan & Huddleston, 1995).

Cystitis	1 in 50–100
Pyelonephritis	1 in 50–100
Urolithiasis	1 in 200
Acute appendicitis	1 in 1500
Acute pancreatitis	1 in 1000–10 000
Intestinal obstruction	1 in 2500–3500
Acute fatty liver of pregnancy	1 in 10 000–15 000

The general impression is that appendicitis occurs more frequently during pregnancy than outwith it, in association with the previously mentioned gastrointestinal changes (To *et al.*, 1995). However, Moawad (1990) states that pregnancy does not affect the incidence, estimates of which vary between 1 in 800–6600 pregnancies (To *et al.*, 1995). The significance of appendicitis in pregnancy derives, therefore, not from an increased incidence, but from diagnosis and prognosis.

Unquestionably the principal diagnostic feature is abdominal pain. During the first trimester this may present in the usual position, often known as McBurney's point, in the right lower abdominal quadrant (Guzinski, 1990; Blendis, 1994). This diagnostic indicator becomes less

reliable as pregnancy progresses, giving rise to, despite falling incidence, increasing mortality (Baskett, 1985). The pain of appendicitis,
and the extreme local tenderness accompanying it, are located higher in
the abdomen in advanced pregnancy. As well as pain and tenderness,
the usual picture of abdominal guarding and rigidity may be absent due
to enlargement. The other symptoms that often accompany appendicitis, such as nausea, vomiting and urinary frequency, are not uncommon features of pregnancy, further confounding the diagnosis.

In a series of 31 pregnant women with appendicitis, To *et al.* (1995)
report four miscarriages and one neonatal death following premature
birth. As well as perinatal risks, ruptured appendix and peritonitis occur
at least twice as frequently in pregnant women as in their non-pregnant
sisters (Durham & McCain, 1993). Thus, accurate diagnosis of
appendicitis appears to be crucial to reduce perinatal and maternal
mortality and morbidity. The differential diagnosis of the 'acute abdomen' in pregnancy includes pregnancy-related conditions, such as
abruptio placenta, together with gastrointestinal conditions, such as
Crohn's disease (Blendis, 1994). The importance of 'proper assessment' of pregnant women experiencing abdominal pain emerged from
a retrospective study, which found that, of women between 20 and 37
weeks' gestation complaining of abdominal pain, the majority were
never diagnosed (Impey & Hughes, 1995). These researchers argue
that, in the absence of tenderness, guarding, peritonism or a positive
urine culture, hospital admission is unnecessary. Considering the
serious implications of hospital admission for the woman's family relationships (MacDonald, 1991), caution about admission is appropriate.

Pain of cardiovascular origin

Changes in the cardiovascular system which cause pain during pregnancy include varicosites at various sites and thromboembolic conditions. The former is the subject of much advice (Jamieson, 1993) which
tends not to be research-based. Because both of these conditions cause
more and more serious problems postnatally than during pregnancy
(HMSO, 1991; HMSO, 1996), I focus on them in Chapter 10 under
'Haemorrhoids' and 'Thromboembolic pain'.

Musculoskeletal problems

Pain associated with musculoskeletal problems is regarded and treated
with varying degrees of seriousness.

Back pain
Often denigrated by being called backache, back pain features in labour
and the puerperium as well as pregnancy. The prevalence of back pain

in pregnancy emerged from the somewhat limited epidemiological research by Meyer and colleagues (1994). 'Backache', as they termed it, was identified in 45% of women at booking, rising to 69% by 28 weeks and almost maintaining that level. This figure may be compared with the 23% of non-pregnant women experiencing back pain. These data are modest in comparison with Kristiansson *et al.*'s more authoritative finding that 76% of their sample (n=200) reported back pain at some time during pregnancy (1996).

The cause of back pain remains unclear (Kristiansson *et al.*, 1996), but the hormone relaxin, produced by the corpus luteum and named for its effect on the interpubic ligaments of laboratory animals (Klopper, 1991), seems instrumental. Its role in initiating labour has, in physiological terms, overtaken its other effects. Relaxin's other functions may, however, matter more to the pregnant woman, as they include increasing laxity of the pelvic ligaments and, hence, enlargement of the pelvic diameters and easier birth. This increasing laxity is due to more relaxin production as pregnancy progresses and is responsible for greater risk of 'trivial trauma' (McNab & McCulloch, 1990). The sacro-iliac joint is particularly vulnerable to trauma because of its relatively great weight-bearing load; the pain associated with such damage is described as 'radiating around the greater trochanter and down the anterolateral aspect of the thigh' (McNab & McCulloch, 1990: 107).

Further to its well-known effects on the pelvic ligaments, relaxin has been shown to allow increased spinal mobility, which has been blamed for the vulnerability of the spine to damage during pregnancy (Calguneri *et al.*, 1982). Similarly, increased mobility may be associated with greater spinal instability, which may develop into long-term back pain (Porter & Jiang, 1990). The major effects of relaxin are ordinarily reversed within three months of the birth (Roman & Artal, 1986).

Another, less well-researched, explanation of the development of back pain in pregnancy relates to the 'strain' imposed by the growing uterus (Dutro & Wheeler, 1991). Such strain can only be aggravated by the alteration in posture or lordosis which the pregnant woman assumes to maintain her balance. Research refutes this long-accepted assumption, because the incidence of back pain peaks at 24–28 weeks, that is well before abdominal growth reaches its maximum (Meyer *et al.*, 1994; Kristiansson *et al.*, 1996).

Dutro and Wheeler (1991) recommend that one solution to back pain is to 'maintain' muscle tone through a programme of yoga-based physical exercise. The benefits of physical exercise in pregnancy are often proposed (Brayshaw, 1993; Halksworth, 1993), but ascertaining the basis of these recommendations is not easy. Lokey *et al.* (1991) undertook a meta-analysis of research into the effects of physical exercise on pregnancy outcomes. Disappointingly, they found no significant differences between those who exercised and the 'couch potatoes'. These researchers wisely indicated the upper limits of 'safe' exercise programmes, taking account of duration and frequency of sessions and the increase in pulse rate.

Although we have an established picture of how common back pain is in pregnancy, it is only relatively recently that attempts have been made to measure the intensity of the 'backache' that women encounter (Kristiansson *et al.*, 1996). These researchers identified the 'great difficulties with normal activities' which back pain causes to 30% of pregnant women.

Carpal tunnel syndrome

Like many bodily changes during pregnancy, carpal tunnel syndrome (CTS) is usually assumed to be hormonally caused, but there may be other factors involved. Accounts of the incidence of CTS vary according to the diagnostic criteria employed; while over 20% of pregnant women may encounter symptoms (Rosenbaum & Ochoa, 1993), in only 2.3% are they sufficiently serious to warrant medical attention (Ekman-Ordeberg *et al.*, 1987).

Recognised by the woman as a painful condition of one or both hands, CTS features tingling, numbness and 'pins and needles'. The area affected gradually extends to include the palmar surface of the thumb and three fingers innervated by the median nerve (index, middle and radial half of ring finger). If the condition does not limit itself, by the ending of the pregnancy at birth, this condition may ultimately result in median nerve atrophy (Maldonado & Barger, 1995). Occasionally the condition begins soon after the birth (Wand, 1990).

CTS is thought to be caused by the entrapment and compression of the median nerve by the surrounding tissues as it passes through the tunnel created by the carpal bones; in pregnancy oedematous soft tissues cause pressure. A further aetiological factor is traction on the median nerve due to displacement of the shoulder girdle, attributable to lordosis of pregnancy (Blackburn & Loper, 1992).

In a prospective study, Ekman-Ordeberg and colleagues (1987) found that 2.3% of pregnant women developed CTS, a small majority of whom were nulliparous. The women were treated conservatively by the use of a back-splint at night. This treatment resolved the condition in all but 10 of the 56 women; of these, 3 underwent surgery to free the entrapped nerve, one had labour induced and one underwent surgery postnatally. The remaining 5 received symptomatic care until the imminent birth.

This condition deserves to be taken seriously, not only because of the risk of permanent nerve damage, but also because of the disruption which sleepless nights cause and the emotional trauma of being unable to lift the new baby.

Leg cramps

Painful spasm of the calf or gastrocnemius muscle is a common problem in pregnancy. Estimates of the incidence vary from a low of 5% of pregnant women to almost 50% (Dahle *et al.*, 1995; Bracken *et al.*, 1989). The problem is due not only to the painful nature of these cramps, but to their frequency and the disturbance in lifestyle due to their nocturnal occurrence. In their study, Dahle *et al.* found that 88% of 73 pregnant sufferers in their sample experienced them only nocturnally, but for the remainder cramps happened in the daytime too. The median frequency was alternate nights, showing the high level of disturbance. These cramps increase towards term but are unrelated to other complications or to perinatal morbidity.

Admitting that the cause is unclear, Bobak and Starn (1993) suggest precipitating factors. They identify that reclining posture is a factor and link this with the gravid uterus compressing nerves supplying the legs; 'pointing toes when stretching legs or walking' is also blamed. These authors mention the chemical imbalance, especially serum calcium and phosphorus levels, which has given rise to pharmacological intervention. Probably linked to the latter point, they suggest that excessive milk intake (over 1 litre/day) may be responsible.

On the basis of a literature review, Bracken and colleagues (1989) recommend that simple remedies 'are surely worth trying'. Such remedies include massage of and heat over the affected muscle, as well as stretching the muscle by standing on the affected limb (Bobak & Starn, 1993). As mentioned above and detailed by Bracken *et al.* (1989: 508), 'The cause and mechanism of these cramps are still not clear'; unfortunately this has acted as a stimulus rather than a deterrent to the introduction of pharmacological remedies. Quinine and vitamin D are among the plethora of pharmacological preparations that have been recommended and, presumably, administered (Bracken *et al.*, 1989)

Because leg cramps resemble hypocalcaemic tetany, the main pharmacological intervention has involved mineral supplementation, including both calcium and magnesium. The trials of calcium administration especially appear to be riddled with methodological weaknesses (Bracken *et al.*, 1989). The study by Dahle and colleagues (1995) addresses some of these issues, and suggests that hypomagnesaemia may be the cause and supplementation the solution. Unfortunately these researchers, although randomising affected women into supplemented and non-supplemented groups and measuring serum magnesium levels in both, failed to include a pregnant group not experiencing leg cramps. Thus, lifestyles are likely to continue to be disrupted by this pain of unknown origin.

Round ligament pain

The round ligaments' role declines markedly with conception and they may cause pain during pregnancy. These ligaments comprise non-striated fibromuscular and connective tissue (Andrews & O'Neill, 1994) and maintain the non-pregnant uterus in its stable anteverted anteflexed position to facilitate conception. As they originate at the cornua and extend through the inguinal canal and are inserted into the deeper tissues of the vulva (Stalheim-Smith & Fitch, 1993), they must increase in length as the gravid uterus enlarges; this is achieved by a combination of stretching and hypertrophy (Olds *et al.*, 1996). The groin pain which the pregnant woman may experience is due to contraction of muscle fibres in the round ligaments and to tension on them as they stretch. Andrews and O'Neill describe round ligament pain as 'painful twinges' or it may be a more intense, 'grabbing' sensation.

In the event of round ligament pain being recognised, the woman is given information and advised to avoid posture causing further traction on the ligament (Bobak, 1993). Andrews and O'Neill's study involved 25 women experiencing round ligament pain, which was assessed using the McGill Pain Questionnaire and treated by pelvic tilt exercises (1994). Recruitment was impeded by some women's physicians disagreeing with the diagnosis of the cause of pain but suggesting neither alternative causes nor remedies. The women acted as their own controls. The researchers describe comprehensively the adverse effects of this pain on the women's lifestyles and relationships. The reduction in the women's pain after a week of exercises did not reach statistical significance, but on the basis of this study the researchers recommend that pelvic tilting should be taught antenatally. Although Andrews and O'Neill's study is inconclusive, it demonstrates a low-tech approach to round ligament pain, which may be relevant to other pain experiences.

Conditions aggravated by pregnancy

In the previous section I discussed some painful health conditions which make their first appearance during pregnancy and disappear after the birth. In this section I focus on conditions that are likely to pre-date the pregnancy and which are aggravated and possibly made more painful by pregnancy.

Genitourinary system

Clearly, because of its function and site, the genitourinary system is markedly affected by the pregnancy and the woman experiences certain changes which are potentially painful.

Braxton Hicks contractions
Just as the myometrium contracts rhythmically and usually painlessly throughout a woman's reproductive life, it is minimally active during

pregnancy. These contractions are usually known by the name of the person who first described them in the last century – J. Braxton Hicks (Mulder & Visser, 1987). Braxton Hicks contractions are weaker than the contractions of labour, peaking at 15 mmHg (Llewellyn-Jones, 1973). Those nearer 15 mmHg are palpable by an attendant. Whether the woman is aware of these contractions, however, is less certain, as is whether and to what extent she feels them painful (Thomson, 1993; Olds *et al.*, 1996).

Braxton Hicks contractions are significant for a number of reasons. First, in my experience, some women do feel them as painful for a large proportion of the pregnancy; for this reason the woman may appreciate being taught coping strategies. Second, these contractions are only qualitatively different from those of labour (Thomson, 1993). The diagnosis of labour may, thus, be confounded; perhaps the transition from Braxton Hicks to labour contractions may only be identified with hindsight. This often-mentioned confusion illustrates the intensity of some Braxton Hicks contractions. Third, the purpose of Braxton Hicks contractions is often described in terms of a 'practice' (Kitzinger, 1987a: 211), suggesting that the uterus is preparing itself for labour. Alternatively, as mentioned above, they may present the woman with opportunities to practise her coping strategies prior to the onset of labour. Fourth, Mulder and Visser (1987) demonstrated a more important function of these contractions. Their research project, involving 14 healthy nulliparous women, showed the marked positive correlation between fetal movements and Braxton Hicks contractions. While careful not to attribute causation, these researchers illuminated an important facet of the process by which the woman comes to know her fetus as a distinct individual. Fifth, and most significantly physiologically, Braxton Hicks contractions assist the circulation of blood through the placental intervillous spaces. In this way, by intermittently increasing the pressure of blood behind the placenta, fetal oxygenation and nutrition are facilitated (Hytten & Chamberlain, 1991).

Thus, Braxton Hicks contractions, which have been subjected to minimal research attention, may be perceived negatively as seriously painful. Alternatively, they may be regarded as a learning opportunity, a chance to relate to the baby or as a fetal growth enhancer.

Urinary tract infection
In the same way as Braxton Hicks contractions may confound the diagnosis of the onset of labour, the woman with a painful urinary tract infection (UTI) may have difficulty differentiating the intermittent pain of renal origin from uterine contractions. An accurate diagnosis may prove similarly elusive for her carers, as when distinguishing between the pain of UTI, premature labour and placental abruption (MacDermott, 1994). Also, like labour, UTI pain may present in various forms and of varying

intensity, depending largely on the location of the infection in the urinary system. Additionally, one form of UTI, asymptomatic bacteriuria (ASB) is, by definition, only diagnosable on urinary microbiological examination (Brettle *et al.*, 1986).

Even covert UTIs have the potential for serious maternal and fetal morbidity (Cunningham & Lucas, 1994). Through a retrospective cohort analysis of the records of 25 746 childbearing women, Shieve *et al.* (1994) established the relationship between UTI, hypertension, anaemia and amnionitis. The fetal effects, however, of maternal UTI are less clear. Schieve *et al.* (1994) accept the association between UTI and premature labour/birth, but are uncertain whether the link is direct, through amnionitis, or indirect, such as through occult renal abnormalities (p. 409). The positive correlation between UTI and low birth weight is better-established (Kass, 1978; Schultz *et al.*, 1991).

While their shorter urethra tends to be blamed for women's increased vulnerability to UTI (Higgins, 1995), the increased incidence of UTI during pregnancy is usually attributed to physiological changes in the urinary tract. Baylis and Davison (1991) discuss the extent to which these changes, especially the dilatation of the ureters, are hormonally determined or are due to obstruction of the ureter by compression against the pelvic brim. The link between this radiologically obvious dilatation and reflux predisposing to infection is difficult to challenge. Superimposed on their anatomical and physiological disadvantage, certain groups of women, such as those in lower socio-economic groups, show additional vulnerability to UTI (Wang & Small, 1989; Cunningham & Lucas, 1994).

Although a descending route of infection occasionally occurs, ascending infection is more common (Higgins, 1995). Perineal commensal organisms enter the urethra and proceed, via the pathways already mentioned, to infect the bladder and/or kidneys. The widely recognised phenomenon of certain women experiencing repeated UTIs is explained by the adhesive attraction between certain organisms and the woman's uroepithelium. Whereas the adhesive substances, or adhesins, carried by most organisms are weak and are carried away by the fluid in the urinary system, certain organisms carried by a minority of people have developed more secure attachments. An example is P-fimbriated *Escherichia coli*, vulnerability to which is linked with certain blood groups (Cunningham & Lucas, 1994).

The symptoms of UTI usually include pain. In cystitis, which comprises an inflammation of the bladder lining, dysuria presents as stinging when voiding urine as well as suprapubic pain (Higgins, 1995; Nathan & Huddleston, 1995). Dysuria features in the majority of confirmed UTIs (MacDermott, 1994). The pain is due to acid urine irritating inflamed tissues. In addition to dysuria the woman with pyelonephritis, an infection of the renal pelvis, experiences pain in the lumbar area or flank, with the pain radiating round into the upper and lower abdominal quadrants (Wang & Small, 1989: 537; Nathan & Huddleston, 1995).

Depending on the severity of her condition, antimicrobial drugs, intravenous fluids, anti-emetics and analgesic medication may be prescribed on the basis of microbiological examination of the urine. The woman's pain may be amenable to simple remedies, such as heat over the painful lumbar area, or she may require analgesic drugs, which should be prescribed for administration by injection if she is nauseated. The woman may benefit from advice relating to the prevention of further UTIs, such as perineal hygiene, avoiding bladder irritants and precautions relating to sexual activity (Olds *et al.*, 1996). For centuries cranberry juice has been justifiably recommended to prevent and limit the severity of UTIs (Nazarko, 1995); the action of this fruit juice is to reduce the adhesion of pathogens to the uroepithelium (Swanberg, 1979).

Much research has focused on UTI in pregnancy because of the fetal risks. It is necessary to consider the possibility of UTI being caused during treatment or iatrogenically. Catheterisation is widely, even routinely, used in labour and birth (Miller & Callander, 1989), which is surprising in view of the 10–27% post-catheterisation UTI rate in the general hospital population (Editorial, 1991). Statistics of post-catheterisation infection among new mothers are hard to locate, but such information should be available to maternity staff, if for no other reason than to provide feedback on their aseptic technique.

Cardiovascular system

Cardiovascular changes during pregnancy are attributable to hormonal changes (de Swiet, 1991). In association with these physiological phenomena potentially painful conditions may develop; because the effects of these physiological changes persist into and tend to become more problematical in the postnatal period, I consider them in Chapter 10.

Sickle cell disease

The management of pain during a crisis is but one of the major issues raised by sickle cell disease (SCD). SCD is a family of blood disorders (Midence & Elander, 1994: 5), which, together with the thalassaemias, comprise the haemoglobinopathies. They are inherited through an autosomal recessive gene, making SCD most common in sub-Saharan Africa and among people who have migrated thence. It also occurs among peoples who originated in the countries surrounding the Mediterranean, and further east in the Indian sub-continent and Albania (Davies, 1994).

Responsible for the transport of oxygen, haemoglobin (Hb) is the iron-rich pigment in red blood cells (RBC). Ordinarily in adult blood haemoglobin is described as Hb A, but in SCD Hb S is present in varying proportions (Singer, 1985). Although genetic constitutions vary, people who are homozygous (having two genes or alleles for Hb S) are said to have sickle cell disease. People who are heterozygous (having one gene for Hb S and one for Hb A) are said to have the less serious sickle cell trait (Midence & Elander, 1994).

In hypoxic conditions, the RBCs of a person with SCD are seen microscopically to distort into a crescent or 'sickle' shape (Mueller & Young, 1995). This is because in people with SCD a miniscule difference in an amino acid chain causes a unique reaction between the molecules within Hb S. Hypoxia causes the molecules to form a rigid structure which produces the sickle shape, although the majority resume their biconcave shape when reoxygenated (Mueller & Young, 1995). It is this 'sickling' which causes both the acute and long-term problems which the person with SCD faces. First, the RBC's cell membrane is damaged by sickling, leading to faster breakdown and a haemolytic type of anaemia. Second, sickled RBCs are less malleable and block small arteries, depriving those tissues of oxygen and leading to infarction and necrosis (Mueller & Young, 1995). Third, the immediate impact of these 'microscopic areas of infarction in bones and tissues' includes pain, and constitutes a 'sickle cell crisis' (Koshy, 1995).

The crisis is the principal cause of morbidity among people with SCD, accounting for 90% of SCD-related hospital admissions (Brozovic *et al.*, 1987). Crises vary in severity from mild discomfort for a few minutes to severe generalised pain lasting for weeks, often requiring admission for treatment with opioids (Anionwu, 1996). Additionally, crises are unpredictable in their occurrence.

'Pregnancy carries an increased risk for a mother with SCD and for the fetus' (Koshy, 1995: 158). The risks are largely due to the greater frequency of sickle cell crises (Konotey-Ahulu, 1991), which in the UK increases both maternal and fetal morbidity and mortality (Howard *et al.*, 1995a). This research involved 81 pregnant women with SCD and a control group comprising 100 women of similar ethnic background with no haemoglobinopathy. The SCD group experienced two maternal deaths and a perinatal mortality rate of 60/1000. The SCD group was also significantly more likely to develop anaemia and have low birth weight babies.

Rest, hydration and analgesia are crucial during a pain crisis in pregnancy, together with reassurance of the transience of the episode (Koshy, 1995). Koshy, like Howard *et al.* (1995a), discusses the role of exchange transfusion in pregnancy. Koshy links infection in a range of sites with the precipitation of a crisis, an argument also advanced by Konotey-Ahulu (1991), who suggests that UTI, rather than pregnancy, is the precipitating factor.

Certain political and organisational issues are raised by SCD, which apply equally during pregnancy. Anionwu (1996) highlights staff attitudes to people experiencing a sickle cell crisis and the ensuing mutual distrust. This relates to the possibility of opioid analgesia causing addiction or facilitating drug dealing. Anionwu's observations are supported by a research project into the perceptions of patients and staff about the treatment of crisis pain (Waters & Thomas, 1995). These researchers demonstrated ignorance among staff as well as the difficulty of translating such knowledge as existed into practice. Dyson *et al.* (1996a,b) report similarly uninformed findings in antenatal care and identify midwives' educational deficits.

While recognising the risks to woman and baby in maternal SCD, both Koshy (1995) and Howard *et al.* (1995a) emphasise that the outcome correlates positively with the standard of care. Although all pregnant women of Afro-Caribbean origin are routinely screened for SCD, in case general anaesthesia is indicated, there is no evidence of routine counselling about the effects of neonatal/infant SCD (Phoenix, 1990). Eboh and van der Akker (1994) discuss the topics which may be raised with prospective parents and the childbearing decisions necessary if both parents are SCD carriers.

Discussing neonatal screening for SCD, Stirk (1991) reminds us of the relative frequency of SCD compared with a condition which, unlike SCD, is routinely sought – phenylketonuria (PKU). Whereas PKU, which is more common in white people, appears in only 10–12 per 100 000, SCD is found in 500 per 100 000 black people. On the basis of these figures, she sympathises with the black community who interprets this resource allocation as racist. Perhaps this interpretation could be extended to include the general care of people with SCD.

Conditions unique to pregnancy

There are certain painful conditions that only occur during pregnancy. Probably to a greater extent than the painful conditions mentioned already, these present a threat, if not to the continuation of the pregnancy, at least to maternal and fetal/neonatal health. For this reason the pain which features in these conditions is regarded more as a diagnostic or prognostic tool than a problem in itself.

Miscarriage

Although not without problems, the term 'miscarriage' is now preferred to 'spontaneous abortion'. The purpose of this change in terminology is partly to differentiate this form of loss from the widely-used 'abortion', to mean termination of a pregnancy (TOP) by artificial means. The woman may draw comparisons between her experience of TOP and miscarriage; as an informant for Marck (1994) reported, it was 'the exact same pain' (p. 124). This woman went on to consider the way in which each of these experiences facilitated her personal growth and her eventual motherhood. Despite this, the issues associated with TOP tend to focus even less on the associated pain and, for this reason, I give it no further attention here.

Miscarriage is the spontaneous expulsion of a pregnancy before the fetus is independently viable. In the UK the legal limit of viability under the Stillbirth (Definition) Act (1992) is 24 weeks. In the process of miscarriage the woman may seek help at one of a number of stages; that is, when the miscarriage threatens, when it becomes inevitable, or when the miscarriage becomes either complete or incomplete (Gould, 1990). When miscarriage threatens, it is necessary for ectopic pregnancy and hydatidiform mole to be excluded, as both of these conditions carry serious physical implications for the mother in addition to the emotional burden which miscarriage invariably carries (Mander, 1994b). It is necessary at this point to mention the different types of pain associated with miscarriage. The pain of grief following miscarriage is now more widely and appropriately recognised (Iles, 1989), but its physical pain is less significant. The relationship between physical and emotional pain is discussed in Chapter 2.

Vaginal bleeding is almost invariably the first symptom when miscarriage threatens (Oakley *et al.*, 1984) and, perhaps for this reason, tends to be regarded as a more significant feature. It may be that the relationship between the appearance of bleeding and the onset of pain indicates an ectopic pregnancy, but this sequence is of little value when ultrasound is available to assist diagnosis. Nevertheless, pain is experienced by 96% of women with ectopic pregnancy, whereas in only 75% is vaginal bleeding a symptom (Oakley *et al.*, 1984).

Guzinski (1990) compares the pain of miscarriage with that of menstruation, in that the pain is intermittent and cramp-like. She describes the pain as mild initially and becoming more intense, as the uterine contractions strengthen. This information is of little help to women who have experienced neither menstrual nor labour pain. The experiences of ten women who had miscarried in the first 15 weeks of pregnancy contribute to a more useful account (Bansen & Stevens, 1992), describing graphically the pain's significance to the woman. These mothers regarded the pain, together with their fear of death, as 'the most notable' findings; one reported 'I thought I was going to die – the pain was incredible'(p. 87).

For those who provide care, the pain of miscarriage is more important as a predictor of the outcome of the miscarriage. Roberts and Evans (1991) found that 95% (n=221) of general practitioners in the west of Scotland regarded complaints of pain as foretelling loss of the pregnancy. Similarly, Everett *et al.* (1987) report a sample of 1290 Wessex general practitioners, of whom 93% associated uterine pain with a poor prognosis. Such concern that pain may predict pregnancy loss is also reflected in research by Fleuren *et al.* (1994). These Dutch researchers sought midwives' (n=241) and general practitioners' (n=313) reports of their care of women with an 'imminent' miscarriage. Details of the duration and nature of the pain was sought by 93% of practitioners and used to decide on transfer to obstetric care. It is clear from these research reports that the pain of miscarriage is considered by the carers to be of little significance in itself; neither does it deserve any attention or remedy. Its significance lies more in its value as a prognostic tool and to determine the management of the woman and her pregnancy. Unfortunately, as shown by Bansen and Stevens (1992), this view does not correspond with the woman's.

Placental abruption

The premature separation of a normally implanted placenta or placental abruption (Saftlas *et al.*, 1991) is a condition of pregnancy in which the seriousness of the clinical picture and the risk of morbidity and mortality vary hugely. Sometimes referred to as 'accidental' antepartum haemorrhage to differentiate it from the 'inevitable' haemorrhage of placenta praevia, in only placental abruption may the haemorrhage not be revealed vaginally (Baskett, 1985). In this situation the woman would be likely to experience greater pain because of the retention or concealment of blood in the retroplacental space and its infiltration between the fibres of the myometrium. Nathan and Huddleston (1995) attribute the lack of any revealed bleeding to the absence of an escape route for the blood loss. Such an extreme condition involves 'an acute abdomen with profound shock. There is severe and continuous abdominal pain. The uterus is woody hard and tender all over' (Baskett 1985: 61). This account, however, ignores the range of intensity of pain which the woman may experience. In the series recounted by Manolitsas *et al.* (1994), the pain varied from none, through uterine tenderness, to abdominal pain which increases in intensity with haemorrhagic episodes, presumably as the retroplacental clot accumulates and increases in size within its confined space. Nathan and Huddleston (1995: 57) describe the pain as 'sharp, tearing or burning' and they emphasise its 'unrelenting' nature. The contractions of labour may be superimposed on the continuous pain, but whether the onset of labour is due to extravasated blood irritating the myometrium into activity or whether there is fetal chemical involvement is uncertain (Fraser & Watson, 1989).

Placental abruption is such a significant condition because of its contribution to both perinatal and maternal mortality, as well as morbidity. Perinatal loss is due to that portion of the placenta which has separated being non-functional. In the UK maternal deaths due to placental abruption are steady at 1–2 per annum (Department of Health, 1996). Death is usually associated with coagulation failure followed by heart or liver failure. This mortality is particularly disturbing in view of the likelihood that the woman is likely to be young (Ananth *et al.*, 1996).

Because of the mortality risks the incidence of this condition is monitored closely and attempts made to identify aetiological factors (Pritchard *et al.*, 1991; Saftlas *et al.*, 1991). These researchers, working in different areas, report decreasing and increasing incidence respectively. Unfortunately, limited attention is given to diagnostic problems which may 'result in poor comparability between published series' (Fraser & Watson, 1989: 597). The problem of diagnosis may be of even greater significance clinically, where the diagnosis is made in 0.5–1.5% of births. The accuracy of diagnosis is questioned in view of changes indicating abruption being found in up to 4.5% of placentae (Fox, 1978).

For these reasons, the treatment tends to be symptomatic: 'In moderate to severe placental abruption maternal resuscitation and analgesia are priorities' (Fraser & Watson, 1989: 598). The intensity of the woman's pain, and its effect in aggravating her shock, are likely to require the use of opioids, despite their hypotensive effects (Rankin, 1993).

Unlike most of the conditions of pregnancy which we have considered, the problems of the woman with placental abruption do not end with the birth. The coagulation defects and anaemia which began antenatally are likely to be corrected most effectively by blood transfusion; however, coagulopathies may actually be aggravated postnatally due to myometrial damage and reduced contractility, caused by extravasated blood (Egley & Cefalo, 1985). Thus the woman who has experienced placental abruption and its dreadful sequelae is also vulnerable to postpartum haemorrhage and further morbidity.

Severe pre-eclampsia

Although the condition that precedes it has undergone reclassification and a name change, eclampsia is still 'the state of having or having had an eclamptic convulsion' (Pickles, 1987). Eclampsia is usually, but not invariably, preceded by pre-eclampsia which, in turn, is commonly preceded by pregnancy-induced hypertension (PIH) (Chesley, 1978). PIH comprises a rise in blood pressure during pregnancy, unless proteinuria is present, in which case the diagnosis becomes one of pre-eclampsia (Pickles, 1987). In both conditions, the clinical picture comprises only signs, to the extent that the woman feels well. It is only when pre-eclampsia becomes severe and eclampsia is impending that the woman may begin to complain of symptoms and begin to feel unwell. At this time she may experience pain and visual disturbances. Her pain is typically experienced in the right upper abdominal quadrant and as headache. The abdominal pain is described as epigastric pain and is thought to be due to changes in the liver, such as oedema. Alternatively, the hepatic changes may involve either liver necrosis or subcapsular haemorrhages (MacGillivray, 1983). Rupture of the liver is the ultimate hepatic change, although MacGillivray argues that this may be iatrogenic, resulting from the treatment rather than the disease. The differential diagnosis is heartburn or dyspepsia, for which medical practitioners may prescribe antacids, having failed to measure the woman's blood pressure (Barry *et al.*, 1994). The epigastric pain has also been described as 'tenderness' (Department of Health, 1996: 27). Although these accounts suggest a mild pain, this was not so for a woman who presented herself for admission complaining of severe abdominal pain and who subsequently died of 'eclampsia and heart failure, for which she had received no treatment whatsoever' (Department of Health, 1996: 27).

The Report on Confidential Enquiries into Maternal Deaths in the UK (Department of Health, 1996) also describes women in whom an eclamptic fit was heralded by 'feeling unwell' and headache. The headache characteristic of fulminating pre-eclampsia has been described as being severe, persistent and frontal or occipital and accompanied by visual disturbances caused by retinal oedema. A woman recently described her fulminating pre-eclamptic headache to me as 'like a migraine only ten times worse'. The onset of eclamptic convulsions has been attributed to 'focal cerebral vasospasm, yielding ischaemic areas from where abnormal electrical activity arises' (Ramsay, 1993). Thus the headache may result from either spasm of the cerebral vessels or the associated ischaemia.

The significance of severe pre-eclampsia lies in its unpredictable nature combined with its potentially dire prognosis for both woman and baby. The fact that 'Most obstetricians in Europe and North America rarely see a case of eclampsia' (Ramsay, 1993: 90) only serves to aggravate these problems. In the UK approximately 25 women per year die of eclampsia or pre-eclampsia (Department of Health, 1996), whereas the figure worldwide is likely to be near 50 000 (Duley, 1994). A major collaborative trial has recently demonstrated the international significance of eclampsia and its treatment (Chalmers & Grant, 1996). The collaborative eclampsia trial identified the crucial role of the local midwife in initiating appropriate treatment (Duley, 1994). This treatment was found to be magnesium sulphate, rather than diazepam and phenytoin, to reduce the recurrence of seizures and minimise morbidity (Chalmers & Grant, 1996).

This research demonstrates our limited knowledge of eclampsia. Little is known of the woman's experience of this potentially devastating condition, especially relating to her disappointed expectations of healthy childbearing. Additionally, knowledge is lacking concerning how health care personnel cope with the possibility of conditions such as eclampsia which appear like 'a bolt from the blue' (Ramsay, 1993). It is not only the unpredictability of such conditions which may be hard for staff to bear, but also the possibility that they may incur maternal as well as fetal loss.

Conditions coincidental to pregnancy

So far in this chapter we have been focusing on conditions that are affected in some way by pregnancy. We began with those that in young women are often attributed to pregnancy, then moved on to conditions that are aggravated by pregnancy and, in the last section, considered those that are unique to pregnancy. In this section, we concentrate on a small group of long-term and painful conditions which, in the context of pregnancy, raise important issues.

Rheumatoid arthritis

Rheumatoid arthritis is an autoimmune condition involving long-term inflammation of synovial joints, such as the knees, interphalangeal and metacarpophalangeal joints (Lowery, 1995). Vulnerability to rheumatoid arthritis is genetically determined, and women are three times more likely to be affected than men. Rheumatoid arthritis typically presents with pain in the form of morning stiffness, joint tenderness and pain on movement (Olds *et al.*, 1996).

For a majority of pregnant women with rheumatoid arthritis, pregnancy alleviates some of the painful symptoms (Carty *et al.*, 1986). The bad news manifests itself in the first trimester as 'overwhelming' fatigue and postnatally as an exacerbation or 'flare up' of the condition. As Carty and colleagues observe, the pregnant woman with rheumatoid arthritis has a fine line to tread between sufficient exercise to maintain mobility and excessive activity aggravating fatigue. This line becomes even more difficult to identify postnatally with the demands of a new baby.

The medication regime, which is the mainstay of treatment, is modified prior to conception in a planned pregnancy to reduce the risk of drug-induced fetal damage. In the event, however, of unplanned pregnancy the woman may be up to eight weeks pregnant before the regime is modified. Opinions differ on the teratogenicity of medication used to treat rheumatoid arthritis, and this prevents reassurance being offered to the woman with an unplanned pregnancy (Carty *et al.*, 1986). This point should be discussed with the woman with rheumatoid arthritis in the context of family planning counselling. The questionable medications include non-steroidal anti-inflammatory drugs (NSAIDs) like indomethacin (Campion, 1990) as well as the immunosuppressants, penicillamine and gold. Corticosteroids in low doses are considered safe, but the risk of neonatal adrenocortical insufficiency persists. Because of their link with platelet dysfunction, low birth weight and stillbirth, salicylates are avoided in pregnancy (Carty *et al.*, 1986).

Thus, it is apparent that the woman with rheumatoid arthritis would benefit from counselling about the risks involved in childbearing before the conception, both for her own sake and that of her child. Canadian research into childbirth education for the woman with rheumatoid arthritis suggests that neither counselling nor information relating to sexuality or contraception is available (Carty & Conine, 1983). These researchers suggest that this omission is amenable to midwifery intervention (Carty *et al.*, 1986).

Systemic lupus erythematosus

Like rheumatoid arthritis (see above) systemic lupus erythematosus (SLE or 'lupus') is an autoimmune condition presenting as a collagen tissue disease (Jones, 1994). Unlike rheumatoid arthritis, which is tissue specific, SLE affects a multiplicity of body systems (Lowery, 1995). These two important conditions are further similar in their likelihood of causing joint pain during pregnancy, although the issues surrounding them differ markedly.

SLE is a complex disease which is influenced by hormonal, genetic/racial and environmental factors (Jones, 1994; Lowery, 1995); it involves production of antiphospholipid autoantibodies causing inflammation and tissue damage in a variety of bodily sites, which result in its typically varied features (Khamashta & Hughes, 1996). The feature that makes SLE relevant in the present context is the arthritic joint pain which is experienced by 90% of people with this condition (Lowery, 1995). Other characteristic features are splenomegaly, thrombocytopaenia, nephritis, thrombosis and skin changes.

During pregnancy the progress of the disease is not affected; similarly the maternal risks are limited to pre-eclampsia unless there is gross renal or vascular impairment (Jones, 1994; Khamashta & Hughes, 1996). Like rheumatoid arthritis, SLE is thought to go into remission or at least stabilise during pregnancy, although the antibodies survive in the woman's circulation; the tendency for a postnatal exacerbation also bears comparison with rheumatoid arthritis. The treatment of SLE is dependent largely on corticosteroids and immunosuppressive therapy, but during pregnancy Jones (1994) recommends a drug regime of aspirin, heparin and prednisone, in that order and only when necessary. It is admitted, though, that there is some difficulty in identifying the effective drug regimes that are associated with minimal fetal harm. A recent research project attempted to identify the most appropriate drug regime (Ruiz-Irastorza *et al.*, 1996). These researchers described the preconceptual advice given in a multidisciplinary 'lupus clinic'. They found that exacerbations ('flares') in pregnancy most frequently involved musculoskeletal and/or cutaneous symptoms. This finding confirms the importance of pain for this woman during pregnancy. Ruiz-Irastorza and colleagues conclude that pregnancy increases SLE activity significantly, activity being worst in the second trimester, and that exacerbations are unaffected by prednisolone.

Unlike other conditions which we have considered, the serious significance of SLE lies not in its effect on the mother's health nor in the adverse effects of medication on the fetus, but in the effect of the disease, that is maternal antibodies, on the fetus. While the maternal–fetal passage of antibodies in the form of immunoglobulin G (IgG) may be beneficial to the neonate in conferring passive immunity, it may also be harmful. The transplacental passage of Rhesus antibodies in Rhesus isoimmunisation is well-known and interventions are usually offered to prevent their ill-effects. Similarly, the autoantibodies in the circulation of the mother with SLE have the potential to adversely affect the fetus/neonate. Obviously these antibodies will disappear from the neonate's circulation in due course, hopefully having caused no permanent damage. Unfortunately, in SLE such damage is a distinct possibility. This damage is likely to take the form of neonatal lupus erythematosus (NLE; Jones, 1994), which varies hugely in the extent of the harm that it causes. The neonatal effects of the pathogenic maternal autoantibodies may be as benign as discoid lupus, which is short term and harmless. On the other hand, at the opposite extreme there may be hepatosplenomegaly, blood dyscrasias, skin changes and congenital complete heart block (CCHB). The size of the problem is that CCHB occurs in 5% of babies of women with SLE, and proves fatal in 25% of these.

In addition to the risk of neonatal lupus erythematosus, the woman with SLE who is contemplating pregnancy must also consider that her pregnancy may not reach the neonatal stage, because there is a 25% risk of fetal/perinatal loss (Jones, 1994). This level of loss is unrelated to the severity of the maternal condition, but rather related with the level of activity of the disease. Histological changes have been identified in the placentae of women with SLE and these changes may be responsible for the high rate of fetal/perinatal loss. Disconcertingly, there is also a high rate of fetal loss among women who subsequently develop SLE, suggesting preclinical changes affecting placental function.

The childbearing decision by a woman with SLE clearly needs particularly serious consideration. While Ruiz-Irastorza and colleagues discuss the place of preconception counselling and contraceptive advice to facilitate the most appropriate timing of a pregnancy, Jones (1994) raises the question of continuing the pregnancy and the possibility of termination of pregnancy.

Cancer

Perhaps because we live in a pronatalist society in which cancerophobia prevails, the woman who is pregnant and has cancer is likely to encounter diametrically conflicting responses both in herself and in others. While pregnancy engenders optimistic pleasure, cancer induces pessimistic horror (Shepherd, 1990). Even though such reactions may be unjustified in epidemiological terms, cancer in pregnancy focuses the mind of the woman and those nearby on the future. The extent to which fear of cancer is justified may be judged from the incidence of cancer in pregnancy being about 1 in 1000–1500 live births (Morrow *et al.*, 1993).

Cancer in pregnancy may present in any one of a number of sites; the tissues that are most commonly affected include the breast, the cervix, the skin and the thyroid, where the tumours are reported as being painless (Hacker & Jochimsen, 1986; Harris, 1990). On the other hand, in pregnancy cancer of the gastrointestinal tract, the lung, the ovary, the brain and bony tissue does tend to cause pain of variable intensity (Moore & Martin, 1992; Morrow *et al.*, 1993). Although rarely seen in pregnancy, bony tumours, such as sarcoma, are likely to be 'very painful' because the associated myelitis may involve nerve roots (Disaia & Creasman, 1984).

The issues around this topic are many and complex and mean that the pregnant woman with cancer and those near to her will be faced with many hard decisions; thus, they need accurate factual information in a supportive caring environment (Harris, 1990).

Because of the physiological changes throughout pregnancy, the diagnosis of certain tumours, such as breast cancer, is problematical; in this site the problem is partly due to hypertrophy impeding palpation and partly to the density of the tissue obscuring mammography. Diagnostic difficulties may be further compounded by certain risks involved in investigations, such as the haemorrhage caused by cone biopsy (Disaia & Creasman, 1984: 433; Harris, 1990). The effect of the pregnancy on the progress of the cancer is a crucial question, which generally warrants a reassuring response, but which is impossible in the case of melanoma (Shepherd, 1990).

In deciding the method of treatment of the cancer, the effect of treatment on the fetus and the timing of treatment need consideration. Clearly, one factor affecting this decision will be the urgency of treatment in view of the rate of growth and risk of spread of the tumour. That cytotoxic drugs and ionising radiation have teratogenic effects is widely known, possibly requiring such interventions to be delayed to avoid fetal harm. The continuation of the pregnancy may also need to be considered in terms of, first, the possibility of termination of pregnancy and, later, fetal viability is considered if premature delivery is indicated to permit therapeutic interventions.

Despite fetal vulnerability to adverse effects of certain therapies, the fetus is surprisingly well-protected from the adverse effects of the tumour. This is largely due to the placental barrier's effectiveness, which minimises the risk of fetal metastases; the exception is melanoma, which is responsible for 50% of placental metastases and 90% of fetal metastases (Hacker & Jochimsen, 1986). In obstetric terms, the presence of a pelvic tumour or genital scar tissue impeding birth may be crucial in deciding the route of delivery.

When considering the pain associated with cancer in pregnancy, the pain directly attributable to the tumour and its effect on nearby structures is not the only aspect. As Cherny and Portenoy (1994) remind us, on top of this pain must be superimposed that caused by diagnostic investigations and by therapeutic interventions. Additionally, the inevitable emotional pain should not be underestimated.

Summary

It is clear from this chapter that, as at other times in a woman's life, pain in pregnancy is not uncommon. We have also seen that that pain is variable in both its intensity and its significance. It is necessary to teach the woman to recognise when her own coping strategies are adequate and when others' interventions are likely to be helpful. It has become apparent that on certain topics there is little research or education; this may be because the attraction of researching or teaching about non-life-threatening conditions is limited. The result is that many untested remedies have been introduced; as Bracken *et al.* observed: 'the most prevalent and discomforting symptoms of pregnancy have received such little study in properly controlled trials' (1989).

What has also emerged from this chapter is that the pain *per se* tends to be regarded by researchers and by medical attendants as of limited significance. Because, through medicalisation, pregnancy has been transformed into a 'medical problem' (Oakley, 1980) rather than an 'altered state of health', those who provide care accept that, as with many health problems, some discomfort or pain is inevitable. Pain in pregnancy tends only to be taken seriously when it indicates a life-threatening condition in either the woman or the fetus; even then, with the exception of placental abruption, the pain itself is not considered sufficiently important to deserve treatment, but rather it is hopefully resolved as the underlying condition is treated.

PART III
The Journey

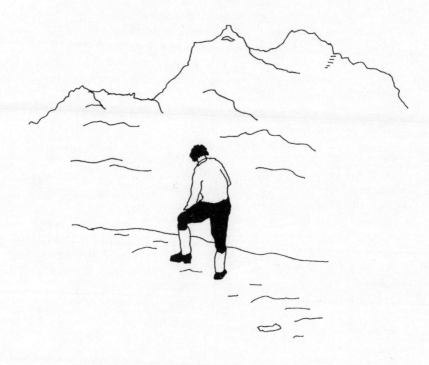

Chapter 7
Labour Pain

While it may be becoming more tenuous, as interventive pain control becomes more prevalent and effective, the link between labour and pain still holds. There persists a perceived inevitability about labour pain, even if it is only as a concept which exists to persuade the mother to contemplate her preferred pain control method. Before looking at childbearing as a continuing journey (Halldorsdottir & Karlsdottir, 1996), in which women regard labour as the major component, comprising 'pain and hard work', I consider here the nature of the journey. As well as issues that may influence our attitudes to the experience of labour pain, this involves examining ideas relating to the physical origins of labour pain, in both uncomplicated labour and in the labour that features some problem.

Issues

In contemplating labour pain, questions about its existence barely warrant a mention. Despite this, questions continue to be resurrected, perhaps endorsing the persistent 'misunderstanding' between some medical practitioners and the women for whom they provide a service (Mander, 1994a). Bonica (1990a: 1314) quotes 'proponents of natural childbirth' early this century as arguing the cultural construction of labour pain. Bonica then utilises his own unpublished data to demolish this highly tenuous argument and, with it, criticisms of obstetric anaesthetic intervention.

The rationale for the existence of labour pain, and particularly for such severe pain, is frequently questioned, bearing in mind that pain ordinarily indicates real or potential damage (Chapter 2). Bonica (1990a) answers this question in terms of the twin requirements to alert the woman to the forthcoming birth and for her to prepare for the child. The plausibility of this rationale is unconvincing. So too is Melzack and Wall's framework (1991), which comprises either prevention of serious injury or learning opportunities to avoid further injury, as well as a 'purposeless pain' such as phantom limb/body pain. It is likely that, in evolutionary terms, a balance has been reached between the minimum viable size/maturity of the human fetus and the most intense pain that women can endure (Niven & Gijsbers, 1996a). These researchers further blame human cerebral development and the reduced pelvic capacity associated with bipedal posture.

As mentioned already (Melzack & Wall, 1991), the link between pain and pathology is pervasive, which is counterproductive in the context of labour, because it labels this physiological process as 'illness' (Niven & Gijsbers, 1996b). Such labels require involvement and intervention by those specialising in treating illness – our medical colleagues.

The intensity of labour pain has been objectively established by researchers on both sides of the Atlantic (Melzack & Wall, 1991; Niven, 1992: 45). When compared with other well-known pain syndromes, as measured by a Pain Rating Index (PRI), the intensity of labour pain, particularly the second stage, far exceeds the disease conditions (Niven & Gijsbers, 1984a). Such research is necessary because labour pain, as with any, is a fundamentally personal, private, unshared and unshareable experience. Although a mother may assume that her experience of pain corresponds with other women's, this is unknowable, establishing the significance in labour of the well-known quotation: 'Pain is whatever the experiencing person says it is, existing whenever [s]he says it does' (McCaffery, 1979). Despite McCaffery's observation, there are certain factors that have been shown to be associated with greater labour pain (Niven, 1992). These factors include a larger baby, primiparity, smaller maternal stature and obstetric intervention such as amniotomy, raising the spectre of iatrogenesis. The impact of factors like labour duration are of uncertain significance.

The contribution of control in the woman's experience of pain is becoming more apparent. Control has broadened its meaning from just 'self-control' (Kitzinger, 1996) to a range of woman-centred orientations (Mander, 1992b). Its crucial importance, however, lies in the person's feelings of being able to act to control her situation (Lefcourt, 1982). Such action is likely to involve certain coping strategies, such as relaxation, which the person has learned prior to the onset of the pain (Melzack & Wall, 1991).

The effect of the woman's feeling of control in different places of birth is related to her perception of her pain (Kitzinger, S., 1989). The findings of Kitzinger's volunteer-based study support the general impression gained through anecdotal reports of home births in Holland (Mander, 1995b). She relates this experience to the empowering nature of home birth, which in turn helps the woman to reinterpret her labour pain positively. A more authoritative study (Morse & Park, 1988) was undertaken to compare the perceptions of labour pain of home birth parents (n=282) and hospital birth parents (n=191). The perceptions of pain were significantly higher among the parents who gave birth in hospital. These researchers admit their neglect of the reality of labour pain and suggest that research focusing on that area is needed.

A factor that may influence the pain of labour but which is rarely mentioned is the meaning of the birth. Newton and Newton (1972) ask whether the significance of the experience affects the woman's pain. This point is reminiscent of Melzack and Wall's (1991) suggestion that the meaning of the pain affects its acceptability and the person's ability to cope with it. Their example is phantom limb pain, which is totally negative and achieves nothing. In the context of labour pain Newton and Newton suggest that local attitudes towards childbirth, that is whether it warrants celebration or requires purification, influence the woman's coping ability. It may be that if pain is viewed on a 'continuum of productivity', phantom limb pain is at the opposite extreme from childbirth. Kitzinger (Kitzinger, S., 1989) quotes mothers' positive comments about labour pains, describing them in terms of mountains climbed and prizes won. Even Niven and Gijsbers eventually admit that positive aspects may be included: 'labour pain [while severe] is not often experienced as intensely aversive. Indeed, some women consider that pain is a desirable part of childbirth' (1996a: 141). Elsewhere these authors recognise that the unique feature of labour pain is its positive connotations (1996a), in that it is a more productive pain than many others.

In examining the meaning of pain in general terms and its influence on coping skills (Taylor, 1983), three themes emerged as fundamental to identifying a meaning of pain. The first theme comprised a 'sense of coherence' or purpose for life events, during which the person attempted to fit the pain experience into their overall view of life. The second theme that Taylor identified, and which has been already mentioned in childbearing, was the need for a sense of control over the experience. The final theme, also relevant to childbirth, comprised the individual's seeking to feel good about him- or herself by using the experience to achieve self-fulfilment or personal growth. Taylor goes on to describe how the person in pain is likely to use 'illusions' to identify the meaning of and thus cope with pain. Such tactics would involve the reinterpretation of noxious stimuli as less unpleasant or even pleasurable.

Origins of labour pain

Our understanding of the physiological factors that cause labour to be painful is less than adequate and tends to rely on the variably authoritative work of Bonica (1990a).

Pain in uncomplicated labour

As McCrea discusses (Chapter 4, 'Pain and overt bodily responses'), labour pain is usually attributed to stretching, pressure and tearing of local structures. Although different characteristics are attributed to pain at differing stages of labour (Moore, 1997), it is uncertain whether these characteristics are determined by pain assessment, by the woman's emotional state or by the interventions of carers.

Pain in complicated labour

In labour which begins as uncomplicated, the mother may encounter other superimposed pain. The additional pain, probably with other signs and symptoms, may indicate complications which may threaten the wellbeing of the baby, the mother or both.

'OP labour'

The pain of labour with the fetal head in an occipito-posterior (OP) position is part of midwifery folklore. This is because the care of this woman challenges all of the midwife's skills, as well as constituting even more of a challenge to the woman's endurance. An OP labour, or North American 'back labour', is due to the most common fetal malposition, occurring in 25% of labours (Oxorn, 1986; Lowdermilk, 1993). The incidence is complicated by the difficulty of diagnosing OP position in early labour and the likelihood that by the time labour becomes established the head may have started to rotate anteriorly.

The incidence of OP labour bears an interesting relationship to the pain control method which is most appropriate to this woman's care. Epidural analgesia is undoubtedly most suitable for a woman with an OP labour, as I learned in the 1960s when caring for an unsupported and frightened young woman whose baby was lying posteriorly. An epidural was suggested, she agreed and thereafter was able to appreciate and learn about becoming a mother. While an epidural may appropriately be used to control the pain of OP labour, it may also contribute to the development of such malpositions. This has been identified as part of the 'cascade of intervention', the existence of which is supported by UK and Finnish studies (Jouppila et al., 1980; Williams et al., 1985). This phenomenon may be associated with epidural-induced neurological changes which cause pelvic floor relaxation and malposition of the fetal head. Oxytocic drugs, administered to overcome delay, are a cause of fetal hypoxia, manifested as fetal distress (Yudkin, 1979; Keirse & Chalmers, 1989), for which interventions to expedite the birth may become necessary. Thus, the solution to the problem may also be its cause, as well as the cause of further morbidity.

A symptomatic remedy, perhaps similar to acupuncture, for low back pain in labour is intracutaneous or intradermal injection of sterile water (Simkin, 1996). Dahl and Aames (1991) found that the pain relief lasted for 79 minutes +/– 15 minutes in their three-group controlled study. A significant reduction in VAS scores for over 90 minutes when compared with a randomised placebo group was identified by Ader *et al.* (1990).

The challenging nature of this labour complication lies, first, in the nature of the pain, which is 'unremitting' (El Halta, 1996), allowing minimal respite. The constant pain is thought to be due to the pressure of the fetal occiput against the maternal sacrum (Lowdermilk, 1993). Second, the duration of the labour, if the head rotates anteriorly, is markedly increased. Because of the duration of this unremitting pain, the woman's condition may deteriorate and dehydration and ketosis may develop.

Pearl *et al.* (1993) found that the problems for the woman experiencing an OP labour did not end with the birth. Morbidity for the mother, in the form of perineal trauma associated with instrumental birth and/or a large presenting diameter, was increased. Neonatal morbidity was also higher due to instrumental intervention, manifesting itself as facial (Bell's) palsy or Erb's palsy. On the basis of Pearl *et al.*'s data, Symes (1994) suggests that a new challenge has developed for midwives, which only indirectly influences the woman's pain. It comprises the midwife preventing this malposition by encouraging maternal action which facilitates rotation of the presenting part. This intervention utilises the principle that the fetal back, being heavier, is likely to rotate anteriorly if the woman adopts a leaning forward or hands and knees posture (Sutton & Scott, 1994; El Halta, 1996). Thus, it is necessary to ask whether the woman and the midwife working together may prevent a problem caused or aggravated by other practitioners.

Rupture of the uterus
Although in this section I concentrate on complications of labour which present with or prominently feature pain, uterine rupture or dehiscence may constitute an exception. While we expect that if rupture happens it will be during labour, it rarely happens before the onset of labour.

The pain of uterine rupture is variable and its prominence depends on the severity of the accompanying signs and symptoms, which in turn is due to the extent of the rupture (Baskett, 1985). The pain of uterine rupture, including tenderness, is characteristically persistent, continuing supra-pubically, between contractions. The degree of maternal shock and fetal involvement depend on the timing, suddenness and extent of the rupture. The influence of more interventive methods of pain control on the occurrence was detailed by Molloy *et al.* (1987), who found an increased incidence of uterine rupture when epidural analgesia was used.

Factors predisposing to uterine rupture include excessive uterine activity, previous myometrial damage and traumatic birth. Currently, active management of labour (O'Driscoll & Meagher, 1986) and the frequency of uterine surgery, such as caesarean section or hysterotomy, may combine to increase the significance of this complication. It is the potential for uterine rupture that produced the adage 'Once a caesarean, always a caesarean' (Craigin, 1916). Risk of rupture of the uterus and adherence to this adage feature in the debate on vaginal birth after caesarean section (VBAC), which rages more acrimoniously in North America due to the higher caesarean section rate there (Nolan, 1990).

Uterine inversion

Like rupture, uterine inversion is a catastrophe of labour which endangers the woman's life. Unlike uterine rupture, inversion is most likely to occur during the third stage of labour (Oxorn, 1986). There are a number of predisposing factors, including various forms of misman-agement, such as 'improper fundal pressure and traction on the cord' (Oxorn, 1986: 547).

As with uterine rupture, inversion varies in its severity and, hence, in the degree of pain that the woman experiences. Her pain is due to traction on the broad, round and ovarian ligaments, which support the uterus through their attachments of the cornua to the side-walls of the pelvis. The pain is serious, not only in itself, but also in its aggravation of the hypovolaemic shock which may supervene if the placenta has become separated (Baskett, 1985). Thus the woman's shock is far more severe than the blood loss would indicate.

Approaching pain

Throughout this book I seek the widest possible interpretation of childbearing-related pain. Despite this broad approach, it is necessary to accept the link, mentioned already, between labour and pain. Thus, in examining the remedies for pain in Chapters 8 and 9, I focus mainly on labour pain in terms of who or what accompanies or helps the woman on her journey. Additionally, other (non-labour) pain in childbearing is often pathological; this requires resolution of the pathology alongside dealing with the pain engendered. This in no way reduces the relevance of the approaches mentioned in these chapters to non-labour pain. Many of these remedies are likely to be used by the mother and by her carers in non-labour situations, but I discuss specific interventions when considering the various causes of such pain.

Because of the range of methods available to assist the mother in coping with the pain of labour it is helpful to categorise them using a theoretical framework. Medical writers tend to use objective frame-works; examples are the pharmacological/non-pharmacological divide (Chalmers *et al.*, 1989), or mode of action (Simkin, 1989) or frequency of use (Steer, 1993). Other frameworks may be chosen, such as according to who controls the method or the extent to which maternal choice features (Mander, 1997c). In the following chapters, however, I combine various approaches by initially distinguishing the non-pharmacological methods and then subdividing them, using Melzack and Wall's categorisation (1991), into physiological mode of operation. For each method I consider the mother's input, describe the mode of action and then the application in childbearing. Next, drawing on research data, I identify the relevant issues for those involved in the utilisation of each method; this will include the mother, the fetus/neonate (or 'baby' when differentiation is unnecessary), the midwife, and any others who make a contribution or are affected.

Chapter 8
Non-Pharmacological Methods of Controlling Pain

In her brief account of the history of childbearing analgesia, Simkin (1989) recounts reasons for women choosing non-pharmacological remedies since the nineteenth-century introduction of pain control medication (Smith, 1979). She identifies three parallel phenomena which fuelled the interest of childbearing women. First is the disillusionment that increasing awareness of medication's adverse side-effects produced. Side-effects are perceived differently by the different contributors to childbirth; for example, chloroform's side-effect, uterine inertia, provided obstetricians with opportunities to intervene to stimulate the iatrogenically slowed labour (Mander, 1996). Simkin, next, shows how women assumed responsibility for treating their own childbirth pain. Although referring specifically to 'over-the-counter' remedies, her observation applies equally to non-drug pain control. Women's attempts to assume autonomy in many aspects of childbearing are reflected in the 'trend towards non-professional self-treatment of pain' (Simkin, 1989: 894). Thus, these spin-offs from the self-care movement constitute the third influencing factor (Kickbusch, 1989).

As becomes apparent in the scrutiny of the individual methods, research into non-pharmacological pain control is plentiful. The quality and authority of this research is, however, another matter. Following a nursing-oriented meta-analysis of these interventions, Sindhu (1996) concludes that, despite being 'intuitively appealing', 'it remains to be ascertained whether they are effective in the management of acute pain' (p. 1158).

Psychological modulation of pain

According to Melzack and Wall (1991), the use of psychological methods to counteract pain derives from research showing the significance of the psychological contribution to pain. The introduction, however, of psychological methods such as 'natural childbirth' and psychoprophylaxis long pre-dated the research. The interconnectedness of the various psychological methods is clear. For example, relaxation constitutes a basic component of many methods, such as hypnosis, biofeedback and guided imagery (Sheikh & Jordan, 1983: 394). Thus the distinctions may be academic, but, as they are likely to exist in the mind of the woman using the method, reflecting on them is worthwhile.

Relaxation

Relaxation is the method of pain control allowing the woman the greatest input. Her contribution is necessary in her decision to use this method, in her choice of whether and where to learn the chosen technique and in her decision regarding whether and for how long to continue its use in labour. The only non-maternal inputs comprise her teaching during pregnancy and reinforcement from her labour companion (Schrock, 1988).

According to Steer (1993: 49), relaxation is the most frequently used non-pharmacological method of pain control in the UK. In the study which he reports, 34% of women used relaxation (Chamberlain *et al.*, 1993). This frequency lags some way behind the use of Entonox (60%), but is not far behind the second most frequently used method, pethidine (36.9%).

Together with education and breathing exercises, relaxation has been a cornerstone of prepared childbirth since Dick-Read first introduced it (1933). The theory underpinning the use of relaxation during childbirth lies in the physiology of the autonomic nervous system (ANS; Schrock, 1988). The ANS is that part of the peripheral nervous system which maintains homeostasis within the individual's internal environment (Chapter 4); thus, these functions rarely reach consciousness-level and there is little, if any, voluntary control (Sherwood, 1995). In stressful or potentially stressful situations the sympathetic component of the ANS swings into action by increasing the blood supply, and hence oxygenation and function, of those organs likely to be needed, as well as increasing the functioning of other crucial structures. This reaction has become known by the unfortunately memorable title of 'fight or flight response' (Cannon, 1932). The relevant organs are dually innervated and, in more vegetative circumstances, the parasympathetic component serves to increase the restorative functions of the body. During childbirth education, the woman learns to minimise the functioning of the sympathetic and to increase the activity of the parasympathetic component. This breaks the escalating fear–tension–pain cycle first described by Dick-Read and subsequently endorsed by McCaffery and Beebe (1989). Thus, the woman may reduce her pain by diminishing the sensation of pain and by controlling the intensity of her reaction to it (Edgar & Smith-Hanrahan, 1992). The technique which the woman learns may involve focused or 'progressive relaxation' (Jacobsen, 1938) or more meditative relaxation techniques (Benson *et al.*, 1977). Other forms of relaxation also bear the name of the originator, such as Wolpe or Bradley. Childbirth educators recommend practising relaxation during 'classes' and at other times, preferably with the intended labour companion (Schrock, 1988).

Research projects probing the effectiveness of relaxation in childbirth are confounded by the multiplicity of other educational inputs during pregnancy. As mentioned already, relaxation is unlikely to be taught without breathing and other potentially helpful topics. Thus, the authoritative research studies have not focused purely on relaxation, but have ranged more widely; examples are the study by Timm (1989) who researched 'prenatal classes of a standard format' and Enkin *et al.* (1972) who studied 'psychoprophylactic preparation classes'. Perhaps research projects on childbirth education omitting such wide-ranging topics would not be ethically permissible. Relaxation alone has, however, been researched in a range of other conditions, which have invariably been chronic and pathological, such as insomnia and hypertension. An example is Philips' study (1988) involving an experimental relaxation group (n=24) of headache sufferers and controls (n=22). Induction of relaxation over 20 minutes was found to significantly reduce the sensory component of pain. Of particular importance in the present context is Philips' finding that the emotional component of pain was equally lowered. Thus, the aggravating effect of anxiety was shown to have been reduced by relaxation, authoritatively supporting Dick-Read's longstanding but unsubstantiated hypothesis.

Generally we should question the relevance to childbirth of the evaluation of relaxation in pathological conditions, but a small study of acute pain may bear comparison (Parsons, 1994). This study showed the benefits of teaching the Benson Relaxation Technique to orthopaedic surgical patients who were being weaned off systemic analgesic drugs. The relaxation group showed lower distress scores, lower pain scores and suffered less from insomnia than the control group. This research suggests that in a comparable acute pain episode relaxation is beneficial.

While it is difficult to imagine that the techniques of relaxation have any adverse side-effects, it may be that failure of the method is sufficiently disconcerting for the woman to justify this description. This may be prevented by beginning teaching early, emphasising the need for the woman and her partner to practise techniques and allowing time for practice in classes (Schrock, 1988).

Hypnotherapy

The high media profile which hypnosis has attracted for centuries contrasts with its infrequent use (Steer, 1993: 50). In his sample, only four women chose this method (0.07%). Although distinctive in its method of induction, hypnosis is just another way of achieving relaxation (Wideman & Singer, 1984; Orner *et al.*, 1986). Further confusion arises from the unclear distinction between hypnotherapy and hypnosis, but Booth (1993a) defines hypnotherapy as the use of hypnosis to induce a compliant and suggestible trance-like state in the treatment of conditions with a large psychological component. Although poorly-authenticated, reports indicate that hypnosis has been used since time immemorial (Stanway, 1992); modern hypnotherapy, and the bad press which has bedevilled it, date from the meteoric yet unfortunate career of Anton Mesmer (1734–1815) (Booth, 1993a).

The mode of action of hypnosis remains uncertain. Advocates compare it with the 'mesmerising' effects of boring activities such as motorway driving or 'highway hypnosis' (Booth, 1993a), or with 'runner's high' (Puskar & Mumford, 1990). Explaining hypnosis, Hilgard (1973) suggests that an individual's consciousness comprises several levels of awareness, which permit functioning at levels other than that at which pain is perceived, resulting in reports of no pain. Simultaneously, a 'hidden observer' maintains awareness of all activities and permits total recall as well as the perception of pain when the hypnotic trance ceases. Alternatively, according to the gate-control theory, hypnosis closes the 'gate' comprising the inhibitory interneurons in the substantia gelatinosa of the dorsal horn (Melzack & Wall, 1965). Detractors, on the other hand, regard hypnosis as a conspiracy resulting in the subject's 'exaggerated role-play in compliance with the hypnotist's suggestion' (Conduit, 1995: 253). That hypnosis acts to enhance the placebo effect of other remedies is still propounded (Melzack & Wall, 1991: 248). Woods, however, argues that the mode of action of hypnotherapy matters less than 'that the individual believes in his experience' (1989: 38). This is likely to be influenced by the individual's 'hypnotisability', which has aroused some concern and much research about the relevance of hypnotherapy in childbirth (Spanos *et al.*, 1994). Baram (1995) states that only 15% of the general population are 'highly suggestible and easy to hypnotize'; an equal proportion are 'difficult to hypnotize' and the remainder vary.

Hilgard and Hilgard (1986) showed that involuntary aspects of pain, such as tachycardia and rising blood pressure, are unaltered, even during deep hypnosis. These researchers observed, however, that the more voluntary components of pain, such as crying or facial expression, are reduced. In childbirth, self-hypnosis is the method of choice, in preference to post-hypnotic suggestion. If used then, like relaxation, the only non-maternal input is that of the hypnotist. Unlike relaxation, however, learning self-hypnosis during pregnancy is time-consuming and militates against its use (Baram, 1995). The training regime comprises weekly sessions during the first and third trimesters with three-weekly sessions mid-trimester (Crasilneck & Hall, 1985).

During childbearing, hypnosis is thought to allow the woman to reinterpret the pain of uterine contractions as benign sensations. In this way the 'gates' in the substantia gelatinosa are prevented by descending impulses from opening and allowing the perception of pain. As with relaxation (see above) the autonomic stress response is reduced and the stress hormones, which ordinarily increase pain perception in labour, are not secreted (Simkin, 1989).

Unrealistic claims have been made of the benefits of hypnotherapy in labour, such as more effective labour, better neonatal condition and better postnatal recovery, supposedly based on research. Baram (1995) reminds us, however, that many studies were undertaken in the USA when any method was likely to produce better outcomes than the heavy sedation or anaesthesia employed in conventional obstetrics. Werner *et al.* (1982) attribute these unrealistic claims to poorly-conducted research, in which the results may owe more to the enthusiasm of those involved than to the effectiveness of hypnotherapy.

Following their review of three randomised controlled trials (RCTs), Spanos *et al.* (1994) conclude that research has failed to establish that hypnotherapy reduces labour pain. These authors ignore, however, an RCT by Freeman and colleagues (1986) involving 82 women. While Freeman *et al.* demonstrated no significant reduction in the mothers' use of pharmacological analgesia, the number of assisted births (forceps/ventouse) was lower, albeit not significantly. More importantly, though, and achieving statistical significance ($p=0.08$), was Freeman's observation that 52% of the hypnotherapy group were 'very satisfied' with their labour, whereas this applied to only 23% of the controls. Whether this finding in any way reflects any beneficial contribution of hypnotherapy must be questioned in view of the impossibility of conducting such a trial 'blind'; the possibility of the Hawthorne effect cannot be ignored.

While Woods claims that hypnosis carries 'no risk or side effects for the woman or child' (1989), others are more cautious. Booth (1993a) warns that a woman with severe mental health problems might become disturbed by attempts to induce hypnosis. In contrast, Arthurs (1994) alerts us to the possibility of hypnosis being 'too effective' to the extent that the woman may not notice pathological pain and miss appropriate care. As mentioned above, hypnosis has always been vulnerable to 'a bad press'; hence the 'alleged sexual improprieties' (Simkin, 1989) may be a further deterrent. Hypnosis, however, is 'like a gun – it's not the tool, but the operator who makes it dangerous' (Olsen, 1991).

Imagery

Guided imagery involves the woman using imagination to control her pain. This is by creating images which either decrease the severity of her pain or which comprise a more acceptable and non-painful substitute (McCaffery & Beebe, 1989). Because of the mother's crucially active involvement in this technique, she may develop a sense of being in control of her pain which, in turn, facilitates relaxation (Edgar & Smith-Hanrahan, 1992).

Just as hypnosis is compared with the trance-like states associated with boring activities, imagery is compared with day-dreaming (Steffes, 1988). Such similarities gave rise to the name 'oneirotherapy', which is derived from the Greek for dream, and has been termed 'waking-dream therapy' (Sheikh & Jordan, 1983). The essential difference, however, relates to guided imagery's 'purposeful' creation of an image for a specific reason, such as relieving pain. The guidance may be by the woman, or she may be assisted by another person or a recording (Mobily *et al.*, 1993).

Melzack and Wall (1991) discuss imagery alongside the distraction that underpins many of the coping strategies used to deal with painful and otherwise unpleasant experiences. These writers suggest that more vivid images facilitate more effective pain control. Their example comprises the well-known pleasurable beach image, whereas Steffes discusses more precise, if neutral, images, such as hanging numbers on a curtain. Her instructions require that the person in pain should not only attend to the details of the numbers (1–100) but also note the details of the hands positioning them.

The effect of guided imagery on dental pain using a tape-recording (Horan *et al.*, 1976) was studied, involving an experiment group, an uninstructed group and a 'neutral' imagery group. Horan showed that the guided imagery group encountered significantly less pain than either the uninstructed or, more importantly, the neutral imagery group.

Although it may be difficult to believe that harmful consequences follow this form of relaxation, certain psychological impediments may ensue. These include withdrawal from everyday life, insomnia and hallucinations (Benson *et al.*, 1974). Thus, it is recommended that imagery should be avoided in people who are at risk of developing psychoses and that there should not be more than two imagery sessions of 20 minutes per day. On the other hand, Steffes (1988) claims that 10 000 guided imagery tapes have been purchased with no reported ill-effects.

Biofeedback

Unlike hypnotherapy, biofeedback is a recent addition to the repertoire of pain remedies, having first been reported in 1970 (Blanchard & Ahles, 1990). Like relaxation, however, much of the research on bio-feedback has focused on the treatment of headache sufferers. Again it is necessary to question the relevance of research into a method that focuses on chronic conditions, bearing in mind the acute nature of labour pain. The appropriateness of such methods may be increased by the time during pregnancy when the woman prepares herself, by learning techniques, to use her chosen method during the acute experience of labour.

Biofeedback is defined as: 'a process in which a person learns to reliably influence physiological responses ... which are not ordinarily under voluntary control' (Blanchard & Epstein, 1978). Thus, the success of biofeedback depends on the individual's ability to learn to control autonomic functions. This learning comprises two stages utilising classical conditioning (Marcer, 1986; Conduit, 1995). The first learning stage introduces the person to the subtle and minute changes in her bodily functioning, such as blood pressure, and then to her own ability to control these functions. A crucial component of the first learning stage is the 'biofeedback machine' which measures the relevant bodily activity, such as blood pressure, and gives instantaneous information or feedback by either a visual or an auditory signal (Jessup & Gallegos, 1994). Using this external feedback loop (Fig. 8.1) the person learns the responses that alter the physiological activity in the desired direction, such as relaxation lowering the blood pressure. The person develops, perhaps independently or with others' help, strategies which achieve these changes; such strategies might include engendering feelings of warmth, peace or calm (Wallace & Fisher, 1987). Clearly biofeedback training involves some improvisation of strategies to cause physiological change, largely on a trial and error basis.

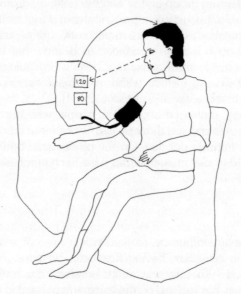

Fig. 8.1 The external feedback loop in biofeedback.

The biofeedback machine is obviously crucial in the first learning stage. The person, however, having become competent in making the desired physiological change, learns next to dispense with the machine. This is by, in the second learning stage, utilising her increasing bodily awareness to pick up and respond to her internal cues in preference to the machine's signals.

The apparatus used in the first learning stage may be the sphygmo-manometer, as shown in Fig. 8.1, or the galvanic skin response (GSR) may be assessed or muscle tension by using an electromyograph (EMG; Marcer, 1986). No objective measure of pain is yet available which could be used in childbirth, so a proxy measure is necessary. Addi-tionally, the instruments mentioned may be less than appropriate in reducing sympathetic activity and facilitating relaxation in labour. For these reasons temperature feedback is likely to be employed for child-birth. Marcer (1986) reports that devices incorporating a 'highly sen-sitive thermistor' use changes in finger temperature to reflect altered sympathetic activity; he indicates that while these devices are suitable for clinical use, their inherent weaknesses render them inappropriate in research.

Although a basic tenet of biofeedback is the person's ability to control her bodily functions without relying on the biofeedback machine, women in labour who use this method do continue to rely on their machine during labour (Bernat *et al.*, 1992). Thus, it appears that another contributor in the form of the machine is involved. An account of biofeedback in childbirth (Di Franco, 1988) discusses the use of instruments, including the 'labor coach', who provides feedback on the woman's state of relaxation using visual and tactile observations.

As with so much research into pain control, research on biofeedback has been hampered by weak design and overenthusiastic researchers. An example is the study by Gregg (1978) which compared the pain medication use in the labour of Lamaze-prepared with Lamaze-/bio-feedback-prepared multiparous women. There were no unprepared controls among this sample of private patients. Only 45% of the Lamaze/biofeedback women sought pain medication, whereas 100% of the Lamaze-only women did so. The latter figure is surprising, but the funding of the research by the manufacturer of the biofeedback machine is disconcerting. Suitable controls were involved when primigravidae were taught biofeedback in pregnancy and used the biofeedback machine in labour (Duchene, 1989). The experiment group reported that they experienced significantly less pain prior to the birth, during the birth and through to day one.

In a four-group controlled study, St James-Roberts *et al.* (1982) sought to assess the value of biofeedback for 'ordinary' women without the high levels of specialised support provided in Gregg's study (1978). One of the biofeedback groups was taught and employed skin conductance level (SCL) and the other electromyography (EMG) to assess their level of relaxation. Each biofeedback group had its own controls. All of the women received the standard childbirth education and relaxation classes. The EMG women were able to achieve a 'profound level of muscle relaxation', but the SCL group found it ineffective. In terms of duration of the first stage of labour, dosage of anaesthetic drugs and women using epidural analgesia there were no significant differences between experiment and control groups. The researchers conclude that EMG is more effective in early labour, but that to be effective throughout labour more intensive training would be necessary, making it unsuitable for routine use.

In their review of the literature on biofeedback, Blanchard and Ahles (1990: 1726) maintain that they have not located any 'reports of untoward side-effects'. They observe that any unexpected side-effects are beneficial, such as improved sleep and reduction of other problems. Complications, they suggest, arise if people using medication for diabetes or hypertension learn biofeedback without adjusting drug regimes.

Psychoprophylaxis

Among the psychological methods for coping with labour pain, relaxation has featured prominently and consistently. Lamaze (1970) followed Dick-Read's earlier work (1933) by applying Pavlovian concepts to relaxation in childbirth and introduced the term 'psychoprophylaxis', meaning preventing pain by psychological methods. In the USA Lamaze's name replaced the term that he introduced (Sloane, 1993). Although differing in some aspects, both approaches to childbirth education, like others, focused on four areas (Melzack & Wall, 1991; Sloane, 1993):

(1) Information-giving – to reduce anxiety
(2) Relaxation training – to reduce tension arising from and aggravating the pain of uterine contractions
(3) Coping strategies – to provide distraction from the pain
(4) Breathing exercises – to facilitate relaxation and distraction, and perhaps assist the birth.

In this section it has become apparent that other, less orthodox, approaches to pain control may also be introduced into childbirth education, such as hypnotherapy and biofeedback. Although neglected in the lists of childbirth education activities (see above), group interaction and mutual support are crucial to 'the classes' (Edwards & Nichols, 1988). Group interaction results in the women and partners learning and benefiting not only from the childbirth educator's knowledge, but also from each others'.

Of the four components of psychoprophylaxis listed above, information-giving is irrelevant here and relaxation has been dealt with separately. The two remaining components, coping strategies/distraction and breathing, may be tautologous (Sloane, 1993). This demonstrates a dismissive attitude to breathing as a form of pain control, which may equally be applied to other non-drug methods, an attitude that may not be helpful to the woman choosing to use them.

Alternatively, it may be helpful to recognise that distraction may make a contribution to pain control in labour. Melzack and Wall (1991) remind us of the well-known phenomenon of injuries passing unnoticed in the heat of battle. This 'battlefield analgesia', though, is associated with other non-pathophysiological benefits that accrue from such injuries which render the soldier less than sorry that they have occurred. The effectiveness of distraction, however, applies if the pain begins slowly and becomes stronger (Melzack *et al.*, 1963). This is what typically happens in uncomplicated labour, increasing the relevance of distraction in this context. Examples of distraction include effleurage (Sloane, 1993), but domestic activity may be a more appropriate example in that the woman continues her ordinary activities as her labour progresses. This broad view of distraction is endorsed in a nursing context by Mobily *et al.* (1993), who maintain that distraction strategies 'are limited only by the creativity of the nurse in combination with the creativity, abilities and preferences of the patient'.

Paced breathing techniques, mentioned already, have long been a mainstay of psychoprophylaxis. Rose and Hilbers (1988) indicate that this has resulted in huge variations in the breathing techniques that women are taught and similar variations in the names applied to techniques. These authors regard this confusion as problematic. However, more of a problem is the risk of hyperventilation and the metabolic and cerebral changes that may ensue in association with hypocapnia (Sherwood, 1995). Research by Melzack and colleagues (1981) investigated the benefits of women learning psychoprophylaxis in pregnancy. As well as identifying factors associated with women experiencing greater pain during childbirth, these researchers found that psychoprophylaxis significantly decreases women's total pain scores. This reduction applies to both the affective and the sensory components of labour pain. Despite this significant reduction, though, the pain scores remained comparable with people suffering from cancer. This continuing high level of pain was found, in this North American study, to result in 88% of women using epidural analgesia. The researchers argue that teachers of psychoprophylaxis should seek ways to make their methods even more effective.

Although this study supports the use of psychoprophylaxis, it raises many questions. In the sample, because of the North American system of maternity care, trained women were greatly over-represented (20 untrained and 61 trained). Additionally, a randomised sample is ethically problematical and self-selection in this area of research introduces subject bias.

Summary

The research on each of the psychological methods has generally shown only small benefits to the woman. More encouraging, though, is the tendency of one method to enhance the effect of another used simultaneously, which has been recognised and entitled 'multiple convergent therapy' (Melzack & Wall, 1991: 261).

Sensory modulation of pain

The sensory modulation of pain is by the utilisation of physical interventions to 'close the gate' to pain impulses. This contrasts with the previous section on psychological methods, which are thought to 'close the gate' on pain impulses by using approaches that depend on the power of thought.

Manual therapies

In some of these interventions the use of the hands is crucial, for which reason they are included in the manual therapies (Haldeman, 1994: 1252). The role of the practitioner's hands, however, is not consistent, but varies with the theoretical basis of each method. I consider these manual therapies first, because they have most in common with the psychological methods which have just been addressed (see 'Psychological modulation of pain').

Massage

Like hypnotherapy, but more recently, the reputation of massage has suffered from adverse publicity. The seedy and erotic associations of this intervention are explicit in the literature (Maxwell-Hudson, 1990; McConnell, 1995). A further issue, apparent in Steer's research report (1993), lies in the uncertain nature of massage. While 19.3% of the women reported having been given massage to relieve childbirth pain, only 5% of midwives reported having used it for individual women. This discrepancy contrasts with the administration of medications such as pethidine, which was reported by 37.8% of midwives and 36.9% of women. The discrepancy may be due to the intervention, identified as massage by the woman, being regarded as mere 'back rubbing' by the midwife.

This confusion is compounded by authoritative writers such as Simkin (1989) who, discussing the reduction of painful stimuli, describes a 'steady strong force applied to a spot on the low back during contractions, using one's . . . "heel" of hand' (p. 896/7). While Simkin terms this 'counterpressure', it is an accurate account of what I do when I 'rub the back' of a woman in labour. Additionally, Simkin's technique is indistinguishable from 'massage in labour' described by Maxwell-Hudson (1990: 102): 'Apply deep, firm pressure on the sacrum with the heel of one hand'. Does the difference between these interventions lie in the mode of application? Or does it lie in the nature of the practitioner, so that what midwives do is mere back rubbing, whereas other practitioners employ massage or counterpressure? This conclusion is endorsed by Mobily and colleagues (1994) who, in nursing, distinguish 'simple massage' from other forms requiring specialised training.

These distinctions are not helpful in understanding this intervention; for this reason I will here define massage by combining Haldeman's (1994: 1252) and Mobily *et al.*'s (1994: 39–40) definitions:

> 'Massage is the application of hand pressure to soft tissues, usually muscles, tendons or ligaments, without causing movement or change in position of a joint in order to decrease pain, produce relaxation, and/or improve circulation.'

Massage is the 'most primitive pain remedy' (Lee *et al.*, 1990: 1777) and it utilises an innate human reflex to hold, rub or squeeze a hurt body part. Such self-administered massage is less relevant to labour, thus marginally reducing the mother's contribution. In describing massage as a complementary therapy in nursing, Malkin (1994) details the six basic movements that are employed. They are: effleurage, pétrissage, tapôtement, hacking, kneading and cupping. Each is characterised by differing pressure, direction, speed, hand position and movement to achieve different effects on underlying tissues.

The main action of massage is thought to be 'closing the gate' to inhibit the passage of pain stimuli to the higher centres of the central nervous system. Further, the tactile stimulation and positive feelings, developed when a caring and empathetic form of touch is applied, serve to enhance the pain-controlling effects of massage (Ferrell-Torry & Glick, 1993). These authors maintain that the benefits of massage are reinforced by the relaxation response which the experience of massage engenders. They relate the effects of pain alleviation by massage to reduction in anxiety, which may be aggravated by pain (Fig. 8.2).

Simkin (1989) observes that the beneficial effects only last for as long as the massage continues and that, when discontinued, the pain increases. This disadvantage is due to the process of adaptation, by which the nervous system becomes accustomed to stimuli and sense organs cease to respond. The result in this context is the diminution of the pain-relieving effects of massage. Thus, Simkin recommends that

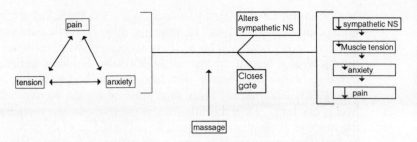

Fig. 8.2 Potential relationships between massage and (cancer) pain.

massage during labour should be intermittent, like back rubbing which typically is used only during contractions, or varied in terms of the type of touch and the location. The techniques recommended by Maxwell-Hudson (1990) might be appropriate; including face massage between contractions using smooth and rhythmic strokes and then firm foot massage.

As mentioned already, the benefits of massage are claimed to extend beyond purely physiological changes; psychological effects may also ensue (Malkin, 1994). A study of massage by nurses caring for cancer patients sought to assess the effects in both physiological and psychological terms (Ferrell-Torry & Glick, 1993). Using well-validated instruments as well as objective physiological data, these researchers measured pain, relaxation and anxiety before and after massage. Their sample comprised nine men suffering from cancer, and these patients' self-reported perceptions of pain, relaxation and anxiety improved significantly after massage. Similarly, physiological measurements reflecting sympathetic activity indicated a reduction in the stimulation of the autonomic nervous system (ANS). Thus, these researchers suggest that massage is used to enhance the effects of pain medication.

The major contraindications to massage relate to its stimulating effect on the circulatory system. For this reason massage for people with health problems such as thrombophlebitic, arteriosclerotic or cardiovascular conditions may be unsuitable. Apart from this, local skin conditions may contraindicate the use of massage; examples are local acute inflammation, acute burn, dermatitis or wounds (Lee *et al.*, 1990; McConnell, 1995). Despite the frequency with which Steer (1993) reports that women receive massage during labour, research into its effectiveness is notable by its absence. This is partly due to the confusion already mentioned about what constitutes massage. As a result, in reviewing the literature, Simkin (1989) regards touch and massage as synonymous. Additionally, a literature review on massage to treat cancer pain identifies the many methodological weaknesses to which such research is prone (Ferrell-Torry & Glick, 1993).

As well as 'basic' massage, more specialised forms, such as reflexology and shiatsu, may be used. The theoretical bases of both of these therapies are related to traditional Chinese medicine (TCM). The limited literature, though, indicates reluctance to use them during childbearing (Booth, 1993b, 1994).

Therapeutic touch

A nursing intervention that, like more specialised forms of massage, may be used to alleviate pain and derives its theoretical framework from the East is therapeutic touch (TT; Daley, 1997). It is necessary to question whether this approach fits into the sensory modulation of pain. Simkin (1989: 900) regards TT as a form of massage, but the similarities are unclear, other than both employing the hands in a less than orthodox approach to pain control.

Although much of the literature on TT suggests its action is more spiritual than physical (Krieger, 1979), others argue that the spiritual aspect is of limited significance (Mackey, 1995). In support of the latter, Samarel (1992) denies that any religious input or professed faith or belief by either practitioner or patient is needed and, additionally, the action of TT in no way involves sensory modulation. This is because, first, no physical contact between the practitioner and 'patient' is involved, hence 'non-contact therapeutic touch' (Daley, 1997). Second, practitioners claim that the TT corrects energy fields, as opposed to neurological activity.

According to its originator Kunz, the action of TT relies on the energy field of which Rogers' Theory of Integrality (1980) states all living things are a part. This concept is similar to the Eastern concept of *prana*, which relates to factors organising life processes, including physiological ones (Krieger, 1979). Health is associated with an abundance of *prana*, whereas a deficit results in illness. A characteristic of *prana* or energy which is crucial to TT is its transferability. Thus, the healthy practitioner's abundance is transferred to correct the patient's deficit. TT utilises the two-way energy flow which comprises each individual's energy field and through the practitioner's hands a direct transfer of energy is made, behaving like a 'conduit' (Mackey, 1995).

Four stages feature in the application of TT, although these may vary (Booth, 1993c). To prepare, the practitioner focuses her mind by 'centreing'. Mackey (1995) describes this as 'silencing the chattering mind', although there are similarities with meditation or trances. Next, 'assessment' involves sensing differences in energy flow by a non-touch technique, known as clearing, in which the hands are moved along the body of the patient, who is clothed, 5–15 cm away from the body. The initial assessment is rapid and may be followed by a recheck. The intervention stage comprises 'unruffling' and redirecting energy. The practitioner aims for a uniform and flowing energy field for the patient in order to induce relaxation and accelerate healing. The practitioner, finally, evaluates the patient's energy field to ensure that flows are balanced. Lothian (1988) maintains that TT may be used to ease anxiety and pain in childbearing, especially for couples who are 'uncomfortable with physical touch'.

The contraindications to and side-effects of TT tend not to be mentioned, but Simkin (1989) concludes that TT is 'apparently a harmless intervention'. It carries the advantages that it is acceptable to labouring women and is easily discontinued if necessary. Booth (1993c) raises more serious concerns about the effects on patients with mental health problems, on the basis of which he states that psychosis is a contraindication.

Although research of varying quality has been undertaken on the effects of TT, research on childbearing women is lacking. A qualitative study of the patient's experience of TT was undertaken using a volunteer sample, the weakness of which was recognised (Samarel, 1992). The data showed the patients' perceptions of changes in their physiological, mental/emotional and spiritual states, suggesting that holistic benefits emerge in terms of personal growth and increased well-being.

While there is no evidence that TT is widely used by midwives or nurses in the UK, the situation differs in North America. The limited research into TT has contributed to the American debate regarding nurses' use of TT. Another factor is the enthusiasm with which TT has been accepted by American nurses, as demonstrated by its endorsement by the National League for Nursing (Booth, 1993c). Thus, TT has become a standard curriculum component in many nurse education institutions. These two factors have combined to cause concern, which is aggravated by a third factor, that is the suspicion that TT may constitute spiritual or faith healing. Such suspicions carry the aura of 'charlatanry' (Booth, 1993c), from which nurse TT practitioners seek to dissociate themselves (Samarel, 1992). These three factors have created an acrimonious debate about the nature and use of nursing knowledge (Oberst, 1995). Nurses cautious about the limited evidence on which TT is based are resentful of its media attention, attention which reflects badly on a serious profession, and augurs badly for the generation of research funds. Thus, it must be asked whether this situation could have been avoided had TT been adequately researched prior to endorsement. This only reinforces Simkin's observation (1989) that 'careful scientific investigations' are needed.

Quasi-manual therapies

I consider two forms of pain control as being on the border between manual and technological.

Acupressure

Having considered the place of massage (see above) in controlling childbirth pain, it is appropriate that we should examine the role of acupressure (also known as shiatsu massage) before moving on to discuss its more invasive counterpart, acupuncture. Acupressure comprises fingertip massage over the acupuncture points (see below; Jungman, 1988; Arthurs, 1994). Like acupuncture, acupressure's mode of action remains uncertain. Two possible explanations are suggested (Simkin, 1989): either local endorphin production is stimulated or, alternatively, acupressure 'closes the gate' to painful stimuli. Research on both the action and effectiveness of this intervention are lacking. The benefits of acupressure may derive not only from its specific analgesic effects, but also from counter-irritation and social reinforcement (Conduit, 1995). Acupressure is more appropriate in labour than acupuncture because it is easily self-administered and particularly beneficial for back pain (Arthurs, 1994).

Acupuncture

The non-maternal inputs into the pain control of the woman who chooses to employ acupuncture are legion. They include the needles themselves, the acupuncturist who positions them and who teaches the woman to stimulate them, but perhaps most significant is the need for the woman to accept the ideological basis of this therapy. Classical acupuncture derives its theoretical basis from 3000-year-old traditional Chinese medicine (TCM; Bond, 1979). The crucial concept is that health depends on a balance between opposing energy forces; thus, ill-health or disease is due to imbalance of energy (Arthurs, 1994). This energy takes two forms: a negative female passive form which is known as '*yin*' and the positive male active '*yang*' (Bond, 1979). Collectively this 'energy' is known as '*Chi*', '*ki*' or '*qi*'. These various names illustrate the problems (WHO, 1991) of communication in this context, due to different nomenclature, dialects, pronunciation and translation.

A person's vital energy is thought to flow through twelve paired interconnected body channels or meridians (Chapman & Gunn, 1990). Although the symbolic names of the meridians relate to organs of the body, such as gallbladder, they do not correspond to Western anatomy. The 365 acupuncture points are sited along the meridians and are recognisable as areas of low electrical resistance. The meridians have been shown to correspond to areas of rapid cell death. Each acupuncture point represents a diseased organ, and puncture there is thought to allow noxious air to escape from that organ and the blood to be cleansed (Bond, 1979).

The conditions for which acupuncture is applied vary with the training and experience of the practitioner (WHO, 1991). There are also variations between practitioners in applying this intervention. The length of the needles used depends on the tissue that is being punctured, shorter needles being used for bonier areas. The individuality of therapists' approaches also becomes apparent in the metal of the needles. Classically the needles are gold or silver (Chapman & Gunn, 1990), but Bond mentions only stainless steel. Mann (1983) recounts how the insertion of the needle, in terms of speed, force and direction, affects the success of treatment. Once the needles have been inserted according to the map of acupuncture points, they are manipulated, which involves moving, twirling or vibrating them in some way, perhaps electrically.

The action of acupuncture has been hypothesised as taking one or more of four forms (Simkin, 1989). First, psychological effects have been identified. These are associated with the cultural components and the need for preparation for acupuncture which is comparable to prepared childbirth (Chapman, 1984). These psychological effects are described by Arthurs (1994: 496) as 'cultural susceptibility rather than individual suggestibility'. Conduit (1995), however, indicates that psychological methods are not the only mode of action, as evidenced by observations that acupuncture works on dogs. Second, the conviction that acupuncture will work has the effect of the higher centres 'closing the gate' to the passage of pain impulses (Melzack, 1975b). Third, Bond (1979) suggests that the needles activate pain-inhibiting mechanisms in the central nervous system, such as endogenous opioid production in the pituitary or brain stem being enhanced by acupuncture. Arthurs (1994) supports this by observations of the sedation that ordinarily occurs 1 hour after the acupuncture session, suggesting that naturally occurring opioids are being stimulated. This is further supported by Narcan/nalorphine, which are narcotic antagonists, reversing the analgesic effects produced by acupuncture (Yang & Kok, 1979). Fourth, the 'closure of the gate' to pain impulses may be by the presynaptic inhibition of sensory fibres at the level of the dorsal horn due to the stimulation of large diameter sensory fibres.

In the course of research on the use of acupuncture in labour, differing perceptions emerged (Abouleish & Depp, 1975). Nine out of twelve women were happy with it, in spite of about eight needles being inserted. In contrast, the obstetricians thought that the insertion of the needles was complicated and 'time consuming', interfered with electronic fetal monitoring and caused immobility for the woman. Such inconvenience to obstetricians begs many questions, but may explain acupuncture's limited use in labour, perhaps making acupressure an acceptable alternative.

The existence of psychological benefits of acupuncture, as mentioned above, is supported by Yang *et al.* (1984), who showed that the analgesic effects lasted only for as long as stimulation was maintained. By comparison the emotional response, that is not being upset by the pain, was longer lasting. In terms of its effects, Chapman and Gunn

(1990) maintain that acupuncture is effective in 50–80% of chronic pain sufferers. This figure should be compared with people who received sham acupuncture, which was 50% effective, and placebo controls in whom 30% found some pain relief.

A limitation on the use of acupuncture, which further supports the significance of the psychocultural component, is its unsuitability for children (Bond, 1979). Another limitation is that the pregnant woman should not have needles inserted below the waist, because this is associated with starting contractions (Arthurs, 1994). This prohibition does not apply during labour, as needles may be inserted during the second stage 'in the perineal body, behind the anus and beside the vagina' (Abouleish & Depp, 1975), although ear points may also be used (Yelland, 1995).

The side-effects of acupuncture include infection due to dirty needles and damage to nearby anatomical structures associated with inadequate anatomical knowledge (Arthurs, 1994). Chapman and Gunn (1990) emphasise these complications, while conceding that problems are rarer than those caused by pharmacological iatrogenesis and by TENS. These medical authors raise the possibility of non-diagnosis or masking symptoms by a non-medical practitioner.

The defensive attitude adopted by these medical writers (Chapman & Gunn, 1990) reminds us of the ongoing power struggle to control the practice of acupuncture. O'Neill (1994) explores the double standard applied by physicians who maintain that 'on the one hand acupuncture is unscientific and should not be used but, on the other hand, if it is used it should be only by physicians'. He compares the medical use of science with the wearing of a phylactery and the safety or danger of interventions such as acupuncture as being more related to the status of the practitioner than to the practice itself. An attempt to reconcile TCM and allopathic medicine was made by Bensoussan (1991). The two traditional camps have comprised, first, the practitioners of acupuncture who accept its functioning and, second, the medical researchers who seek explanations in Western terms. These differences hinder communication between practitioners to the detriment of clients, in whose interests effective communication should be established.

Non-manual interventions

Certain methods of sensory modulation utilise non-manual devices.

TENS (transcutaneous electrical nerve stimulation)

A crucial difference between TENS and other methods of pain control derives from its origins. While most methods have evolved over hundreds or thousands of years, TENS was invented in a laboratory (Wall & Sweet, 1967) following the development of the gate-control theory.

This intervention, however, may be derived from the electric fish, first used in Socrates' era, on which the sufferer stood in order to reduce pain. The action of TENS exploits 'the patient's own in-built neuro-biological control mechanisms' (Woolf & Thompson, 1994: 1191). Thus, in physiological terms at least, TENS permits the woman a large degree of control.

The main action of TENS comprises 'closing the gate' to the passage of pain impulses, which results from a below-pain-threshold barrage of impulses (Sjölund *et al.*, 1990). This barrage is produced by a current generator. The other action of TENS is to stimulate endorphin release (Chapter 4, 'Electrical blocks'). Endorphins serve to modulate the transmission of pain perceptions and, thereby, raise the pain threshold to produce sedation and euphoria (Hawkins, 1994). Thus, the action of TENS is less debated than is its effectiveness.

The equipment needed to administer TENS comprises, first, a pulse generator and amplifier. This is a hand-held unit which combines an on/off switch, an intensity (amplitude) control and continuous/pulse control. This TENS unit is attached by insulated wires to the electrodes, which are made of rubber impregnated with carbon. The electrodes are applied to the skin, using saline gel for contact, and then fixed with tape. The siting of the electrodes is crucial because they must be applied in the segment of the body where the pain is located. This positioning contrasts with acupuncture and acupressure, which is applied extra-segmentally along the lines of the relevant meridians (Woolf & Thompson, 1994). In contrast to this recommendation the siting of TENS on acupuncture points has been investigated non-clinically to increase TENS' effectiveness (Kemp, 1996). In labour the TENS unit is set just below the woman's pain threshold and maintained there between contractions. The woman increases the intensity of electrical stimulation during contractions to compete with their pain (Simkin, 1989).

Contraindications to the use of TENS in labour are few. The presence of an on-demand cardiac pacemaker is an absolute contraindication, but one that is rarely likely to apply in childbearing (Woolf & Thompson, 1994). Localised phenomena, such as skin reactions to the tape (Sjölund *et al.*, 1990), and the risk of interference with cardiotocograph recordings appear to be the most serious side-effects (Simkin, 1989).

In assessing TENS' effectiveness, like other 'complementary' pain control methods, research is fraught with methodological weaknesses. The result is considerable uncertainty about the benefits of TENS in childbirth. One exception to this generally uncertain picture is a double blind RCT involving 150 women (Harrison *et al.*, 1986), which showed that women using TENS were less likely to need any other analgesia, suggesting a weakly beneficial effect, and high satisfaction with TENS.

An example of the problems frequently encountered in TENS

research is found in the work of Hardy (1991). She began an RCT, but the study remains incomplete due to recruitment problems. On the basis of 80 women using TENS and 67 controls and disregarding Entonox use, more women using TENS were found to have used no additional analgesia, albeit not significantly. Whereas the originators of TENS claim that it is beneficial for back pain (Melzack & Wall, 1991), Hardy's work did not support this. The midwives' tendency to assess the TENS users' pain as more severe than the women's assessment and more severe than the controls' pain leads Hardy to ask whether midwives find it easier caring for narcotised women. It has been suggested that TENS' high intensity electrical impulses affect the fetal heart's conducting system. Bundsen and Ericson (1982) found that with a maximum current density of 0.5 $\mu amp/mm^2$ (even when applied to the supra pubic area as opposed to the usual para-vertebral position in the lumbo-sacral area) there were no adverse perinatal effects.

A further benefit of TENS was identified postnatally, as women who used TENS were significantly more likely than those who used pharmacological methods to be breast feeding at 6 weeks (Rajan, 1994). It may be that this was due to the 'type' of woman who uses TENS. Alternatively, as Rajan argues, these babies' behaviour may not have been negatively affected in the way that, as she also identified, the babies of women who have received drugs like pethidine are affected.

Women's use of TENS raises many issues for midwives (Hardy, 1991; Cluett, 1994). Since 1991 adequately instructed midwives have been permitted to 'encourage, advise on and use TENS equipment to relieve labour pain' (Ralph, 1991). Whether any practitioner should be 'encouraging' the use of any analgesic intervention, even less one based on such inconclusive research evidence, is questionable. Other midwife-related issues include the training of staff, the uncertain availability of TENS units and the organisation of a TENS service – all of which constitute new challenges to midwifery services (Hawkins, 1994).

In summary, TENS is non-invasive, cheap and portable, with few side-effects. Its favourable reception by women may compensate for lingering doubts about TENS' effectiveness. The consensus appears to be that TENS is appropriately regarded as one of a repertoire of pain control methods, one or more of which any woman may consider using (Simkin, 1989; Sjölund *et al.*, 1990).

Music

Although music is often heard in the labour ward, I am uncertain whether it is anything more than aural wallpaper. If it has a purpose, who benefits? Is it intended to help the hearer relax or is it used, as I have found necessary, to disguise other less acceptable sounds (Hanser *et al.*, 1983)? Audioanalgesia includes both music and other forms of purposeful sound, such as 'white sound', but the latter has attracted little attention since its

1960s' heyday (Moore *et al.*, 1965). Music therapy is used to treat chronic conditions that feature emotional disturbance (Hanser & Thompson, 1994), but its use in childbirth is less well-publicised. The action by which music may help the woman to cope with her labour pain may lie in its distraction and its ability 'to make one lose track of time' (Livingston, 1985). Sammons (1984) recounts the 'uplifting effects' of music and its ability to promote positive relationships.

As well as these rather general environmental effects, more significantly, in this context, music may 'energize and bring order through rhythm' (Sammons, 1984); thus music of an appropriate tempo assists the woman in regulating her breathing (Di Franco, 1988). More specifically, Sammons suggests that music decreases the patient's discomfort and need for anaesthetic drugs in dentistry and surgery. She links the mechanism for achieving this to the gate-control theory, by which impulses triggered by musical stimuli override the pain impulses carried by smaller-diameter nerve fibres.

While the cassette player/transistor radio features universally in the labour room, this may not be the most appropriate equipment by which to deliver music therapy. This is not only because of the variation in individuals' musical tastes, but also because of the woman's limited control over, for example, the volume. A personal stereo would 'allow for exclusion of all other sounds', thus facilitating the woman's therapeutic concentration on her chosen music (Livingston, 1985; Zimmerman *et al.*, 1989).

The benefits of music therapy were established by Hanser and Thompson (1994) in the context of the care of depressed elderly people. This controlled study involved 30 community-based veterans who volunteered. The two treatment groups showed significant improvement in their depression, anxiety, self-esteem and mood, which continued over a nine month follow-up.

The effects of relaxing music on cancer patients' need for narcotic analgesics were studied in an RCT (Zimmerman *et al.*, 1989). Forty patients were allocated to music or no-music groups, with the former listening to relaxing music with positive suggestions of pain reduction. Of the McGill Pain Questionnaire's seven scores, six were significantly lower in the music group, suggesting that music decreases the intensity of chronic pain. The effect of music on acute obstetric/gynaecological pain was researched using matched samples of postoperative patients (Locsin, 1981). The experimental group listened to music for 30 minutes before each second hour for 48 hours postoperatively. The experiment group's physiological and pain assessment data on overt pain reactions showed significant benefits, but autonomic alterations were less marked. The music group used less analgesic medication. The author concluded that music is beneficial postoperatively, leading to the question of whether it has a place during labour.

The acceptability of music therapy during childbirth was studied by an RCT involving a volunteer sample of 54 women attending childbirth education who either received or did not receive music 'rehearsals' antenatally (Sammons, 1984). Data, collected by a postnatal postal questionnaire, showed no significant differences between the groups, although the small proportion who used music in labour stated that they would do so again. Apparently the childbirth educator avoided 'selling' music therapy too strongly during the classes, reducing the distinction between the two groups. This reflects a weakness in the research design, as the author comments: 'Effectively informing pregnant women of the option of music use must involve delivery of a more emphatic statement than was made in the class series described here' (1984: 270). This is another example of what has been observed throughout this section, in that poorly designed research impedes conclusions being drawn about complementary interventions. Yet another example is Durham and Collins' study (1986) which identified a reduction in the use of analgesic medication in their randomly allocated sample. Unfortunately, though, the antenatal/labour music group and the no-music group comprised only 15 women.

The literature suggests that this harm-free intervention has the potential for enjoyment by all present. The general acceptance of music into the labour room, though, has been poorly thought-through and may constitute an example of a potentially helpful intervention being introduced while ignoring the research data. The result is that women and midwives find themselves listening to local commercial radio stations whose output satisfies no-one. Accurate information should be available to women based on authoritative research; only this could change the role of music in labour from environmentally polluting to therapeutic.

Hydrotherapy

Water to comfort or heal is longstanding and commonplace; in spite of this huge variations persist in recommendations about the water's application, in terms of flow, direction, force and temperature. Using water during childbearing, however, is a more recent development (Brown, 1982), and has been widely publicised (Odent, 1983). Giving birth in water (waterbirth) has attracted much publicity and some notoriety, but here I focus on water being used to help the woman to cope with the pain of labour, conveniently referred to as 'hydrotherapy' (Simkin, 1989: 898).

The increasing popularity of hydrotherapy is reflected in the difference between the 1990 data reported by Steer (1993) and those reported by Alderdice *et al.* (1995) relating to 1992/3. In Steer's sample of 6093 women, none used water for pain control, whereas Alderdice *et al.* found that only 5 out of 219 (2.3%) provider units had not used water for labour.

According to Garland and Jones (1994) the benefits of hydrotherapy are attributable to two phenomena. First, 'hydrothermia', resulting from water being a conductor of heat, releases muscle spasm and, hence, relieves pain. Second, 'hydrokinesis' abolishes the effects of gravity, together with the discomforts associated with pressure on the pelvis and other structures. Hydrothermia and hydrokinesis combine to assist relaxation and, hence, reduce anxiety and fatigue.

As mentioned above, the recent interest in hydrotherapy in childbearing has resulted in an increasing number of midwives and maternity units offering labour in water (Alderdice *et al.*, 1995). This development is due to women using commercially hired pools, with maternity units making suitable pools available and midwives encouraging women to use traditional baths in labour.

The risk of perinatal death due to asphyxia following waterbirth has been widely publicised, but the risk of maternal death due to water embolism less so. The former has been associated with the practice of holding the baby beneath the water for a prolonged period (Kitzinger, 1992b). The likelihood of maternal water embolism is thought to be reduced if the woman leaves the pool for the third stage, although Balaskas and Gordon (1990) maintain that this is unnecessary.

A traditional rationale for discouraging the woman from bathing in labour is vaginal contamination leading to maternal and/or perinatal infection. With the increasing significance of blood-borne infections, the risk to carers and other pool users has also emerged. Using a retrospective design, Waldenström and Nilsson (1992) investigated the problem of infection following bathing. Their sample comprised 89 women who bathed after their membranes had ruptured spontaneously (SRM); the control group consisted of 89 women who did not bathe after SRM and whose SRM-delivery interval was similar. Like Eriksson *et al.*'s larger study (1996) and a smaller UK study (Hawkins, 1995), Waldenström and Nilsson found no statistical difference between the two groups' incidence of neonatal or maternal infection. They did, however, identify a trend among the bathing group towards experiencing other health problems, such as the significantly lower five minute apgar scores among the 'bathing' babies if the membranes had been ruptured for over 24 hours.

In terms of their medication use, the women who bathed required less augmentation with oxytocin, which was significant in the second stage. The pain experience of the 'bathing' women seems to have been similarly positively affected; their use of analgesic medication was consistently lower, with pethidine and Entonox use being significantly lower.

Because of the media hype associated with waterbirth and the medical response to the 'aquatic fanatics' (Loeffler, cited in Beech, 1995b: 1) much research has been undertaken. A literature review by

McCandlish and Renfrew (1993) summarises the findings of seven controlled studies, including two RCTs. The results show variations in terms of the risks and benefits. Waldenström and Nilsson's finding (1992) of less analgesic medication for bathing women was not invariably supported.

A more recent RCT (Cammu *et al.*, 1994) involved 120 low risk primigravid women who spent an hour in a bath in which the water was 50 cm deep. When the pain was assessed after 25 minutes, the bathing group's pain had increased less markedly than the bed group's; at 1 hour there was no difference. Thus, the authors identified that bathing has a pain stabilising rather than a pain relieving effect. The women commented favourably on bathing's soothing and relaxing effect. The contribution of this study to the debate needs to be questioned, however, in view of the local obstetricians' aggressively active approach to the management of labour. Despite each of the sample women having been identified as 'low risk', all underwent elective artificial rupture of the membranes and application of a fetal scalp electrode before the cervix reached 5 cm dilatation. Robinson (1994) questions the effect of such aggressive intervention on the woman's experience of pain.

Although not widely available in the UK, whirlpool baths (jacuzzis) were compared with opioid and epidural use by an RCT (Rush *et al.*, 1996). The bathing group of 785 women, despite primigravidae being over-represented, used significantly less pharmacological analgesia, experienced significantly fewer assisted births and were significantly more likely to sustain an intact perineum. In those women with ruptured membranes, there was no increase in maternal or neonatal infection.

Hydrotherapy raises many issues relating to the woman's and midwife's autonomy. As Beech observes: 'A woman in a pool is very much more in control of her labour, and it is a great deal more difficult for the staff to intervene. Therein lies the rub' (1995b: 1). This observation certainly applies once the woman is in the pool, but getting there may be challenging. Beech argues that our medical colleagues have attempted to limit the availability of this facility for women on the grounds that the baby may be at risk. Beech reminds us of the uncertain benefits associated with some medical interventions, such as ultrasound, which are similarly unresearched, but which are certainly not denied to women.

Homeopathy

Authoritative data (Steer, 1993) show that 0.4% of women use homeopathic methods to control their labour pain. Unfortunately, this report does not name these remedies as it does allopathic medications. Homeopathy developed from the observation by Samuel Hahnemann (1755–1843) that 'like cures like'. Thus, a substance that causes symptoms in a healthy person may cure those symptoms when part of a disease process (Castro, 1992). Homeopathic remedies work not by curing the disease, but by stimulating the body to heal itself (Kaplan, 1994). On the basis of a homeopathic consultation the practitioner obtains a complete picture of the 'patient's' general constitution, and then, using this picture, selects the appropriate substance to treat the patient holistically (Jones, 1994).

Castro (1992) discusses the contribution of homepathic remedies to the emotional challenges of childbirth, such as aconite to relieve anxiety, fear and panic. To facilitate coping with the pain of labour she recommends a labour kit (1992) which is used unsupervised. It includes remedies such as kali carbonicum to relieve back pain in labour.

It may be assumed that, because infinitesimally small dilutions of substances like sea salt are prescribed, homeopathy is invariably safe. Castro (1992) warns against this assumption by illustrating how continuing treatment beyond the point of cure may cause a relapse. Kaplan (1994) admits that while homeopathy may be beneficial in some conditions, such as viral infections, there are other situations where it has no place, such as appendicitis. The reported research into homeopathy has little relevance to childbearing, but it establishes its efficacy in rheumatoid arthritis and hay fever (Gibson *et al.*, 1980; Reilly *et al.*, 1986).

Although some women choose homeopathy to help them cope with the pain of labour (Steer, 1993), Nicholls (1988) is pessimistic about the likelihood of the longstanding conflict with allopathic medicine being resolved. This conflict dates back to Hahnemann's original self-imposed experiments as alternatives to potentially lethal medical interventions such as purging and blood-letting (Castro, 1992). [These are appropriate examples of allopathic medicine, which seeks to 'cure by removing or opposing the cause of the disease or to suppress or palliate symptoms' (Nicholls, 1988: 3).] The gloomy forebodings for homeopathy are attributed to the 'economic constraints of the medical industry, elite control of medical education and the fact that there is no direct financial incentive for doctors [in the UK] to question standard routines of practice' (1988). It is necessary to ask whether these are the very factors that may engender increasing lay acceptance and use of such complementary therapies.

Position, posture and ambulation
Although the benefits of changing the woman's posture have been recognised since the days of William Smellie (McLintock, 1876), they have related more to the progress of labour than to the woman's comfort. In addition to the effects of gravity, the benefits of a non-recumbent or upright posture in labour may be associated with changes in pelvic dimensions. Radiological evidence suggests that squatting, for example, increases the diameter of the pelvic outlet by up to 30% or 2 cm (Russell, 1969). While Pavlik (1988) maintains that a cross-legged sitting position relieves backache, she argues that such positions, as well

as ambulation, permit better alignment of the fetal and maternal spines and the fetal head with the woman's pelvis. Such strategies are particularly appropriate (Banks, 1992) if the woman has back pain due to an occipito-posterior position; then the woman's upright posture facilitates rotation of the fetal occiput anteriorly. Thus, it becomes apparent that alterations in posture which encourage the progress of labour may also help to alleviate pain.

There are few contraindications to changes in posture in labour. Vogler (1993a) states that ambulation is contraindicated if the presenting part is above the pelvis after the membranes have ruptured, increasing the risk of cord prolapse. Similarly, standing or walking may be difficult or dangerous if opioids or epidural analgesia have been administered.

As mentioned already, research focusing on the pain-controlling effects of posture is limited, in that none has been located. The effects of posture on the woman's pain has, however, been addressed in studies concentrating on the effect on her labour. A study by Mendez-Bauer and colleagues (1975) stimulated interest in posture in labour. They found that, in terms of uterine efficiency, standing produces the most favourable outcomes. In their sample of 20 women, however, each acted as her own control and, as well as changing her position half-hourly, was subjected to a vaginal examination at the same time. It is possible that these examinations affected, that is accelerated, the progress of labour.

Mendez-Bauer's less than satisfactory study persuaded McManus and Calder to replicate it (1978). This study refuted the benefits claimed by Mendez-Bauer *et al.* by demonstrating no difference between the upright and the recumbent group. The ambulant group's analgesia use was marginally, but not significantly, greater than their recumbent counterparts'. This study recruited women who were having labour induced; although all women had a cervical score of at least six, suggesting that they were physiologically ready for labour, the maternal response to induction varied hugely and may have influenced the findings. Additionally, minimal information is provided about the postures and positions in which the women actually laboured.

Some of these methodological problems were resolved by Flynn and her colleagues (1978). A sample of 68 women in spontaneous labour was recruited and randomly allocated to a recumbent or an ambulant group. As well as the ambulant women experiencing less medical intervention, they used significantly less analgesia. In the recumbent group, all of the women used pethidine with or without an epidural. Of the ambulant group, 20 women out of the 34 used no analgesic medication. Maternal satisfaction was also shown to have benefited, as did breastfeeding rates. Flynn *et al.* surmise that the benefits of ambulation derive from less intervention, less medication, and gravity, or from a combination of these factors.

More recently a study was undertaken in the USA by Andrews and Chrzanowski (1990). Using a convenience sample of 40 nulliparous labouring women, equal numbers were randomly allocated to a recumbent and an upright group. The researchers assessed maternal comfort and progress of labour during the acceleration phase (when the cervix dilates 4–9 cm). While this phase was markedly shorter in the upright group, there was no reported difference between the mean comfort scores of the two groups; despite this, the upright women used less analgesic medication.

Although these studies indicate no apparent disadvantages to labouring in non-recumbent positions, we are reminded that research-ing these interventions is even more problematic than researching other 'complementary' therapies (Roberts, 1989). The difficulties are asso-ciated with the researcher's inability to conceal the treatment or inter-vention group to which a subject has been allocated. Thus, it is impossible to 'blind' carers and researchers to who is in the experi-mental and who is in the control groups. Because staff and researchers may have their own feelings about particular positions, the potential for inadvertent or even deliberate bias is increased. Alternatively, the ability of an individual woman to maintain the position or posture to which she has been allocated may be difficult. This is particularly likely to happen if the woman becomes sleepy due to medication or tired due to her labour.

Posture and ambulation in labour are determined by the prevailing culture and non-recumbent postures have been associated with 'primi-tive peoples all over the world' (Dening, 1982: 440). The cultural implications and benefits of posture and ambulation became apparent to me when a labouring woman decided to practise her belly dancing. This involved complex pelvic movements, which might otherwise have been erotic, but for her assisted in realigning of the fetal head. The recumbent posture has been attributed to the advent of male midwives in Western Europe (Tew, 1995). An analogy links the woman's recumbency denoting her 'weakness, inferiority and submission', compared with the 'strong superior obstetrician ... who stands before her' (p. 143). The issue of power appears in Banks' historical account of posture in labour (1992). She observes that the upright woman is able to develop a 'better relationship' with her carers, presumably because she is, at least physically, on their level. Banks then argues that recumbency is secure and convenient for the carers, to the extent that other positions may threaten the carers' control. These observations are endorsed by our medical colleagues: 'nursing patients in bed simplifies important aspects of management, such as fetal monitoring and fluid therapy' (McManus & Calder, 1978: 74). Thus the consensus is that the woman's preference should determine her posture and position in labour (Roberts, 1989); this is reminiscent of William Smellie's recom-mendation that the woman should 'consult her own ease' (cited in Arney

1982: 68). The woman's contribution appears supreme. It is necessary to question, though, whether entrenched attitudes about 'the normal practice of conducting labour with the woman in bed' (McManus & Calder, 1978: 74) are likely to influence her preference. In this context, as in other situations, the woman's choice may be more 'illusory than real' (House of Commons, 1992: Para 51; Mander, 1993a).

The environment of labour

In considering the link between the woman's environment and her pain control I interpret 'environment' very broadly. Thus, I include the physical environment or place where she labours as well as the emotional environment, particularly the woman's relationships with those nearby. The woman in labour is supported by the formal care providers, such as the midwife, as well as the informal carers, such as her family. The research literature is unhelpful because research on midwives' support has addressed the woman's *complete* childbearing experience, rather than just her labour, in an effort to improve continuity (Flint, 1989; Davies, 1993). The research on labour support, however, has been undertaken in settings barely comparable with the UK (Sosa *et al.*, 1980; Kennell *et al.*, 1988).

Describing the nature and action of interventions to control labour pain is ordinarily straightforward. Describing support in labour, however, is more challenging in view of the various forms that it assumes. Examples are physical contact, such as hand holding, or conversing or adopting a certain attitude. The crucial prerequisite appears to be, however, simply the presence of another person (Keirse *et al.*, 1989). Perhaps the only strength of the aggressive active management practised in Dublin (O'Driscoll & Meagher, 1986) is that it details the woman's support, albeit often by unqualified personnel. The nature of physical contact is stated, as is the emotional rapport, through eye contact and the informational component. This regime has been criticised for the difficulty of evaluating the various parts, as well as the likelihood that support is the only effective feature (Thornton & Lilford, 1994). Unfortunately, the uncertain acceptability of an intense relationship with an unqualified, possibly male, stranger is ignored by this regime's advocates.

A research-based and comprehensive description of professional support provided the framework for Hodnett and Osborn's study (1989). They defined support according to four categories: the first was 'physical comfort measures' including cooling cloths, positioning and massage. The second was 'emotional support' including reassurance, encouragement and continuity of care. Information/instruction was third and included coaching breathing, information-giving about labour's progress and advice about pushing. The fourth, qualitatively different, category was 'advocacy'; this comprised 'interpreting woman's needs to other staff members, acting on woman's behalf and supporting woman's decisions' (1989: 181). Thus, varying levels of complexity of support become apparent.

The research on support in labour has focused largely on the partner's role and on the non-professional companion or 'doulah'. The effect of the partner's presence on the woman's labour pain was that she perceived him beneficial in that her pain was easier to cope with (Copstick *et al.*, 1985); the two groups' pain ratings did not, however, support the women's positive perceptions. The research on doulahs (Sosa *et al.*, 1980; Kennell *et al.*, 1988) demonstrates highly favourable results, but their applicability to the UK is doubtful. This limited relevance is associated with it having been undertaken in countries whose maternity services differ hugely from the UK. This criticism may apply to the Dublin regime (O'Driscoll & Meagher 1980) more than the Canadian study (Hodnett & Osborn, 1989). The Dublin protocol disregards the partner's presence and prevents the flexibility that informal carers' presence requires. Hodnett and Osborn (1989), however, adopted 'the community midwife' model for their 'monitrices', employing lay midwives in a DOMINO-like arrangement. Women in the experiment group were significantly more likely to require no pain control medication. Unfortunately, the rapidly changing maternity care situation in Toronto at the time prevents evaluation of the monitrice's contribution.

Two studies have attempted to correct the limited applicability of previous work. First, a prospective RCT was undertaken in a deprived suburb of Johannesburg, where women were ordinarily single and unaccompanied (Hofmeyr & Nikodem, 1996). Women (n=92) were allocated a companion who, though unqualified, was comforting, reassuring and praising. The control group comprised 97 similar women. The improvement in physical outcomes such as duration of labour in the supported group did not reach statistical significance. In contrast, the improved psychosocial outcomes were highly significant, such as state of anxiety, self-esteem, impressions of labour and parenting skills at 24 hours and 6 weeks.

Another study (Table 8.1) was undertaken in a Westernised setting by Kennell *et al.* (1991). The sample comprised 412 healthy first-time mothers who were allocated randomly to a supported or an observed group. A control group was recruited retrospectively. Major interventions such as epidural analgesia were significantly lower in the supported group compared with the observed group. Likewise, differences were clear between the experiment groups and the controls, which also applied to other interventions and pathological outcomes. These data confirm that the presence of another person improves the woman's experience, which is further enhanced if that presence is supportive. Despite such encouraging findings it is still necessary to consider the

Table 8.1   Intervention rates in the Kennell *et al.* (1991) study.

	Supported	Observed	Controls
	n=200	n=212	n=204
LUSCS	8%	13%	18%
Epidural	7.8%	22.6%	55.3%

LUSCS, lower uterine segment caesarean section.

applicability of this research to the UK, where 'one-to-one' midwifery care is better established than in other countries.

A local study which better illuminates the contribution of professional support was undertaken by Niven (1994). Reporting the retrospective phase of her study of 51 Scottish women coping with labour pain, she identified the important role of 'trusting the staff'. This trust emerged in the women who felt that the (midwifery) staff controlled the situation and were happy with this. It may be that Niven's 'trust' corresponds with a perception of being supported. Niven found that 'trust' was associated with significantly lower levels of pain on seven assessments. The differences in pain perception between the trusting or supported women and the others (those who did not consider the staff to be in control or those who thought the staff were in control but were unhappy about it) were also highly significant.

There were positive correlations between 'trusting the staff', effective analgesic medication, effective non-pharmacological pain control and attendance for childbirth education. Niven suggests that childbirth education encourages positive relationships between the midwife and the woman, perhaps due to earlier non-threatening encounters with midwives prior to the stress of labour inhibiting new impressions. A factor that Niven ignores is the likelihood of a common socio-economic background between the midwife and the woman who attends childbirth education, which in itself may engender trust (Perkins, 1980). Regardless of the reason for trust, the women who trusted the staff were more likely to employ a range of coping strategies. Niven argues that these effective strategies, such as relaxation, are more easily attempted and utilised successfully within a trusting, supportive environment.

The significance of the socio-economic background, which was neglected by Niven, is endorsed by the findings of a prospective study of the birth experience of 59 first-time mothers (Quine *et al.*, 1993). These researchers established correlations between socio-economic background, perceptions of being supported and reports of less pain during labour.

A systematic review of support identified 11 trials, some of which, as mentioned already, bear little relevance to developed Western states

(Sosa *et al.*, 1980; Kennell *et al.*, 1988; Klaus *et al.*, 1986; Hodnett, 1994). Hodnett's review does, however, suggest that doulah-type support in labour is associated with shorter labour, less need for pharmacological analgesia and reduced risk of assisted birth or low apgar scores at 5 minutes. Although this review allows Hodnett to recommend organisational changes, she neglects alternative routes to effective intrapartum support, such as enhancing midwifery care. It is necessary to further question why our North American colleagues are so keen to introduce untrained and unqualified personnel into the labour room. Perhaps, as well as being low-cost, their threat to the established order would be minimal, unlike the relatively well-educated midwife.

Thus, it is clear that support modifies the alien physical environment which the labouring woman all-too-frequently encounters (Kitzinger, 1992a). Keirse and colleagues (1989) contemplate the woman's physical environment in terms of its unfamiliarity and its isolation, not to mention potentially invasive interventions. The debate on the place of birth often mentions Dutch women giving birth at home and links this with their decreased use of analgesic medication (Mander, 1995b), but no causal relationship between these phenomena has yet been shown. A Danish study, which examined pethidine use in labour, does show the moderating effect of an alternative birthing centre (ABC; Skibsted & Lange, 1992). The researchers studied 295 women who chose to give birth in either an ABC or an obstetric ward. While 18% of the women in the ward used pethidine, only 4.8% of the women in the ABC did so. This difference is partly explained by the differences in the women themselves, as the women in the ABC were older and of higher socioeconomic status and parity. The influence of the environment is clear, however, in the 24 women refused ABC care due to lack of 'accommodation' who gave birth in the ward. These women shared the characteristics of the ABC women but the pethidine use of the ward women.

It may be that, although the physical environment is an aspect of labour that greatly influences her pain, it is the one over which women in the UK currently have least control.

Other interventions and strategies

This account of non-pharmacological pain control methods is in no way exhaustive, because some methods are used infrequently and/or have not yet been published. Included in such methods may be the 'idiosyncratic strategies' recounted to Niven (Niven & Gijsbers, 1996b). Of her 51 interviewees, 31 employed pain control strategies which could not be categorised using an orthodox framework; examples are reversal of affect and 'time limiting' to convince herself that 'it will all be over by tomorrow'.

A coping strategy that has been widely neglected is 'shouting'

(McCrea, 1996), which may alternatively manifest itself as crying or moaning. Midwives' attitudes to the woman's articulation of her pain are mentioned elsewhere (Chapter 12). McCrea found that midwives discourage 'making a noise' by persuading the woman that energy is being wasted (1996) or that other women would be upset. Although these arguments may be appropriate, a feeling persists that staff encounter difficulty with pain vocalisation. Perhaps because many women seem to find it helpful, McCrea concludes that the 'value of moaning or shouting should be investigated'.

Forms of pain control are constantly developing and attitudes change, making them more or less significant. This dynamic situation may cause difficulties for the practitioner trying to keep abreast of new approaches to pain as well as for the writer trying to describe them, but it can only be of benefit to the woman, who is able to choose the methods best attuned to her view of labour.

Conclusion

In this chapter it has become clear that many non-pharmacological methods of pain control are inadequately researched or incompletely understood. It is necessary to question whether this justifies abandoning interventions that often appear satisfactory to women. Additionally, the question emerges of whether a double standard is operating – with particularly rigorous criteria being applied to less orthodox methods, which are not applied to standard interventions. The answer to the latter question may become apparent in the next chapter on the pharmacological methods of pain control.

Chapter 9
Pharmacological Methods of Controlling Pain

As with many aspects of health care, the 'magic bullet' to 'solve' the problem of labour pain is elusive. A single-action remedy would be widely welcomed. Our knowledge of the disadvantageous side-effects of the current analgesic repertoire is constantly increasing, the iatrogenesis being both short-term and long-term. The existence of some iatrogenic effects is disputed; hence, the extent to which those administering these interventions accept and give the woman such information emerges in this chapter.

Before examining its various pharmacological forms, we should recall the meaning of 'analgesia'. Defined as 'a decreased or absent sensation of pain' (Anderson, 1994), analgesia is sought through various pharmacological and other techniques. We should distinguish this reduction or removal of pain from the intervention with which it is closely pharmacologically linked; anaesthesia is 'the absence of normal sensation' (Anderson, 1994) and is ordinarily achieved by medication. The distinction between analgesia and anaesthesia is significant in childbearing for two reasons.

The first reason relates to the pharmacological effects of the agents themselves. Certain drugs, such as nitrous oxide, at one dosage or concentration produce analgesia, whereas at a higher dosage or concentration anaesthesia results. Second, the intent underpinning administration may appear too obvious for words, but may become blurred in the minds of those involved. Whereas certain techniques may be administered initially to achieve analgesia, they may later in the labour be used for anaesthesia. An example is epidural analgesia, which may be established or 'sited' for a woman with difficulty coping, but it also increases her risk of an instrumental or operative birth (Greiff et al., 1994). So, although the woman requests, consents to and has administered epidural analgesia, the ultimate intention, unbeknown to her, is that it will be in position in the increasingly likely event of anaesthesia being required.

144

Inhalational analgesia

Analgesics have been inhaled for as long as human beings have been able to create and breathe fumes from naturally occurring substances, such as opium poppies. Simpson's introduction of anaesthesia/analgesia into childbearing in 1847 took the form of chloroform administered by inhalation. Various inhaled analgesics have been or are used in childbearing, including methoxyflurane (0.35%), trichlorethylene (0.25–1%) and different concentrations/combinations of nitrous oxide (Bonica, 1994: 634). In the UK premixed nitrous oxide and oxygen (50% N_2O and 50% O_2) delivered by the Entonox apparatus is currently permitted for use by a labouring woman supervised by a midwife. A major principle, which enhances inhalational analgesia's safety, is self-administration. The woman is prevented from overdosing on the gas by excessively high intakes causing sleepiness and the face mask or mouthpiece falling away, thus preventing further intake. The woman learns, ideally during pregnancy with reinforcement in labour, the principles of self-administration to maximise pain control.

Nitrous oxide achieves analgesia or anaesthesia by limiting neuronal and synaptic transmission in the central nervous system (CNS), by increasing the threshold for the firing of the action potential (Trevor & Miller, 1992). The popularity of Entonox derives from it being 'moderately effective without causing significant maternal or neonatal depression' (Bonica & McDonald, 1990: 1334). The potential for fetal hypoxia exists if the woman hyperventilates to control her pain while using Entonox. Gamsu (1993), however, questions the likelihood of this, because no behavioural changes have been observed in neonates whose mothers used Entonox. Further potential disadvantages have emerged in the lowering of maternal and fetal central vascular resistance (Polvi *et al.*, 1996). Although not yet a problem clinically, the risk of cerebral haemorrhage in preterm babies may be increased.

Due to its low lipid solubility, nitrous oxide quickly reaches analgesic levels in the maternal circulation (Dickersin, 1989), and analgesia ends equally quickly when inhalation ceases. Slight delay in it taking effect means that the woman should begin self-administration '10 to 15 seconds before the painful period of each contraction' (Bonica & McDonald, 1990: 1334). This regime provides 60% of women with good analgesia and a further 30% with partial analgesia. Unfortunately, these authors omit their evidence supporting these effectiveness rates.

Being self-administered, Entonox allows the woman to control its administration. Its effectiveness, however, is less controllable, dependent as it is on her having been given and being able to follow instructions about self-administration. Another advantage of nitrous oxide and oxygen, also relating to its administration, lies in its low cost, as no medical involvement is necessary and supervision by the midwife is minimal following initial instruction.

Entonox is the most widely available agent used for controlling labour pain in the UK, being provided in 99% of maternity units (Chamberlain *et al.*, 1993). These researchers have probably underestimated the use of nitrous oxide and oxygen, because the portable 500l cylinder is accessible to the woman giving birth at home. Steer (1993) maintains that this agent is used in 75% of labours. The frequency of its use falls when epidural analgesia is easily available, but the rate still remains above 50% of labours. Steer relates the pain control method to the 'mode of delivery'. He notes that over 80% of women who used non-pharmacological methods, pethidine or Entonox gave birth spontaneously. This applied to only 50% of women who received epidural analgesia. Steer argues, however, that it is the nature of the labour and birth that determine the pain control method, rather than vice versa. But his data fail to establish causation. The noisy blue cylinders with white quartered tops are disappearing as more labour areas ensure a continuous supply by piping Entonox from a central depot. Entonox is administered via a two-stage valve system; the first reduces the gas pressure and the second comprises an on-demand valve which opens in response to the negative pressure of the woman's inspiration.

Although it is relatively safe for the woman and baby, concerns have emerged relating to Entonox's potential for harming staff. Teratogenic and other pathological effects on reproductive performance have been reported among staff frequently using nitrous oxide, such as dentists and midwives (Newton, 1992; Ahlborg *et al.*, 1996). A study of 14 midwives showed that their exposure levels to nitrous oxide greatly exceeded those stipulated in countries where legislation controls upper limits. This finding is endorsed by a more authoritative study of 242 midwife shifts (Mills *et al.*, 1996). The extent of midwives' overexposure to nitrous oxide is shown in Table 9.1. Newton concludes that midwives should take 'personal responsibility' for their safety when Entonox is being administered. Mills, however, advocates that operating theatres' high standard of ventilation and scavenging should also be installed in birthing rooms.

Despite its widespread use and anecdotal reports, research-based evidence about the effectiveness of nitrous oxide and oxygen is lacking. A large study of childbirth pain led Wraight (1993) to conclude that 85% of women were satisfied with this agent. She notes, however, that their satisfaction did not derive from the pharmacological effects, which are impeded by the woman's difficulty in implementing the regime of administration. Wraight maintains that women's satisfaction derives from Entonox 'as a distraction and an activity which assisted in relaxation and breathing exercises' (1993: 80). Perhaps the pharmacological effect is further enhanced by the woman's feel-

Table 9.1 Midwives' overexposure to nitrous oxide in two labour wards (from Mills *et al.*, 1996).

Maximum approved level		Frequency	
Sweden	100 ppm		
USA	25 ppm		
UK (proposed)	100 ppm		
Exposure levels over	500 ppm	3%	7 midwife shifts
	100 ppm	23%	56 midwife shifts
Maximum recorded level	1638 ppm		
Background level in the labour ward	22 ppm to >100 ppm		

ing of control over this agent. The 15% of women in Wraight's sample who were not satisfied with nitrous oxide and oxygen is likely to have included those who disliked either the 'mask' or the psychotropic effects of this drug; these latter effects gave it its original name 'laughing gas' which, I occasionally find, may actually be appreciated by the woman.

Opioid analgesia

Although the terms are often used interchangeably (Melzack & Wall, 1991), opioids and narcotics are subtly different. Opioids are derived, naturally or synthetically, from the opium poppy, but narcotics are all substances that cause sleepiness or ultimately narcosis, that is insensibility. The opioids used in labour are also narcotics. 'Narcotics' have become associated with illegal drug use, especially in the USA. Partly for this reason and partly because of its imprecision, the term has fallen into disuse; it has been replaced with 'opioids' when referring to the legal therapeutic use of these drugs, to which the controlled drugs regulations apply (Way & Way, 1992).

Frequency of use

Their powerful pain-controlling action makes the strong opioids appropriate during labour; the weak opioids, such as codeine, have no place in childbirth (Twycross, 1994). In a UK-wide study of 6093 labouring women, 2247 (36.9%) women received pethidine, 128 (2.1%) received diamorphine and 107 (1.8%) received meptazinol (Steer, 1993). Thus, 41% of women were administered opioids during labour. This proportion, though a minority, is significant because opioids are second only to Entonox in frequency of use.

Actions

The actions of the opioids, especially pain control, result from their ability to bind with receptor sites in the CNS. Physiologically these receptors respond to endogenous opioids, sometimes known as 'endorphins' (Chapter 4, 'Electrical blocks'). The receptor sites include the mu, kappa, sigma and delta sites and their heterogeneity reflects the range of effects of these substances; the kappa receptors, however, are primarily responsible for analgesia (Way & Way, 1992).

The receptor sites where the opioids are active are located in two main areas in the CNS. First, in the substantia gelatinosa of the dorsal horn of the spinal cord, there are high concentrations of opioid receptors. Second, in the midbrain a system of periaqueductal grey matter, together with thalamic and hypothalamic nuclei, indirectly inhibit the transmission of pain impulses to the cerebral hemispheres. These two groups of receptor sites enhance each other's activity in limiting the transmission of pain impulses to the higher centres (Melzack & Wall, 1991).

The role of the higher centres is less clear than that of the areas in the cord, brain stem and thalamus. Perception of pain in the cerebral hemispheres is assumed to occur in the functional areas of the frontal cortex. This assumption arose from similarities observed between the action of opioids in reducing the individual's concern with pain and responses following some forms of psychosurgery (Way & Way, 1992).

While opioid activity is initiated at various receptor sites, the action at cell level is to reduce the release of neurotransmitters by affecting the presynaptic neurone. Neurotransmitter release, involving serotonin, acetylcholine and noradrenaline among others, has been shown to be inhibited. In the same way as the variety of receptor sites is partly responsible for the wide ranging effects of the opioids, the variety of neurotransmitters affected may be similarly responsible.

Effects

Because few health care interventions produce only one single effect, we usually consider their main and side-effects. The main effect, or reason for the intervention, is invariably regarded as beneficial. The side-effects or by-products, however, are variably advantageous and less significant, even disregarded. Here I first consider the main effect or reason for opioid administration and then look at the side-effects.

Main effect

The prime reason for opioid use in labour is analgesia, which derives from two sources: alteration of, first, the perception of pain and, second, the reaction to it. Opioids raise the pain threshold (Way & Way,

1992) and personal accounts show the effect on the woman's reaction to pain: 'I felt pethidine helped relaxation.... [It] made me mentally dopey and out of control and less concerned with the pain' (Steer, 1993: 51).

Side-effects
Whereas the main effects of interventions are supposedly beneficial, the side-effects may not be, inasmuch as they range from being appreciated to being life-threatening. Despite this, rather than classifying them as beneficial or harmful, the individual woman should decide whether a side-effect is acceptable to her. The actions of the opioids, including side-effects, are either depressant or excitatory. In humans the depressant effects tend to predominate, as evidenced by the frequency of sedation. The side-effects which feature excitation are caused by opioid-induced depression of inhibitory pathways (Cox, 1990).

Considering the use of opioids in controlling cancer pain, Twycross (1994) distinguishes clinical pharmacological problems from those relating to laboratory-based investigations. While we may safely assume that the experience of cancer pain is essentially different from pain in childbearing, the intensity of these forms of pain is comparable (Melzack & Wall, 1991). It may be, therefore, that the methods employed to control each of these forms of pain are also comparable. Thus, research into the side-effects may be transferable.

Respiratory depression
All opioids have been shown experimentally to induce respiratory depression through their inhibition of the brain stem respiratory centre (Way & Way, 1992). The main feature of this depression comprises inhibiting the response to rising CO_2 levels, knowledge of which is significant for two reasons: first, the woman in labour is protected from opioid-induced respiratory depression because 'pain acts as a physiological antagonist to the central depressant effects of morphine' (Regnard & Badger, 1987). Second, risks of neonatal respiratory depression are aggravated by the ease of opioid passage transplacentally (Way & Way, 1992). While the mature blood–brain barrier limits opioid transport into brain tissue, perinatally its effectiveness is reduced by immaturity, even in term babies. Thus, opioid-induced respiratory depression threatens a baby whose mother has recently been administered these drugs and this prospect determines their use, although Cawthra (1986) questions whether this applies to pethidine.

Euphoria/dysphoria
The psychotropic or mind-altering effects of opioids probably explain their popularity as drugs of abuse for over 6000 years (Cox, 1990). The happier aspects of these effects are described as 'a pleasant floating

sensation and freedom from anxiety and distress' (Way & Way, 1992: 425). Sedation may also result from the depressant effects of the opioids, and while it may be welcomed in labour, the reports of 'dizziness, dysphoria and drowsiness' accompanying it are not (Moore & Ball, 1974). Dysphoria is defined as a 'disquieted state ... and a feeling of malaise' (Way & Way, 1992: 425). Such unwelcome side-effects have serious consequences for the woman (Kitzinger, 1987a) as they 'cause confusion and can make a woman feel powerless to cope actively with labour', thus reducing her control over her situation. As examples, two psychotropic reactions are recounted by Wraight's respondents (1993: 81):

'I had pethidine for the birth of my first baby and felt relaxed and happy during the birth.'
'I was very disappointed with the pethidine as I could not think straight and could not do as I was told. This was because the pethidine made me very sleepy.'

Gastrointestinal side-effects
The excitatory effects of the opioids on the chemoreceptors in the brain stem result in the all too familiar nausea and vomiting. These symptoms may be further aggravated by movement or ambulation, due to opioids' effects on the vestibular apparatus (Way & Way, 1992: 427). Because of this side-effect, it is usual to administer an anti-emetic prophylactically with the opioid.

The opioids are responsible for aggravating the more sinister delay in gastric emptying (Park & Fulton, 1991), which underlies Mendelson's syndrome (maternal acid aspiration, Chapter 9, 'General anaesthesia'). This condition's continuing significance is evidenced by the current maternal mortality figures due to Mendelson's syndrome having only improved slightly since the 1950s (Vanner, 1993).

Cardiovascular side-effects
While not exerting any direct effect on the heart, the opioids engender a mild degree of hypotension in a cardiovascular system that is already stressed. While the reason for this hypotensive effect is uncertain (Way & Way, 1992), it may occasionally be utilised therapeutically.

Tolerance and addiction
Staff anxiety about the possibility of engendering opioid dependence has resulted in the underprescription and underadministration of therapeutic opioid analgesics and has caused immeasurable unnecessary suffering (Twycross, 1994: 947; Chapter 2, 'Traditional observation'). While caution is necessary in comparing childbirth pain with that for

which nurses treat patients, it may be that midwives who originated as nurses bring these anxieties with them.

Tolerance of a drug or intervention comprises a decreased response, in terms of the desired or main effect, requiring increasing doses (Hollister, 1992). Research involving 1000 patients with advanced cancer showed that only 5% developed any degree of tolerance to long-term opioids (Twycross, 1994); this suggests that in childbearing this phenomenon merits no consideration.

Addiction, or more correctly drug dependence, has been shown to constitute a rare side-effect of cancer patients' opioid therapy. A study of 12 000 hospital patients being treated with strong opioids showed that only one person became dependent on these drugs (Porter & Jick, 1980). Like tolerance, addiction does not deserve consideration when making decisions about pain control in childbearing.

The place of opioids in childbearing

Having examined some general issues relating to their use, we now consider what opioid drugs currently offer to the woman in labour. This is partly because Steer's research (1993) and observations appear to contradict Bonica's scant and scathing mention of opioids (1994). Presumably on the basis of 'my own observations in various countries' (p. 633), Bonica indicates that 'in many parts of the world where anaesthetists are not available, the midwife or obstetrician must rely on the use of . . . simple methods of drug induced analgesia' (1994: 633/4). This suggests that opioids are used only where other methods are unavailable and they have no other contribution in controlling a woman's labour pain. As with most medical and other interventions, the woman may need information to help her to scrutinise the balance between costs and benefits. Increasing knowledge is giving rise to concern about the effects of opioids on more general outcomes, as well as longer-term neonatal, infant and even adolescent behaviour (Mander, 1992b).

Effectiveness

Authoritative research into the analgesic effectiveness of opioids began by focusing on pethidine. A prospective randomised double-blind trial involving 1100 labouring women showed pain scores falling for 90–120 minutes following intramuscular pethidine (Morrison *et al.*, 1987). These researchers were appropriately critical of its poor effect.

These concerns about the effectiveness of opioids resulted in a Swedish study of morphine and pethidine (Olofsson *et al.*, 1996). Unfortunately this small study provides a rallying point for those advocating other pain control methods (Reynolds, 1997b). Olofsson recruited and randomly allocated 20 nulliparous women in labour. Each was then given three doses of either pethidine or morphine intravenously (IV). Each woman received, by UK standards, niggardly weight-related doses of opioid over the duration of three contractions. Pain intensity and sedation were assessed using visual analogue scales. Data presentation is crude with little detail except to claim 'no significant change' (p. 969) and the researchers conclude that opioids have no analgesic effect, just sedation. Thus, even the analgesic effectiveness of opioids is uncertain (Mander, 1997a).

Breastfeeding

The benefits of breastfeeding and particularly early breastfeeding are becoming increasingly apparent, but the possibility of problems when opioids have been administered has emerged (Freeborn *et al.*, 1980). Researchers measured opioid (pethidine) levels in the neonatal circulation and saliva and, unsurprisingly, found that the opioid had been transferred transplacentally. Babies given infant formula excreted the opioid rapidly, resulting in an elimination half-life of approximately 30 hours. In a stark and disconcerting contrast, breast-fed babies demonstrated a significant increase in salivary opioid in the first day, followed by a gradual reduction in the second 24 hours. The conclusion was drawn that the opioid was transferred during breastfeeding, and the woman who receives an opioid in labour and breastfeeds puts her baby in double jeopardy.

Canadian research utilised a specially designed Infant Breast Feeding Assessment Tool (IBFAT) to identify the woman's perceptions of her baby's breastfeeding at each feed (Matthews, 1989). The sample comprised multiparous women, 18 of whom had received no opioid in labour and 20 who had. The data collection ascertained when effective breastfeeding became established. Babies in the medicated group were found to initiate effective breastfeeding hours, or even days, later than those in the unmedicated group.

A further attempt was made to compare the effects of opioids on breastfeeding using IBFAT in a small sample incorporating new and experienced mothers (Crowell *et al.*, 1994). These researchers also showed the unhelpful effects of opioids on the initiation of breastfeeding. Their conclusions, however, are confounded by differences in reactions to labour pain and medication use as well as previous infant feeding experience. Crowell *et al.* did find, though, that the breastfeeding of babies whose mothers received an opioid within an hour prior to the birth was less affected by the drug than those who had it administered 1–3 hours before birth; these findings were supported by a more recent study by Nissen *et al.* (1997). It may be that the babies with the shortest dose-delivery time interval were given a narcotic antagonist to counteract respiratory depression; this may also have lessened more general opioid-induced depression, thus facilitating the initiation of breastfeeding. On the basis of their findings, Crowell *et al.* suggest that better support in labour and postnatally prevents the need for opioids and the ensuing neonatal problems, respectively, and encourages perseverance with breastfeeding. Crowell *et al.*'s mention of perseverance with breastfeeding reminds us of the limited research attention given to the effects of opioids administered in labour on the woman's continuation, or all too frequently discontinuation, of breastfeeding.

Effects in adolescence
The long-term effects of opioids may also give rise to concern (Robinson, 1995). Swedish research suggests that diamorphine given during labour is associated with a greater risk of drug addiction when the 'baby' reaches adulthood. Thus, not only are the woman's control and neonatal well-being jeopardised when opioids are administered, but also the autonomy of the one to whom she gives birth.

Dystocia
The effects of opioids on the progress of labour have been assumed to be beneficial (De Voe *et al.*, 1969), but a pilot RCT on directed versus spontaneous second stage pushing produced unexpected findings. It identified a positive correlation between the length of the first and second stage of labour and the amount of pethidine that had been administered (Thomson & Hillier, 1994). In the sample of 32 women, 14 had not received pethidine and 18 had, in doses totalling up to 250 mg. There were no differences in ethnic origin, gestation, haemoglobin, other drug use or baby details. Significant differences were identified between the two groups' duration of the first and second stage. For the unmedicated women the mean length of the first stage was 7.7 hours, whereas for the medicated women it was 11.7 hours. The difference in the length of the second stage was similarly significant. That pethidine interferes with efficient uterine contractions is further supported by the observation of increased third stage haemorrhage. The authors admit, though, that this may be associated with the increased incidence of instrumental assistance for the birth in the medicated group. The researchers' literature review found no evidence to contradict their findings. They are critical of the low-quality data on the effects of this frequently used drug, stating that the side-effects have 'not been adequately assessed'. Contemplating further research, the authors discuss the ethics of an RCT which would deprive some women of their chosen method of pain control. It is necessary to further question, though, the ethical basis of widespread administration of a drug whose effects are inadequately researched and whether the woman should be expected to make decisions about pain control on the basis of incomplete information (Mander, 1993a).

Opioid drugs

Steer (1993) identified three opioids which are most commonly used in labour in the UK (see 'Frequency of use'). I now examine their main features.

Diamorphine

Due to its chemical structure, diamorphine has greater lipid solubility than morphine, allowing faster penetration into cerebral tissue. This rapid diffusion permits an equally rapid conversion into morphine, the active agent (Park & Fulton, 1991). Diamorphine is less likely to cause gastrointestinal upsets than morphine and the psychological benefits are more intense. Intramuscular (IM) administration of diamorphine results in the drug taking effect within 5–10 minutes and lasting for 3 hours. The recommended dosage varies between 2.5 and 7.5 mg (Moir, 1973; Park & Fulton, 1991), although this seems inadequate for a woman in labour.

Pethidine

A synthetic analgesic, pethidine is metabolised in the liver; this is significant because the neonatal liver is immature, thus prolonging pethidine's neonatal effects (see 'Breastfeeding'). With IM administration the analgesic effect begins within 15 minutes and is supposed to continue for 2 hours. The recommended IM dosage is from 50 to 150 mg (Royal Infirmary of Edinburgh, 1995).

Meptazinol

Meptazinol may be preferred to pethidine because neonatal respiratory depression is less marked (Park & Fulton, 1991). The analgesic action begins within 15 minutes and continues for at least 4 hours (Knights, 1986). The recommended IM dosage is from 75 to 100 mg (Park & Fulton, 1991).

Summary

In attempting to describe the opioids' place in the control of labour pain, the woman and her attendants must take account of the disadvantages of these agents as well as their benefits. In this section I have shown that the costs may be long-term as well as immediate and that although any benefits accrue mainly to the woman, the baby carries the burden of costs through respiratory depression and breastfeeding difficulties. The woman's control over these drugs is clearly non-existent once she has consented and they have been administered. However, even before she consents, her input may be limited by the lack of information that is available to her, which in turn is limited by the lack of research about issues that concern her, such as the effect of these drugs on her labour.

Before the question of opioids' relevance may be answered definitively, though, it is necessary to examine the alternative. When considering the pharmacological approaches to controlling labour pain, the only effective alternative to opioids is epidural analgesia, which is examined next.

Regional analgesia/anaesthesia

Methods of regional analgesia/anaesthesia which have been used during childbearing are legion, varying hugely in extent but involving the administration of a local anaesthetic, opioid or combination. Opioids' mode of action is described above. Local anaesthetics act by affecting the plasma membranes of excitable cells, that is neurones. The resting potential of the cell membrane is unaffected by these drugs, but they prevent transmission of the action potential. This inhibition is due to the interruption of the first part of the action potential, the rapid inflow of sodium ions, by the displacement of membrane-bound calcium and the constriction of the sodium channels. Receptors for local anaesthetics, which are sited on either the neuronal membrane or within the sodium channel, initiate this response (Steinberg *et al.*, 1996). Additionally, there is a decrease in the rate and degree of the depolarisation phase of the action potential, resulting in failure to reach the threshold potential. Thus, a blockade of conduction is achieved (Gillies *et al.*, 1986; Covino, 1993: 216).

Regional analgesia/anaesthesia varies in extent from perineal infiltration for episiotomy to the spinal block which is likely to engender 'not only numbness but also paralysis of the lower limbs' (Bonica, 1990a: 1336). Epidural analgesia, however, is the regional approach which is widely used to control labour pain, as opposed to techniques used to facilitate specific interventions (Steer, 1993). Despite this, I refer briefly to spinal anaesthesia for completeness' sake.

Spinal anaesthesia

Spinal anaesthesia is sometimes indicated because it carries certain advantages compared with other anaesthetic or analgesic approaches, such as epidural to which it is similar (Shergold, 1986). The advantages include easier introduction, lower dosage, speedier onset and shorter action. These advantages, though, must be balanced against the higher risk of hypotension. Additionally, because the subarachnoid space is accessed, the likelihood of cerebrospinal fluid leakage is increased (Bonica, 1990a). These considerations result in spinal anaesthesia being utilised for a large majority of caesarean sections (Scottish Office Home and Health Department, 1996).

Epidural analgesia (and combined)

A surgical technique not unlike lumbar puncture facilitates the injection of slow-acting local anaesthetics, such as bupivicaine, or other analgesic into the lumbar epidural space. The cannula, for delivering the drug, is sited and the initial injection administered by an obstetric anaesthetist. The administration may be on an intermittent or 'top up' basis, by a suitably trained midwife given written instructions by an anaesthetist. A 'patient controlled analgesia' (PCA) delivery system or continuous infusion may be used instead. A shorter-acting local anaesthetic, such as lignocaine, is injected as a test dose or opioids may be administered epidurally.

Effects

Epidural analgesia blocks the transmission of pain impulses via the afferent spinal nerves that traverse the epidural space and transmit pain impulses from organs such as the uterus to the CNS. The efficient binding of bupivicaine with maternal plasma proteins prevents any more than 20% being transferred transplacentally.

Incidence

Because of the serious maternal risks associated with this form of pain control (Scott & Tunstall, 1995), the maternity units offering it are limited. The proportion of maternity units with the resources, that is suitably trained personnel, to provide a full 24-hour on-demand epidural service correlates inversely with the proportion of small maternity units in a region (Morgan, 1993a). The proportion varies from 100% in the Oxford region to 28% in Wales.

In the UK epidural block is used to control pain in 19.3% of labours (Steer, 1993). This seemingly low figure conceals wide variations. Epidural rates as low as 14% are reported in Northern Ireland (Morgan, 1993a) and 6% in one maternity unit with full anaesthetic cover (Scottish Office Home and Health Department, 1996). On the other hand, epidural rates of 87% have been reported (Mander, 1995a), but published rates do not yet exceed 67% (Morgan, 1993b). The extent to which these variations reflect women's control is discussed below.

Issues

Obstetric anaesthesia and analgesia

When first introduced for use in labour, epidural analgesia provided effective pain control in well-defined potentially pathological situations, such as a woman experiencing incoordinate uterine action (Moir, 1973). The realisation that epidural anaesthesia could also remedy the abysmal contribution of obstetric anaesthesia to maternal mortality provided the obstetric anaesthetists' excuse for entering the birthing room (Doughty, 1987; Morgan, 1987). In this way our anaesthetic colleagues established a power base, from which they could expand their role and professional status (Mander, 1993b). This expansion involved epidural analgesia in uncomplicated labour being 'fostered directly or indirectly by the professionals' (Hibbard & Scott, 1990). Such 'fostering', 'encouragement' or 'hard selling' has been reported anecdotally (Wilshin & Wilson, 1991; Machover, 1995), but evidence is limited. The result is the wide-ranging rates detailed in 'Incidence'. Despite concerted efforts to persuade that this form of pain control is women's method of choice (Morgan 1984; MacDonald *et al.*, 1988; Reynolds, 1989), the autonomy and information on which this choice is based remain uncertain (Mander, 1994a, 1996).

Effectiveness
An effective epidural unquestionably eradicates the pain of uterine contractions (Howell & Chalmers, 1992) or, as Morgan *et al.* (1982) on the basis of their 1000 women study claimed, 'an epidural is strikingly more effective . . . than any other analgesic method'. The proportion of epidural blocks that are effective, though, is difficult to estimate as data are not readily available. The success rate of epidural analgesia varies between 67% and 90% (Simkin, 1989); this is supported by one of the few, albeit shaky, studies to even mention the risk of epidural failure (Kitzinger, 1987b).

Other problems
Unfortunately, as well as pain impulses, non-pain efferent impulses may also be blocked (Pursey, 1994), causing immobility and the woman to be bedfast for at least the duration of the epidural block. Additionally, sympathetic nerve fibres are blocked, resulting in vasodilatation in the lower body, which causes sudden and potentially life-threatening hypotension. To prevent this, a rapid IV infusion is established prior to siting the epidural and a supine posture discouraged. In 2% of women receiving epidural analgesia the hypotensive episode is sufficiently severe to require stimulation using ephedrine (Ramin *et al.*, 1995).

Together with pain, bladder sensation is removed. This results, in combination with the generous IV fluid intake, in the bladder becoming distended (Williams *et al.*, 1985). Without urinary catheterisation, labour becomes further prolonged.

Dystocia
The tendency of epidural analgesia to prolong labour, particularly the second stage, is long-recognised (Williams *et al.*, 1985). Such delay may be associated with malrotation of the presenting part (Howell & Chalmers, 1992). Chestnut *et al.* (1987) showed that an epidural 'topped

up' after 8 cm cervical dilatation was associated with prolonged second stage and instrumental assistance for the birth. Williams' study involving 85 women of whom 38 chose epidural analgesia demonstrated the increased incidence of a series of obstetric procedures, recognised as the 'cascade of intervention' (Jouppila *et al.*, 1980). This has been identified in obstetric practice and may have been facilitated or aggravated by the introduction of effective pain control (Varney Burst, 1983). The 'cascade' may be associated with neurological changes mentioned above in 'Other problems' which cause pelvic floor relaxation, malposition of the fetal head, incomplete rotation and delay in the second stage. Oxytocic drugs which correct delay are associated with fetal hypoxia (Yudkin, 1979; Keirse & Chalmers, 1989; Evans, 1992). Thus, interventions to expedite the birth, for example application of forceps or caesarean section, become necessary. Of primigravid women who use epidural analgesia in labour, only 46% will avoid such intervention for the birth (Scott & Tunstall, 1995). Research has proposed that the late siting of the epidural (>5 cm cervical dilatation) may reduce interventive births (Chestnut *et al.*, 1994). In view of the limited research on women's views on the costs and benefits of epidurals (Howell & Chalmers, 1992; Mander, 1994a), such a strategy should take account of women's attitudes.

Problems associated with epidurals, such as difficulty bearing down, motor block, malrotation and deflexion, have long been recognised (Scottish Home and Health Department, 1985). For a similar time there has been confidence that 'variations in anaesthetic technique' will resolve them (Scottish Home and Health Department, 1985: 4). An example is the combination spinal/epidurals, introduced to overcome some of the hazards associated with traditional epidural techniques (Morgan & Kadim, 1994). A small study suggests that problems persist to the extent that 47% of women experienced an operative birth (Morey *et al.*, 1994).

After-effects
The problems that the woman encounters after using epidural analgesia have been widely investigated. The occurrence of headache varies in intensity, duration and, hence, treatment (MacArthur *et al.*, 1991). 'Spinal axis syndrome', involving subclinical neurological and orthopaedic damage, has been suggested to explain the symptoms that women experience postepidurally (MacArthur *et al.*, 1991). Of the epidural users in their retrospective sample, 18.9% developed back pain, compared with 10.5% in those women using other analgesia. In a study with a better response rate (MacLeod *et al.*, 1995), those with back pain increased to 26.2%. On the basis of a volunteer sample, these claims have been dismissed as 'amnesia', as some women developed their back pain prior to labour (Russell *et al.*, 1996).

Perinatal and woman-oriented issues
The lack of authoritative data on neonatal and long-term maternal effects has been highlighted (Howell & Chalmers, 1992). The rise in maternal temperature associated with the administration of epidural analgesia (Fusi *et al.*, 1989) inevitably causes fetal changes. If the woman's epidural has been ongoing for over 8 hours fetal tachycardia may result and be misdiagnosed as fetal distress, leading to supposedly appropriate intervention in the labour and subsequently.

The paucity of research into woman-oriented aspects of this form of pain control has been noted repeatedly (Howell & Chalmers, 1992; Mander, 1994a), as has the need for suitably strong and suitably timed research (Chalmers, 1993; Oakley, 1993). The care of the woman in labour involves supporting her in a series of decisions, which are impossible without comprehensive research-based information. Those caring for the woman are responsible for ensuring that such information is made available to her (Mander, 1993a).

Methods of administration

Because certain innovations in drug administration relate particularly to epidural analgesia, I discuss them here. As mentioned in Chapter 8, the woman's control over her use of non-pharmacological methods of pain control tends to be great but variable. Traditionally, there has been less maternal control over the administration of pharmacological methods, because they are prescribed and administered by professional carers. The use of inhalational analgesics may be an exception to this observation.

Feelings of powerlessness inherent in any pain experience are aggravated by dependence on others for analgesia and by uncertainty about its availability and effect (Fordham & Dunn, 1994). The delayed onset of some drugs together with the large doses needed to prolong their effects has been long-recognised as 'roller coaster analgesia' (Sechzer, 1971; Reynolds, 1990), which comprises huge swings in analgesia between the peaks of sedation and the troughs of pain, as illustrated in Fig. 9.1. (Kepes & Claudio-Santiago, 1996).

To overcome these problems in acute pain situations, 'patient controlled analgesia' or 'parturant controlled analgesia' (PCA) systems have been introduced to administer drugs either IV or epidurally (Ferrante *et al.*, 1990; Niven & Gijsbers, 1996a: 143). The pumps employed to administer the drug may permit a background infusion and/or a patient-triggered bolus infusion (Welchew, 1995). The rate of the infusion, the size of the bolus and the lockout period (during which no bolus is obtainable) are programmed by the physician when the PCA is established.

Research undertaken in non-maternity postoperative situations initi-

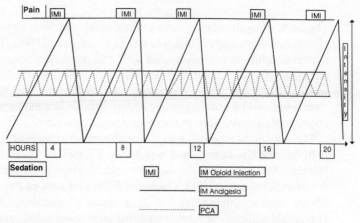

Fig. 9.1 Roller coaster analgesia and patient controlled analgesia.

ally indicated widespread user-satisfaction with opioid PCA systems (Shade, 1992). There is considerable variation in drug intake between users (Bennett *et al.*, 1992), suggesting that PCA does individualise doses; however, this variation tends towards higher drug intake (Rogers *et al.*, 1990). Recent research, however, suggests that other outcomes, such as ambulation, may not be improved or may even be impaired by PCA use (Snell *et al.*, 1997). Snell's study raises the issue of post-operative nausea and vomiting among PCA users which, in my experience, is more prevalent and causes more pain and concern than among women receiving intermittent opioids.

Patient controlled epidural analgesia (PCEA), perhaps supported by a continuous background infusion, has been introduced experimentally in childbearing (Paech, 1996). Postcaesarean local anaesthetic PCEA is not feasible, but opioids may be administered postoperatively epidurally. There is still uncertainty about the acceptability and effectiveness of bupivicaine PCEA in labour. The implications of this method of drug administration for midwifery staffing and practice are clearly immense. Continuous epidural infusion is another technique introduced to avoid 'roller coaster analgesia' characteristic of intermittent administration (Gaylard, 1990). Continuous epidural infusion of either local anaesthetics or opioids may permit fine tuning to meet the needs of the labouring woman. Despite this, it has been reported that occasional top-ups are still necessary (Ewen *et al.*, 1986), suggesting that individualisation of the dose is not yet perfected.

General anaesthesia

General anaesthesia (GA) is not a conventional form of pain control, but it is included here because it is used in maternity care to permit interventions that would otherwise be too painful to contemplate and also because it raises important issues. Used to facilitate the birth of the baby or just the placenta in emergencies, GA is appropriate when there is insufficient time and/or expertise for establishing regional anaesthesia.

GA is used infrequently in maternity; in one series only 238 women out of 6459 (3.9%) were administered GA during labour (Steer, 1993). This small number is probably due to the increasing availability of regional anaesthesia and the serious risks of GA. Thus, disconcertingly, GA is used relatively frequently in small and very small maternity units (<2000 births per annum) (Scottish Office Home and Health Department, 1996).

General, or whole body, anaesthesia involves the patient's loss of consciousness as the brain is exposed to controlled concentrations of reversible medications, which would otherwise be poisonous (Gillies *et al.*, 1986; Brunner & Suddarth, 1992). The crucial characteristics of GA include amnesia and freedom from pain (Boswell & Hameroff, 1996). These writers admit ignorance of the action of the agents used; such ignorance applies to the mechanism as well as the site of action (p. 457).

Morgan (1987) relates the dreadful history of the contribution of obstetric GA to maternal mortality. The *number* of maternal deaths due to or associated with GA peaked during 1964–1969 (in which time 100 women died thus); however, of greater significance is the *proportion* of maternal deaths that were due to or associated with GA. Despite the rising birth rate then, the number of maternal deaths due to other causes was falling markedly, due to higher living standards, smaller families, better antenatal care and the availability of blood transfusion and anti-biotics. The proportion of direct maternal deaths due to GA, however, rose from a stable level of 2.5–3.5% during 1952–1963 to 13.0% during 1982–1984 (Cloake, 1991).

A majority of maternal deaths due to or associated with GA were caused by the aspiration of acid stomach contents into the woman's lungs during the induction of GA in labour (Mendelson's syndrome; Morgan, 1987). Disconcertingly, Vanner (1993) suggests that the current maternal mortality figures due to Mendelson's syndrome are only slightly improved on the 1950s' figures, in spite of the widespread use of cricoid pressure during the induction of GA.

Unsurprisingly, the possibility of maternal death does not feature in the information given to the woman about to undergo a GA, but the risk of the woman being 'aware' during GA has attracted attention among consumer groups (Beech, 1995a). This 'awareness' results from the likelihood of a light GA being administered to minimise transplacental transfer of anaesthetic drugs, which would cause neonatal respiratory depression. This precaution clearly benefits the neonate, but may mean that the woman is inadequately anaesthetised, causing her to remain conscious but unable to communicate during the operation. The extent of this problem becomes apparent in Beech's quotation of Crawford's estimate of 1% of women being 'aware' during GA; she converts this into 400 women every year (1995a). In the absence of research on this topic, we have to rely on personal anecdotal evidence to indicate the trauma of such an experience. These accounts lead us to question whether the woman should be informed of the possibility of awareness, as she is informed of other adverse outcomes. In their discussion of women's experiences of caesarean delivery, Oakley and Richards (1990) list the all-round benefits of the father's presence during the operation. They explain how the father, having been in the operating room, is able to give the woman who underwent GA an account of the birth. These researchers imply that this 'account' is helpful to the woman who was unconscious for the birth. Is the father ordinarily permitted to be present in this situation? My observation is that the father is excluded on the grounds that the couple are unable to 'share' the birth. I suggest that his presence, far from being unnecessary, matters more if the woman has a GA.

Summary

It is clear that, while our knowledge of the effects of pharmacological pain control methods is more extensive than of their non-pharmacological counterparts, great gaps in our understanding of both interventions persist. These gaps apply particularly to the 'softer', more woman-oriented effects. For this reason, I remain unconvinced that the midwife is justified in encouraging a woman to accept pharmacological analgesia in such familiar terms as 'You don't get a medal for being a martyr' (Langford, 1997).

PART IV
The Journey's End

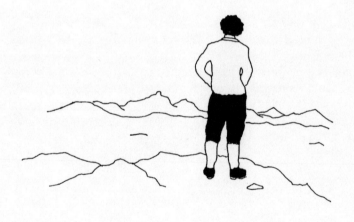

Chapter 10
Postnatal Pain

Postnatal care is held in low regard. On one side of this equation are midwives, who consider that care postnatally is the 'Cinderella' of maternity (i.e. it is undervalued and underresourced), despite the fact that it consumes over half of available midwifery resources (Beard, 1978; Ball, 1991). Is this because it lacks the pregnancy's exciting uncertainty or the high-tech glamour of intrapartum care? Or is it because postnatal care relies so heavily on interpersonal skills, probably the most fundamental of the midwife's repertoire.

The limited significance attached by women to the postnatal period becomes apparent when the woman talks of 'it' being over, meaning the labour, as if the birth ends her childbearing experience. Thus, with such low regard on both sides, it is hardly surprising that the postnatal period may be anticlimactic and, for the woman, aggravated by painful echoes of the birth, labour and even pregnancy.

After observing this low regard in medical textbooks, Dewan and colleagues (1993) surveyed the type and severity of postnatal pain and assessed the effectiveness of therapeutic interventions. They recruited 198 women and interviewed them on the first, second and fourth days postnatally, if the woman remained in hospital. The prevalence of postnatal pain appeared on the first day, when 95% of women complained of at least one type of pain. Its severity is indicated by the proportion (72%) who took analgesic medication.

This study illuminates a much-neglected area and began with a large sample (n=198). The generalisability of the findings are questionable, though, in view of the inevitable loss from the study as women went home. Thus, by day four less than 50% of the women were still responding (n=94). It may be that these women had problems that prevented their transfer home and, hence, were unrepresentative.

Pelvic pain

When contemplating postnatal pelvic pain, the immediate reaction is 'Hardly surprising . . .'. However, birth trauma is not the only cause. In this section I consider first a pain unrelated to trauma, and then move on to three types of pain which are largely traumatic, but which may cause the woman difficulty in differentiating the source. Although urinary tract infection may cause pain postnatally, it is discussed elsewhere (Chapter 6).

Afterpains

As we found in relation to Braxton Hicks' contractions (Chapter 6), women feel uterine contractions painful at particular times in their lives. The postnatal period is another of these times, constituting a painful echo of labour. Usually referred to as 'afterpains', they are 'afterbirth pains' in North America (Bloomfield *et al.*, 1986) or 'uterine cramps' (Niven & Gijsbers, 1996a: 131). Chronologically, afterpains are the woman's first hint that, although her baby is born, her pain may be unfinished, because afterpains may begin during the third stage.

The research and clinical attention focusing on afterpains, like pregnancy-related pain (Chapter 6), is scanty. Thus, I have located minimal evidence on the effectiveness of the remedies used and none on the incidence of afterpains. This disregard contrasts with my observation as a midwife: that some women experience their afterpains as a major burden requiring powerful analgesia.

Textbooks state that afterpains 'occur more commonly in multiparas than in primiparas' (Olds *et al.*, 1996: 1047), which is attributed to the tendency of the multiparous uterus to relax. Afterpains are also associated with breastfeeding through the mediation of oxytocin facilitating the let-down reflex (Royal College of Midwives, 1991). Vogler (1993b) reports the intrauterine pressure during afterpains as 150 mmHg, which is greater than the measurements during labour, which peak at 100 mmHg. The woman's perception of the severity of afterpains, however, has been assessed mainly in two drug trials. Both protocols assessed the woman's pain on entry into the trial. Using a scale of 0–3 to represent none to severe pain respectively, 159 women rated their pain as ranging from 0.09 to 2.53 (Bloomfield *et al.*, 1986). In Norway 64 women completed a 10 cm visual analogue scale extending from 'no pain' to 'pain as bad as it can be'; this produced an average score of just below 60 (Skovlund *et al.*, 1991). These data provide no indication of the incidence of afterpains, because each study recruited on the basis of experiencing afterpains; they do, however, show how severely women perceive afterpains. Because each trial was time-limited they do not indicate the duration of afterpains, but this has been 'guesstimated' at 2–3 days (Olds *et al.*, 1996).

Olds *et al.*'s guesstimate is supported by a Scottish survey which included 'uterine cramps' in the data collection (Dewan *et al.*, 1993). Unsurprisingly, these researchers found that afterpains were felt by more women and more severely on the first day, compared with second and fourth days. Fewer primigravid women felt these pains and felt them less severely than their multiparous sisters. The maximal incidence and severity was when afterpains were felt as moderate/severe by 56% of first day multiparous women. By day four no primigravid women were experiencing them as moderate/severe, but 5% of multiparous women felt them persistently so.

Pharmaceutical companies' obvious interest indicates that analgesic medication is widely used to treat afterpains, and administration has been recommended 'one hour before feeding her infant' (Olds *et al.*, 1996: 1047); such advice raises a host of questions about breastfeeding practice. Vogler (1993b) recommends explanations, warmth, rest, relaxation and keeping the bladder empty rather than medication.

It appears, yet again, that this pain is not considered significant, contrasting with my observation of women's experience. Disconcertingly, afterpains coincide with nipple pain, as both happen during breastfeeding (Niven & Gijsbers, 1996a). This coincidence only increases the risk of the woman discontinuing breastfeeding, as 22% of Scottish mothers do within the first two weeks (Scottish Office, 1995). For this, if for no other reason, afterpains deserve more, and more serious, attention.

The pain of perineal repair

Although postnatal perineal pain has quite rightly attracted considerable clinical and research attention (see 'Perineal pain', below), the pain caused by the repair has been neglected. One exception to this observation arose in a large, wide-ranging and authoritative study of labour (Green *et al.*, 1988). These researchers happened upon women's dissatisfaction with the 'actual suturing' of perineal damage. Only one-third of the women were not caused pain during this procedure. Severe pain was experienced by 19%, to the extent that some women remember it as 'the worst thing about the entire birth' (1988: 6.21).

Additionally, Wraight (1993) refers to the mothers in a large study who were dissatisfied with their pain control during their 'stitching'. She details the pain control methods used (Table 10.1).

These data raise important issues. First, was the epidural analgesia adequate, bearing in mind the usual practice of allowing the epidural to 'wear off' for the birth? This may not have been a problem because of the high proportion of women with epidurals whose birth is assisted and who have a 'top up' in preparation for the birth. Further, a total of 19.3% of women in the study used epidural analgesia (Steer, 1993); this leaves a shortfall of 5.78% of women who had either an epidural and no damage requiring suturing or an epidural and other pain control for the

Table 10.1 Methods of pain control used for perineal repair (from Wraight 1993: 89).

Method	Number	Percentage
Local anaesthetic	1758	45.18
Nitrous oxide and oxygen	1215	31.22
Epidural	526	13.52
None	266	6.84
Don't know	126	3.24
Total	3891	100.00

repair. Greater concern arises from the large proportion of women who underwent this procedure without adequate analgesia. These are the women who used only nitrous oxide and oxygen or nothing at all – a total of almost 39% of the women. These women's problems were impressed on me when I was involved in a home birth prior to midwives being permitted to suture the perineum. The general practitioner who required to be called to suture the laceration declined to infiltrate with local anaesthetic, so nitrous oxide and oxygen was used with inadequate effect. Thus, my impression is that perineal suturing is painful and that effective analgesia is crucial. It may be, though, that if a laceration is small, local anaesthetic causes more problems than it solves. It is to be hoped that this applied to these women. We should question, however, whether a laceration so small that local anaesthetic is not needed really requires suturing.

The issue of non-suturing of perineal lacerations attracts interest, more because of its effect on subsequent perineal pain than the pain of suturing (Cochrane, 1992). A retrospective survey of non-suturing of first and second degree tears suggests favourable outcomes in terms of infection, subsequent pain and resumption of sexual intercourse (Head, 1993). The pain of perineal repair was not assessed.

Tissue adhesives have been introduced in surgery and might render irrelevant the pain of perineal repair. These substances, applied to the wound edges, mimic the final stages of coagulation to form a fibrin clot which is both haemostatic and adhesive (Lasa *et al.*, 1993). Tissue adhesives' value in perineal repair is doubtful, because their main advantage is their cosmetic finish (Keng & Bucknall, 1989), the importance of which is uncertain in this context. Additionally, using these adhesives still requires suturing of the deep layers as the adhesive is applied only to the skin (Adoni & Anteby, 1991; Tarrant, 1993). Having found no evidence on the relative painfulness of suturing these layers, I have difficulty imagining that non-suturing of just the skin would greatly reduce the woman's pain.

Perineal pain

Postnatal perineal pain matters, not only in itself, but also in its effect on the woman's relationships with those close to her. This applies initially to her ability to relax sufficiently to breastfeed (Royal College of Midwives, 1991) and then to her resumption of sexual activity (see 'Dyspareunia', this chapter). The occurrence and severity of perineal pain has been studied in relation to certain interventions, which may resolve birth-related trauma. Additionally, many remedies have been suggested and used to reduce perineal pain, some of which have been researched.

Perineal damage

Following longstanding claims to justify using episiotomy (Banta & Thacker, 1982; Formato, 1985), a major research project sought to ascertain its short-term and long-term effects (Sleep, 1984). A randomised controlled trial (RCT) attempted to distinguish the effects of more liberal and more restrictive use of episiotomy; in the former the midwife endeavoured to prevent perineal laceration, and the latter permitted an episiotomy only if specific signs of fetal distress appeared. The sample comprised 1000 women randomised late in the second stage. No significant differences emerged between the two groups' perineal pain at 10 days or at 3 months, but the women in the restrictive group tended to resume sexual intercourse earlier. While establishing benefits of neither laceration nor episiotomy, this study showed that a restrictive approach to episiotomy is associated with more women giving birth without perineal damage. A follow-up study, 3 years later, sought the long-term effects of the different (restrictive/liberal) policies (Sleep & Grant, 1987a). Again, no clear differences manifested themselves.

Suture technique/material

Since midwives first assumed responsibility for perineal repair in the 1980s they have been in a position to decide the most appropriate suture material and method of suturing. Research into suture materials has measured outcomes such as perineal pain, analgesic medication, need for suture removal, need for resuturing, resumption of sexual intercourse and dyspareunia (Spencer et al., 1986). Similar criteria were also used for the evaluation of non-absorbable sutures (Mahomed et al., 1989). Spencer and colleagues found that chromic catgut was more likely to cause perineal pain in the short term, and to need removal for this reason. Glycerol-impregnated catgut or 'softgut', however, caused even more serious problems, which comprised dyspareunia for up to 3 years after the birth. Grant (1989a) suggests that treated catgut causes a reaction within the perineal tissues, perhaps associated with increased fibrosis.

After reviewing research on the techniques, Grant (1989b) recommended unambiguously the superiority of subcuticular sutures. A prospective study, however, failed to support such enthusiasm (Mahomed *et al.*, 1989); these researchers found that the differences in perineal pain were less and the incidence of dyspareunia in the subcuticular group at 3 months was higher than in women with interrupted sutures. Another RCT sought to clarify this situation by comparing skin closure using interrupted chromic catgut with subcuticular prolene (Doyle *et al.*, 1993). While the day three responses of 199 women indicated no difference, subsequent response rates were too low to permit valid conclusions. Those who recall the trauma for the woman of removing non-absorbable perineal sutures would agree that their reintroduction would be a retrograde step in terms of their removal causing anxiety, if not pain.

The link between suture techniques/materials and perineal pain emerges from a cost effectiveness analysis (Howard *et al.*, 1995b). These health economists drew on two systematic reviews and other sources to analyse the cost effectiveness of perineal repair techniques. The factors affecting costs were analysed according to suture material and technique, and were related to outcomes with cost implications. Valid research on non-absorbable and absorbable sutures relied predominantly on pain to evaluate benefits, such as short-term and long-term pain and dyspareunia. Additionally, analgesic medication use, removal of absorbable material and resuturing had been evaluated. Short-term pain and analgesia use differed markedly, with non-absorbable sutures being associated with pain in 32% of women compared with 22% with absorbable sutures, giving an odds ratio of 0.60. Analgesia use was also significantly different. Howard scrutinised research on continuous and interrupted skin suturing, finding clearly better outcomes in terms of short-term pain with continuous suturing, with an odds ratio of 0.68. Additionally, suture material was more likely to need removal, incurring major costs, because of tightness and/or pain, when interrupted suturing was used. Without specifying it, these researchers introduce an argument persuasive to the reformed UK health care system; this states that greater pain increases health care costs and that such costs are reduced by applying research appropriately.

Local measures

Although bathing has traditionally been recommended as a remedy both for pain and for healing, empirical data do not support this. An uncontrolled study (Sleep & Grant 1988a) found that 93% of women questioned on day ten agreed that bathing had relieved their perineal pain. These researchers, when measuring perineal pain at 10 days and at 3 months, found no difference in pain reports between women who had added salt, Savlon (chlorhexidine gluconate 1.5% wv and cetrimide ph eur 15% wv in an aqueous solution) or neither to their bath water. Replicating this study and including a 'shower' group would clarify the value of bathing, but a 'bidet' group might be necessary to control for the psychological benefits of immersion and flowing water.

Local measures comprise the perineal application of a variety of preparations. Ice packs have been used in 84% of maternity units, but their benefit lasts only while the ice remains frozen (Sleep & Grant, 1988b). The potentially harmful effects on wound healing associated with temporary ischaemia or ice burns should, however, indicate the need for caution. Pharmacological preparations have been marketed, but their benefits have not always been well-established and their impairment of healing has outweighed possible analgesic effects (Sleep, 1991).

Physical remedies

The multiplicity of physical interventions recommended in the postnatal period is underresearched and, hence, of unproven benefit. Postnatal exercises are one example of such an intervention. The effect of pelvic floor exercises on urinary and faecal incontinence was evaluated by Sleep and Grant (1987b). The compliance of the sample women verged on enthusiasm, which makes the findings less valid by raising the spectre of the Hawthorne effect. One group was taught the usual pelvic floor exercises in the usual way, whereas the experiment group received individual tuition by a midwife and kept a health diary for a month. Despite the methodological problems, it is noteworthy that perineal pain was significantly less in the experiment group at 3 months, although there were no significant differences in any other symptoms. Postnatal exercises have had many claims made for them, but pain control is not one; this research suggests that pain control is their only benefit.

The air ring or ring cushion has found its way from nursing elderly people to easing postnatal perineal pain. In both situations the aim is to reduce pressure on a limited area by raising it from the surface. Church and Lyne (1994) argue that the damage hypothesised as occurring in elderly tissues by the displacement of pressure by air rings is unproven. They suggest that new mothers should not be deprived of this potential source of comfort because our nursing cousins have overreacted to a specious argument.

Various forms of energy, such as infra-red light, have been applied to the perineum to assist healing and reduce pain. The effectiveness of two currently fashionable interventions, ultrasound and pulsed electromagnetic energy treatment, was evaluated in an RCT (Grant *et al.*, 1989). No significant differences were found in perineal outcomes in either of the treatment groups compared with the controls.

Systemic preparations
The range of oral analgesics available to remedy perineal pain is immense, but their unwanted side-effects, for both woman and baby, demand careful consideration. Grant and Sleep (1989) observe that this range is available only to treat less intense pain; for this reason the woman for whom these medications are inadequate may be encouraged to resort to the physical remedies mentioned above.

Complementary therapies
The main focus of complementary remedies in postnatal perineal care is on herbal preparations to assist healing, as shown by midwives in a National Health Service (NHS) Trust (Lewis, 1994). Comfrey leaf, lavender flower and calendula flower are infused in water and then used for a sitz bath, which became associated with non-suturing of the perineum (see 'The pain of perineal repair' and 'Local measures'). Because these are 'complementary' interventions and midwives are unlikely to have been taught about their use, comprehensive consultation with recognised herbalists and pharmacists is essential to protect the midwife. Further, regarding knowledge of their effects, herbal interventions should be treated with the same caution that we apply to pharmacological interventions. However, that 'evidence is required that they are both safe and therapeutic' (Sleep, 1991: 8) is a counsel of perfection which has been applied less than assiduously to their pharmacological equivalents.

A search for evidence was made in relation to lavender oil, a form of aromatherapy, which is widely used for its healing and antiseptic properties but may also be added to bath water to reduce perineal pain (Dale & Cornwell, 1994). These researchers' double blind RCT involved 635 women, of whom one group added pure lavender oil to their bath, the second group used synthetic lavender oil and the third used an inert placebo. Six drops were added to the daily bath for the first 10 postnatal days. Data were collected by a visual analogue scale which the woman completed 30 minutes after her bath and which sought information on perineal pain and mood. On the tenth day the woman and midwife completed questionnaires on perineal healing. The data showed that 90% of the mothers reported feeling better after a bath and in 74% the perineum was healed by day ten; these findings, like the women using pure lavender oil having lower pain scores, did not reach statistical significance. That no side-effects were identified suggests the safety of this therapy.

A pilot study into the effectiveness of herbal remedies has begun (Holwell, 1994) involving 20 women. Ten women took one tablet of the homeopathic remedy Arnica Montana 30c 6-hourly for the first 3 days after the birth. Arnica or leopard's bane is intended to stimulate healing and reduce bruising (Sleep, 1991). The number of women experiencing perineal pain in the experimental group was significantly greater at day ten; however, the value of this finding in such a small sample is questionable.

Summary

Since the early 1980s and due largely to one team, midwives' research-based knowledge of perineal damage and associated pain has escalated. Similarly, our knowledge of the causes and treatment of perineal pain has expanded. This important research has, possibly in combination with other developments, resulted in changes in practice. Our attention, however, has been drawn to the inconsistent and idiosyncratic use of research findings in practice (Harris, 1992). She interviewed a sample of 76 practitioners, mainly midwives, about the research basis of their perineal care. Harris found that the questionably relevant ideas on air rings were most frequently quoted. This contrasted with the pertinent and authoritative studies on suture material and technique mentioned above, which were not reported. Thus, Harris identified 'inappropriate' research utilisation.

While certain forms of painful perineal damage, such as episiotomy and laceration, are easily identifiable and hence researchable, others are less so. This means that other forms of perineal damage and the ensuing pain are underresearched. Examples are bruising and oedema which midwives not infrequently observe and seek to advise the woman about, as well as the probably less common haematoma. Sleep's pioneering work needs to be followed up by increasing our knowledge of and improving our care for women with these even less glamorous problems.

Dyspareunia

As emerged in the last section, the woman's ability to enjoy coitus is often used to indicate perineal healing. Thus, we should consider first the pathophysiological factors associated with postnatal dyspareunia, which occurs in a majority of new mothers (Hay-Smith & Mantle, 1996).

A widely recognised factor with the potential to make intercourse painful for a woman is the lack of vaginal lubrication, which occurs at various times in her life. This dryness is associated with 'soreness and irritation' during intercourse or afterwards, assuming that it is insufficiently severe to prevent penetration. Vaginal dryness postnatally, and extending through lactation, is due to oestrogen deficiency. Thus the vaginal wall not only becomes drier, but also thinner, being relatively atrophic (Bancroft, 1994).

Perineal damage has been implicated in changes in sexual function postnatally. While occasionally these changes may be positive (Fleming

& Schafer, 1989; Raphael-Leff, 1991), the reverse is now more widely accepted (Kitzinger, 1995). In a survey involving 89 women, suturing of the perineum was identified as the crucial predictor of dyspareunia rather than the intentionality of the damage (Fleming & Schafer 1989). These researchers did, however, find a significantly higher level of long-term dyspareunia in women who had an episiotomy. They surmise that this is due to the more extensive tissue damage which an episiotomy incurs, which may in turn be due to the incision being made prior to the physiological displacement of muscle tissue.

A study on perineal pain focused on dyspareunia in relation to the suture material (Sleep *et al.*, 1989). Chromic softgut, which was compared with chromic catgut, was 33% more likely to be associated with dyspareunia, even though the timing of resuming sexual intercourse showed no inter-group difference. These findings indicate the significance that women attach to their sexual relationships following the birth and their need to return to 'normal' functioning. This significance reflects the research emphasis on penetrative sex postnatally, resulting in the considerable general concern with female dyspareunia. The lighthearted feminist stance adopted by Kitzinger (1995) reminds us that sexuality is not limited to one particular act between two people of different genders, but includes a range of activities, attitudes and orientations. The woman's attitudes contribute to how comfortable she is to resume sex; for example, erotic/maternal self-conflict and feelings of territoriality of certain body parts such as her breasts and genitalia may inhibit sex (Raphael-Leff, 1991).

Research on postnatal sexuality focuses narrowly on dyspareunia as a problem of the only 'acceptable' sexual behaviour, that is penetration by a male (Ussher, 1996: 177). On this basis a feminist plea is made for a more complete or holistic view of women's sexuality giving due regard to the wide ranging sexual needs of the new mother. Ussher's plea is that the topic of postnatal sexuality should be opened up, by being both more inclusive and more openly discussed. This need for openness contrasts with observations in a medical postnatal clinic that women who dared mention sexual problems had their questions ignored (Porter & Macintyre, 1989). While women may be recommended to seek expert advice about postnatal sexual problems (Niven, 1992), the recommendation that 'couples can be encouraged to express their affection and love through kissing, holding and talking' (Olds *et al.*, 1996: 1082) seems a sensible preliminary. Perhaps adopting new positions for lovemaking in order to avoid tender spots or including the application of a lubricant as part of the foreplay may be an opportunity for the couple to revitalise their sexual relationship.

Until recently the woman was recommended to avoid sexual inter-course until after her 6-week postnatal examination. As a student I was taught that this was to prevent some unspecified 'infection'. It is necessary to question whether this recommendation was to prevent health care providers being asked to advise about painful sexual problems, by delaying the manifestation of those problems beyond 6 weeks.

Haemorrhoids

Haemorrhoids or piles are a problem that is partly due to physiological changes in the pregnant woman's cardiovascular system. In spite of this, I am including it in the 'Pelvic pain' section, rather than with pain in the circulatory system (see 'Thromboembolic pain', this chapter); this is because, in my experience, women find difficulty distinguishing the pain of haemorrhoids from other perineal pain. Although haemorrhoids are often said to present for the first time during pregnancy, they are thought to be aggravated by birth. Women are also said to be more aware of this problem postnatally, and for this reason it is included here rather than with pregnancy pain (Chapter 6, 'Pain of cardiovascular origin').

During childbearing varicose veins affect a number of sites in the woman's body, such as legs, abdomen and vulva, but when the anal canal is affected haemorrhoids result (Widmer, 1978). The incidence of this problem is uncertain, but 'between 8–20% of women' develop varicosities in the legs during pregnancy (Callam, 1994). Although the association with childbearing is beyond dispute, the incidence of haemorrhoids and their development are less certain. De Swiet attributes haemorrhoids partly to the increased venous blood pressure in the dependent parts of the woman's body (1991). Superimposed on this rise in pressure is a 50% increase in the venous distensibility or degree of dilatation at a given pressure, due to placental oestrogens. The development of haemorrhoids has been linked with diet and constipation (Kimmey & Silverstein, 1990; Olds *et al.*, 1996), but the empirical evidence supporting this is unclear. Based on this assertion, women are advised to ensure adequate dietary fibre and a high fluid intake (Jamieson, 1993).

Sturdy differentiates painless internal haemorrhoids from those that prolapse through the anal orifice and 'swell alarmingly' (1990: 87). The pain of haemorrhoids is said to be continuous, being exacerbated by straining, sitting and walking; it is associated with a mucoid discharge and sometimes bleeding, which stains toilet paper and clothing, as well as anal pruritis (Olds *et al.*, 1996).

Local palliative remedies, such as ice or ointments, are recommended to reduce the size and hence pain of haemorrhoids (Sturdy, 1990), but haemorrhoidectomy may be necessary. The literature on haemorrhoids in childbearing tends towards the reassuring; as Olds *et al.* state: haemorrhoids 'usually become asymptomatic after the early postpartal period' (1996). Like other statements relating to haemorrhoids, there is no indication of its research basis. As these authors indicate and is generally accepted, the expulsive efforts of the second stage are thought to exacerbate haemorrhoids, but again evidence is lacking.

Amid this gloomy absence of evidence, MacArthur and colleagues' work (1991) illuminates an albeit limited area. These researchers were concerned only with those problems, including haemorrhoids, that manifested themselves after a particular or 'index' birth. Of the 11 701 women who responded to the questionnaire, 8% (n=931) reported haemorrhoids lasting over 6 weeks for the first time within 3 months of the index birth. In addition to these 'new cases', almost 10% of the women (n=1143) reported a recurrence of haemorrhoids at and for this time. The generalisability of these data is questionable because of this study's low response rate (39%).

While the literature tends to reassure the woman of the transience of haemorrhoids, MacArthur *et al.* found that in only 16% of the new cases had the problem resolved within 3 months. On the contrary, in 70% of women the haemorrhoids continued for over 1 year, and in 67% of women the symptoms had lasted for between 13 months and 9 years. For a large majority of the respondents the symptoms began within 1 week of the birth. These researchers charitably describe the reassurance as 'misplaced' (1991: 167). As well as refuting the misinformation given to women, this research supports some assumptions about the aetiology of haemorrhoids. This includes the positive correlation with greater birthweight, longer second stage, assistance with obstetric forceps and vaginal birth. The use of birthing chairs during the second stage has also been linked with the onset of haemorrhoids (Cottrell & Shannahan, 1986).

While MacArthurs *et al.*'s research may be criticised, it illuminates an otherwise neglected area of care. On the basis of these researchers' findings, I proposed, with a multidisciplinary team, to undertake to seek answers prospectively on the still-outstanding questions about haemorrhoids in childbearing. The funding bodies greeted the research proposal with deafening silence, leading to the conclusion that a problem as fundamental as this holds little attraction for grant-givers. Thus, our lack of authoritative empirical knowledge about this pervasive problem persists and will continue as long as funding bodies direct resources towards acute problems which are amenable to high-tech interventions.

Thromboembolic pain

The pain of thromboembolism is another example, which we encountered in Chapter 6, 'Pain of cardiovascular origin', of pain *per se* being relatively insignificant. Thromboembolic conditions are, rightly, viewed more seriously than the pain that initially indicates their presence.

Following de Swiet's terminology (1995), here I use 'thromboembolism' to denote serious conditions involving thrombosis and/or embolism.

While thromboembolism happens not uncommonly in pregnancy and occasionally in labour, it is most likely to occur postnatally (Baskett, 1985; HMSO, 1996: 48). Baskett's 'guesstimate' that two-thirds of thromboembolic episodes occur postnatally is supported by Confidential Enquiry data which records 35 maternal deaths due to this condition, only 12 of which occurred antenatally (HMSO, 1996). These figures also show the significance of thromboembolism. It is the UK's major single cause of maternal death, being equal in absolute numbers to deaths due to the second and third most common causes of mortality, namely hypertension and haemorrhage, respectively. As well as mortality, thromboembolism contributes to morbidity in the forms of pulmonary hypertension and abnormal lung function (de Swiet, 1995).

Superficial thrombophlebitis

Not warranting inclusion with thromboembolism because it is so benign, thrombophlebitis is still painful. It appears by about day four as swelling over the affected blood vessel, usually one of the superficial saphenous veins (Olds *et al.*, 1996). Warmth, reddening and tension feature due to local inflammation and the woman may have low grade pyrexia and tachycardia. Treatment is by a correctly applied support stocking without limitation of mobility. The woman should elevate the affected leg when stationary to reduce swelling (Ball, 1993). Local heat and systemic analgesics may reduce pain, but anticoagulant therapy is unnecessary. Ball cautions that, although superficial thrombophlebitis carries no risk of embolism, the woman vulnerable to this condition is also at increased risk of deep vein thrombosis (DVT), because she is likely to be older, parous and overweight. Clearly, vigilance is essential.

Thromboembolic conditions

DVT and the embolus that it may release constitute the threat to maternal life with which I introduced this topic.

Pathophysiology

Certain physiological mechanisms protect the woman from excessive blood loss during childbirth. These mechanisms include increased plasma fibrinogen, decreased fibrinolytic activity, increased circulating volume and myometrial contractility (Letsky, 1991). Unfortunately, the first two of these mechanisms may be too effective and put the woman in jeopardy of excessive blood coagulation. Immobility or other factors leading to slow circulation in the dependent body parts, such as pelvis or legs, may be sufficient to initiate haemostasis. Thrombosis begins with the aggregation of platelets in a blood vessel, such as the femoral vein, possibly at the site of endothelial damage. The thrombus thus formed may not threaten health as, outwith pregnancy, fibrinolysis would destroy it (Hinchliff & Montague, 1988). A surviving thrombus, however, grows to occlude the lumen and the blood beyond it becomes static and coagulates, forming a 'tail' of clot, anchored only at its origin. Clearly, portions of this tail may detach forming emboli, which lodge in pulmonary or cerebral arterioles causing dreadful pain and other clinical features (Baskett, 1985).

The commonly mentioned complication of DVT is pulmonary embolism (Baskett, 1985; Bonica, 1990b). The reason for this exclusivity is unclear in view of the 17% cerebral embolism risk (HMSO, 1996). Pulmonary embolism's dire effects are due to the occlusion of the pulmonary circulation by the thrombus, producing hypoxia, acute pulmonary hypertension, right ventricular failure and cardiogenic shock. The local effect of pulmonary occlusion is exacerbated by the production of serotonin, prostaglandins and histamine, which further constrict circulation (Bonica, 1990b). While massive pulmonary embolism causes the woman to collapse suddenly and die, she may survive the initial episode and be transferred for intensive care. She may, however, die in the intensive care unit from an associated condition, such as acute respiratory distress syndrome or multiple organ failure (HMSO, 1996).

In a seriously ill woman, perhaps with a condition such as placental abruption (Chapter 6), coagulation failure is linked with disseminated intravascular coagulation (DIC). This involves clotting throughout the circulation; clotting factors and platelets are consumed, leading to a 'vicious circle' of clotting and 'disastrous bleeding' (Letsky, 1991: 74). In DVT, thrombus formation may be associated with local inflammation, causing pain and tenderness in the affected vein (Procacci *et al.*, 1994). The structures surrounding the affected vein may also be inflamed and painful, including muscles, tendons and other perivascular tissues. These authors indicate the severity of the pain in these other structures by stating that, even after the inflammation of the affected vein is resolved, postphlebitis pain often lingers.

Should pulmonary embolism occur, the pain is comparable with that of myocardial infarction, being deep, retrosternal and crushing (Bonica, 1990b). The crucial difference is that pulmonary embolism pain does not radiate. The pain is thought to be due to the sudden distension of the pulmonary artery. The nature of the pain of cerebral thrombosis depends on its site; if cortical the headache increases gradually, whereas if the sagittal sinus is occluded cerebral hypertension and raised intracranial pressure ensue (Donaldson, 1995).

Risk factors

Although increasing age, excess weight and high multiparity have been incriminated as predisposing to thromboembolism, caesarean section's significant role emerges clearly from the Confidential Enquiries (HMSO, 1996). Of the 17 maternal deaths due to pulmonary embolism within 6 weeks, 13 (76%) of the women gave birth by caesarean section.

Diagnosis

Thromboembolic disorders are initially diagnosed on the basis of the clinical picture, but ultrasound, doppler flow studies and contrast radiography confirm the diagnosis (Baskett, 1985; Ball, 1993; Allotey & Louca, 1997). Pulmonary embolism varies considerably in its effects, depending on the size of the embolism and area of lung affected. Clinical signs indicate the need for radiographic investigations, such as pulmonary angiography (Keep, 1995). The fetal effects of radiological investigations in pregnancy must be balanced against the potentially dire maternal outcome.

Although diagnosis appears straightforward, the techniques commonly employed are inadequate (Baskett, 1985). The tragic outcomes resulting from diagnostic difficulties emerged in the Confidential Enquiries (HMSO, 1996). Women died of pulmonary embolism, having been treated for respiratory infection after complaining to a general practitioner or another of breathlessness or chest pain soon after giving birth. As Robinson appropriately observes, '. . . chest pain . . . was too readily dismissed as 'flu or asthma without further investigation' (1996a: 382). The Confidential Enquiries conclude:

> 'It is recommended that close attention is paid to any woman with chest symptoms who is currently pregnant or recently delivered, to exclude the presence of deep vein thrombosis or potential small pulmonary embolism.' (HMSO, 1996: 57)

Diagnostic difficulties are further hampered by communication problems with women whose first language is not English (HMSO, 1996). A case is reported of a woman 'who spoke no English', who died of undiagnosed pulmonary embolism. Although, in my experience, women with little English find other ways of communicating pain information, her interpreter could not have recognised the significance of the information that she gave him. The argument for professional interpreters who are fluent, health-oriented and trustworthy is irrefutable in this situation (Schott & Henley, 1996). The woman's partner clearly has a role, but it should not be to act as translator (Mander, 1995c).

Treatment

The main approach to thromboembolic disorders is prevention. This comprises pharmacological prophylaxis using anticoagulant therapy in women at risk (Butler, 1995). Prophylactic nursing interventions, such as passive movement and early mobilisation, are particularly significant in this group of women (HMSO, 1996). Ethnic minority users of the maternity services also contribute to thromboembolism statistics in other ways. Problems relating to mobilisation are highlighted by Robinson (1996a). The culture-based belief among Asian mothers of the need for prolonged and complete rest after the birth may make a mother wary of mobilising after an operative birth. To resolve this situation Robinson suggests 'multi-language advice'.

In women with perineal trauma, air rings have been condemned as predisposing to thromboembolism and have been withdrawn. Church and Lyne (1994) question the evidence on air rings, which I have seen many women welcome as a godsend. They conclude that empirical evidence does not justify denying new mothers this comfort.

The emergency interventions in the event of pulmonary embolism focus on oxygenation, medical aid, analgesia and resuscitation, followed by long-term anticoagulant therapy (Butler 1995; Keep, 1995; Allotey & Louca, 1997).

Summary

Although, as I mentioned in my introduction, thromboembolic pain is relatively insignificant, we ignore it at our peril. This doggerel reminds midwives, like our nursing cousins, of the danger:

> A little pain behind the calf
> Just seemed to make the nurses laugh.
> But then to their intense surprise
> I died.
> They didn't realise
> A CLOT
> Was what
> I'd got. (Douglas, 1968: 413)

The pain of motherhood

One way of coping with pain is by ascribing it some purpose (Chapter 1). It may serve as a warning of pathology or, as in labour, alert the woman to the impending birth. Pain postnatally, though, is surprising in its pointlessness (Dewan *et al.*, 1993). It is recommended that women should be prepared for this during their 'antenatal counselling and postnatal care'. I focus here on certain forms of postnatal pain which relate particularly to the woman's babycare.

Breast pain in the non-breastfeeding woman

Women may not breastfeed for many reasons, but the woman who feeds her baby only with formula is still vulnerable to pain due to her breasts becoming full and, perhaps, engorged. In their study of postnatal pain, Dewan and colleagues (1993) identified how many 'bottlefeeding mothers' developed breast pain. While the proportions of primigravid and multiparous women who experienced mild breast pain were similar, Table 10.2 shows that more multiparous women developed moderate/severe pain.

Table 10.2   Breast pain in non-breastfeeding women (from Dewan et al., 1993).

	Primigravid women		Multiparous women	
	Mild	Moderate/severe	Mild	Moderate/severe
Day 1 (n=86)	0%	0%	9%	5%
Day 2 (n=81)	20%	7%	28%	20%
Day 4 (n=41)	28%	32%	31%	56%

Oestrogen preparations have been used historically to impede the action of prolactin and to inhibit lactation. They not only fail to prevent the milk 'coming in' (Niebyl et al., 1979), but also increase the risk of thromboembolic disease (Kennedy, 1978). For these reasons, non-pharmacological methods of inhibiting lactation are widely recommended. Perhaps because by definition there are no commercial interests, the non-pharmacological methods are relatively under-researched (Parazzini et al., 1989). Such ignorance is of particular concern after the woman's transfer home, when her support changes markedly. An exception to the lack of research is a study comparing lactation inhibition using bromocriptine mesylate with three non-pharmacological methods, that is surgical compression binder, standardised support bra and fluid limitation (Brooten et al., 1983). The 68 women in the sample were 'divided' among these four intervention groups. The outcomes (engorgement, pain and leakage) were significantly less in the bromocriptine group, but the binder was associated with the most rapid decrease in pain in the non-pharmacological intervention groups. These findings may be questioned because of the small sample and non-random allocation. The researchers do, however, show that breast pain for the non-breastfeeding woman is greatest from day 3–5. This clearly has implications for our teaching, as this woman is increasingly likely to have transferred home before this pain begins.

More authoritative studies have been undertaken on breast pain in non-breastfeeding women in which the emphasis has been on phar-macological prevention of breast symptoms, such as a study comparing the effectiveness of a non-pharmacological method (breast binder) with a drug intervention (bromocriptine) (Shapiro & Thomas, 1984). These researchers also found that this drug was more effective in controlling symptoms during the first week. Later the balance of effectiveness changed, so that by week three the women experiencing pain were all in the bromocriptine group.

Thus, there is a dearth of evidence relating to the care of the non-breastfeeding woman. Although the oestrogens are no longer admi-nistered, current drug interventions also have problems of rebound lactation and leakage. As Parazzini and colleagues observe, this unsatisfactory knowledge-base is unlikely to improve as long as com-mercial interests control this research (1989).

The pain of breastfeeding

Logically it is difficult to explain why breastfeeding is painful. Why is it that an activity so beneficial to a baby (Inch, 1996) may cause such pain to the woman? It has been argued that pain and other problems asso-ciated with breastfeeding are a result of incorrect care, in the form of ignorance about positioning and misguided hospital regimes, making it another example of iatrogenic pain. Such attitudes have been sum-marised: '... breastfeeding should not hurt at all' (Inch & Renfrew, 1989: 1375). The considerable evidence to the contrary suggests that this statement constitutes a counsel of perfection. One of these authors has since recanted: 'A few mothers feel acute pain as the baby begins to suckle' (Henschel & Inch, 1996: 80). Negative pressure on the milk ducts is blamed by the latter authors for the pain which the woman may experience prior to the 'let down' reflex operating (Lawrence, 1989). Breast massage and expression of colostrum may alleviate this short-term problem.

The frequency of breastfeeding pain has been catalogued by various authoritative sources, beginning with Gunther (1945) who reported 64% of breastfeeding mothers experiencing nipple pain. Drewett and colleagues (1987) recorded the prevalence of nipple pain among breastfeeding mothers as peaking at 65% on day two. A larger study identified an incidence as high as 96% in the USA (Ziemer et al., 1990). Despite these data, breast pain in breastfeeding women is not accepted as physiological.

Nipple pain

The nipple pain which women who are breastfeeding may experience is usually referred to as 'sore nipples'. This term is valuable because, while underestimating the pain, it does recognise its traumatic origin. This pain is due to poor positioning and an inadequate amount of breast tissue being taken into the baby's mouth to form a teat (Woolridge, 1986). The friction caused by this inadequate teat slipping in and out as the baby sucks is graphically compared with 'a heel in an ill-fitting new shoe' (Henschel & Inch, 1996: 81). The emotional distress of nipple pain is demonstrated by Amir and colleagues (1996) who, using well-validated instruments, established the strong positive correlation between nipple pain and postnatal depression.

Sore nipples may be prevented by teaching the woman, either during pregnancy or at the first feed, how to position her baby to minimise friction. If the nipples are damaged various remedies have been suggested, by applying healing agents or by using mechanical aids. A randomised controlled trial (RCT) of interventions to relieve nipple pain found no differences between the application of expressed breast milk, modified lanolin, warm water compresses and education only (Pugh *et al.*, 1996). All of the women (n=177) were taught individually about techniques of positioning the baby and this alone was as effective as any application in preventing soreness.

Nipple shields have been recommended to reduce trauma and pain and to allow healing. An RCT which investigated the treatment of sore nipples showed no significant difference in the rate of healing between a resting group, a nipple shield group and a supervised continued feeding group (Nicholson, 1985). This study did show, however, that the nipple shield was the least acceptable intervention. Such a disadvantage would be exacerbated by the likelihood of the milk supply declining with the use of this device (Inch & Renfrew, 1989). Thus, the crucial role of teaching emerges. Creams, sprays or mechanical aids may not always be harmful, but they are not the complete answer in preventing or resolving nipple pain.

Breast pain in the breastfeeding woman
Breast engorgement is associated with two physiological phenomena which may aggravate each other and which may be further exacerbated by inappropriate care. These phenomena are the increasing blood supply to the breasts, possibly with some degree of oedema, and the secretion of milk within the alveoli (Henschel & Inch, 1996). The limitation of the baby's frequency and duration of access to the breast by misguided policies further aggravates the physiological changes. The secretion of milk operates on a demand–supply principle, so that production ceases if milk is not removed; hence, the serious consequences of uncorrected engorgement for a woman wishing to breastfeed (Inch & Renfrew, 1989). The problem is intensified by the baby's difficulty in fixing on to the full, tense breast and inability to empty it. The physiological nature of engorgement appears in data showing that 40–45% of

breastfeeding women experience it within 96 hours of the birth (Nikodem, 1993).

The pain of engorgement is 'throbbing and aching' and the woman 'can find no comfortable position except to lie flat on her back and very still' (Lawrence, 1989: 193). These words remind us that sleeping is difficult for this woman, as the usual turns and movements awaken her in pain. Engorgement pain was assessed in Dewan and colleagues' study (1993), which showed that primigravid and multiparous breast-feeding women are likely to experience a similar intensity of breast pain, with the most severe pain being experienced by primigravid women on day four (Table 10.3). The pain of engorgement has been shown to correlate positively with nipple pain, arousing suspicions that the same misguided regimes engender both painful conditions (L'Esperance, 1980). Thus, engorgement is yet another example of an iatrogenic pain (Inch & Renfrew, 1989).

Table 10.3 Frequency of engorgement pain in breastfeeding women (from Dewan *et al.*, 1993).

	Primigravid women		Multiparous women	
	Mild	Moderate/severe	Mild	Moderate/severe
Day 1 (n=110)	7%	7%	22%	8%
Day 2 (n=103)	35%	18%	43%	20%
Day 4 (n=51)	28%	44%	37%	37%

While palliative measures, such as a firm bra and hot/cold bathing, may ease the woman's pain to some extent (Lawrence, 1989), the baby's unrestricted access to the breast is most effective in both pre-venting and treating this condition. Although many pharmacological remedies have been studied, their benefits are unclear, unlike their dangers (Inch & Renfrew, 1989).

An innovative palliative approach to engorgement is the local appli-cation of cabbage leaves. Anecdotal evidence suggests that the woman appreciates this low-tech intervention and the risks due to contamination with pesticides are slight. We are reminded, though, that this is nothing more than a palliative and is no substitute for pre-vention by teaching (Johnston & Minchin, 1994). The effect of cab-bage leaves was studied in relation to women's perceptions of engorgement and breastfeeding duration (Nikodem *et al.*, 1993). The leaves were applied for 20 minutes after three feeds per day when engorgement was greatest. In this RCT (n=120) no significant differences emerged, although the experiment group continued breastfeeding for longer.

Mastitis

The nature of mastitis is contentious because it essentially comprises a dynamic process. One of the few consistent features as this condition progresses from blocked ducts, through inflammation to infective mastitis and possibly to breast abcess is pain and localised tenderness (Lawrence, 1989). The mechanism suggested by Gunther (1958) and recently endorsed (Woolridge, 1992; Inch & Fisher, 1996) is that pressure on the duct system of the breast is responsible for initiating this process. The pressure might be either internal, possibly from oedematous tissue, or external, possibly from clothing, manual pressure or poor positioning, and may lead to obstruction of the milk ducts. This obstruction results in a buildup of pressure behind the blockage and milk secreted there is forced into the nearby tissues. The local reaction is an immune response, which is recognised by the woman as painful and tender hardening and reddening, that is inflammation. Damage, such as a cracked nipple, or poor hygiene may allow the ascent of pathogens, such as *Staphylococcus aureus* or *Candida albicans*; this changes the clinical picture to infective mastitis, carrying the risk of breast abcess (Henschel & Inch, 1996: 87–8; Saunders, 1997).

As with the other painful problems of breastfeeding discussed here, teaching the woman to position her baby, to permit the breast to be effectively 'milked' and emptied, is thought to prevent mastitis or to prevent its progression (Inch & Fisher, 1996). This recommendation derives from the research by Thomsen and colleagues (1984) which classified the progression of mastitis not by milk culture which is notoriously misleading, but by leucocyte and bacterial counts. On the basis of these investigations the women with symptoms were allocated to either continue to breastfeed or to additionally express the affected breast after feeding. In the 'blocked duct' group additional expression did not improve the good outcomes of those who just continued feeding. Where non-infectious inflammation had become established, expression significantly improved the outcome and lessened the likelihood of infective mastitis developing. In the group in whom infective mastitis had been diagnosed, the women who expressed were more successful in their lactation and none developed breast abcess; this compared with the 9% of the breastfeeding-only women in whom an abcess formed.

As well as positioning and local phenomena predisposing to mastitis, other factors have recently been suggested. By studying the relation between 'handedness' and which breast is affected, Inch and Fisher (1996) demonstrate the importance of manual dexterity in positioning the baby at the breast. These data reinforce the significance of teaching the woman the manual skills of breastfeeding. Additionally, a Dutch study showed, unsurprisingly, the increased likelihood of a woman developing mastitis if she had had it before or if she had local problems such as breast pain or damaged nipples (Foxman *et al.*, 1994). More interestingly, this study showed that women who were unable to rest during the day were more vulnerable to mastitis. While the prevalence of tiredness for the new mother is generally recognised and particularly for the breastfeeding woman (MacArthur *et al.*, 1991; Herbert, 1994), these findings emphasise the need to identify and utilise sources of support.

Back pain

Although back pain in pregnancy has been given appropriate research attention (see Chapter 6) and the same now applies to certain post-intervention pain (see below), there is a serious lack of data on postnatal back pain (MacArthur *et al.*, 1991). While preparing for a major study, Garcia and Marchant (1993) found that back pain was considered by women to be a minor problem, even though it was reported as having been experienced by 20% of new mothers (n=90) 8 weeks after the birth. To explain the significance of this pain, Garcia and Marchant (1993) remind us of the interaction between physical and emotional aspects of wellbeing, without mentioning the downward spiral which may develop in the absence of either. These researchers illustrate the significance of problems such as back pain; they discuss the inter-dependence of family members, in physical and emotional terms, at challenging times, such as after the birth. In a purely physical sense, MacArthur and colleagues (1991) remind us of the changes in the woman's lifestyle which are likely to influence back pain shortly after the birth. These researchers list child-lifting/carrying, feeding and the demands of extra laundry. Although these examples are physical, they are also fundamental to the maternal role. It may be that a woman's difficulty with them affects her self-perception of herself as a mother.

While considering maternal back pain, it is useful to remember that back pain is also common among those who provide care (Hignett, 1996). While probably still more prevalent among our nursing cousins, changes in obstetric practice may result in this problem affecting more midwives (Mander, 1997b).

Summary

The pain of motherhood is dominated by pain associated with infant feeding, particularly breastfeeding. Although some regard breastfeeding pain as an unnecessary, even iatrogenic, phenomenon, it is the common experience of a large majority of women who breastfeed. The extent to which women should be warned of the likelihood of experiencing pain during breastfeeding is uncertain. On the one hand this information may constitute negative advertising, which may deter women from even attempting breastfeeding (Watson & Mander, 1995). On the other hand, presenting the pregnant woman with too rosy a picture of breastfeeding, or motherhood in general, may foster unreal expectations, which may make it difficult for her to cope when, as a mother, she experiences the contrasting reality.

Postintervention pain

Pain that is experienced postnatally often results from events that began during pregnancy and labour. Afterpains (this chapter) relate to physiological processes, indicating that the uterine growth of pregnancy is being reversed and that the contractions of labour are continuing and reducing the risk of haemorrhage. Other postnatal pain may be due to spontaneous, variably physiological processes, such as the pain, felt as dysuria, resulting from perineal laceration. There are other interventions used during labour and which are thought or known to be associated with postnatal pain, which to a greater or lesser extent is iatrogenic. In Chapter 12, I consider various types of childbearing pain which may be iatrogenic, but because these interventions in labour give rise to postnatal pain, I consider them specifically here.

Postepidural back pain

Although the effects of epidural analgesia on the progress of labour have been recognised for some time (Williams *et al.*, 1985), the findings of MacArthur and her colleagues on the long-term effects of this intervention were disconcerting for obstetric anaesthetists (1991). This retrospective, low-response study showed an increased incidence of new back pain following epidural analgesia in labour; to the extent that 18.9% of women in whom an epidural had been used developed back pain, whereas only 10.5% of women with no epidural did so (Chapter 9, 'Epidural analgesia (and combined)'). This revelation struck at obstetric anaesthetists' very *raison d'être* (Mander, 1993b) and was greeted with hasty attempts at damage limitation by disproving these data.

This damage limitation exercise produced various results, depending on the research method and the sample. One group of studies, such as MacLeod *et al.* (1995), not only endorsed MacArthur *et al.*'s findings, but exceeded them. These researchers identified a new back pain rate of 26.2% among epidural users, compared with 2% among other analgesia users. Thus, these researchers affirmed the causal link between epidural in labour and back pain.

A second reaction is exemplified by Russell *et al.* (1993), whose retrospective study achieved a 63% response rate and findings comparable with those of MacArthur *et al.* These researchers sought to explain away their unwelcome findings with a number of strategies. First, 'psychological' factors were blamed by linking the back pain with depressed state. Second, the validity of the responses was questioned, stating that 'these women were prone to tick boxes' (p. 1302). Third, the back pain was played down by dismissing it as 'postural and not severe'. Fourth, other explanations for the women's back pain were suggested, such as dislocated/fractured coccyx. Fifth, the woman's poor posture was a cause. Sixth, re-entering the realms of psychology, these researchers blamed the woman's projection of her disappointment with her labour onto the epidural. The final explanation which these researchers offer for their findings is the 'self-fulfilling prophecy' (Russell *et al.*, 1993: 1388), due to the media interest in MacArthur *et al.*'s findings. While the latter might possibly apply to Russell and colleagues' data, it is disproved by MacLeod *et al.* (1995) whose data collection pre-dated the media attention and whose findings exceed MacArthur *et al.*'s. Thus, Russell *et al.* deny both their data and their responsibility for this iatrogenic pain by blaming a range of improbable factors. This abuse of research findings causes us to question, yet again, the quality of obstetric anaesthetic research (Mander, 1994a).

Russell *et al.* followed this study with another (1996) in which the concentration of the local anaesthetic was lowered and an opioid was introduced (0.125% bupivicaine or 0.0625% bupivicaine with an opioid). As a result, epidural analgesia was found to have no association with back pain. This finding was achieved after the data were 'massaged' to reclassify 'peripartum' back pain (i.e. in labour) as 'pre-existing', thus reducing the proportion of new cases. The inferiority of this research manifests itself in the researchers' report that informed consent was obtained in labour and that the high level of obstetric intervention was the reason for the epidural, rather than the reverse (p. 1387). These researchers' low regard for the women for whom they provide a service emerges in the feeble excuses offered to explain away the data. This may constitute another round in obstetric anaesthetists' ongoing struggle (Mander, 1994a).

A third group of studies, many of which are North American, have refuted any causal association between epidural and back pain (Ostgaard & Andersson, 1992; Breen *et al.*, 1994; MacArthur *et al.*, 1995). The reasons for this consistency are unclear, although Breen suggests that expectation of back pain is 'a prejudice not as widely held among American women' (1994: 33). This intervention and its potential for causing pain clearly raises many fundamental issues, the essence of which is succinctly summarised by an anaesthesiologist:

'The practice of obstetric anaesthesia is unique in medicine in that we use an invasive and potentially hazardous procedure to provide a humanitarian service to healthy women undergoing a physiological process.' (Bogod, 1995)

Post-general anaesthetic neck/shoulder pain

In their survey of postnatal pain, Dewan and colleagues (1993) encountered a small proportion who complained of neck and/or shoulder pain (Table 10.4). Like MacArthur and colleagues (1991), these researchers related their findings to having had a general anaesthetic (GA). They found a significant difference in the proportions of women experiencing this pain following GA compared with others (64% as opposed to 24%).

Table 10.4 Severity of post-general anaesthetic neck/shoulder pain (from Dewan *et al.*, 1993).

	Primigravid women		Multiparous women	
	Mild	Moderate/severe	Mild	Moderate/severe
Day 1 (n=198)	6%	7%	19%	7%
Day 2 (n=190)	13%	3%	17%	3%
Day 4 (n=94)	9%	2%	8%	0%

When MacArthur and colleagues (1991) examined the association between neck/shoulder pain and GA, they found neck pain to be unrelated. Shoulder pain was, however, marginally more common among women who had had a GA, but the difference was not statistically significant. These symptoms are attributed to the 'postures and manipulations' (p. 123) which are necessary to facilitate intubation, together with the general laxity of ligaments in pregnancy.

Table 10.4 shows the proportion of women with severe pain, which may lead us to assume that it is of short duration. It is necessary to ascertain whether this is the case and whether anaesthetic practice is amenable to change to reduce the incidence of this pain.

Post-caesarean section pain

There is a disconcerting trend towards regarding caesarean section as just an 'alternative method' of birth (Culp & Osofsky, 1989), which is only encouraged by describing it as 'cesarean birth' (Olds *et al.*, 1996: 1084). Despite this, we should recall that caesarean section is major abdominal surgery and carries similar risks (HMSO, 1996).

Research by Hillan (1992a) on caesarean section involved 100 women and a multiplicity of data collection methods. She emphasises the woman's difficulty in coping postnatally with 'the physical and psychological impact of major surgery, which may have occurred on top of a long and exhausting labour' (1992a: 160). These difficulties were compounded by the women's perception that 'the midwives were unaware of the difficulties [the women] had ... in coping with the "aftermath" of this method of delivery' (p. 168). While still in hospital, a majority (68%) were experiencing difficulty with infant care, which related to lifting/handling the baby, moving into and out of bed and finding comfortable feeding positions. Although not explicitly mentioned, it is likely that pain was responsible for these difficulties, especially in view of these mothers' slow recovery (Hillan, 1992b).

A postal questionnaire sent to a larger cohort (n=444) at 12 weeks demonstrated the women's recovery from caesarean section (Hillan, 1992b). The rate of recovery becomes apparent in the duration of wound pain, which for almost half of the women lasted beyond their transfer home. Of the women, 32 were still experiencing wound pain when completing the questionnaire. The wound pain after transfer was sufficiently severe to require prescription of analgesic medication in 52 (11.7% of) women.

The women's perception of their problems being denigrated by staff is supported by the longer term data (Hillan, 1992b) which compared women's experience with medical and midwifery records. Although 43% reported back pain and 12% reported painful haemorrhoids these were recorded in only 8% and none, respectively, of the women's notes. These data lead to the conclusion that the underestimation of the pain of caesarean section may be prevalent among staff.

The woman's reality of experiencing the 'aftermath' of caesarean section contrasts sharply with the medical practitioner's aims (Minzter, 1993). In deciding medication the anaesthetist seeks to ensure analgesia and minimal sedation while ensuring the woman's ability to ambulate. Minzter recommends fast-acting pain control which permits minimal drug transfer during breastfeeding. In achieving this she discounts intramuscular (IM) opioids as providing inadequate analgesia, whereas opioids administered by patient/parturient controlled analgesia (PCA) either intravenously (IV) or epidurally are more effective. Although my experience supports this observation regarding short-term pain control, I have found that nausea and vomiting are problematic for the woman using PCA. This may be due to the 'routine' administration of anti-emetics with IM opioids, but not with PCA administration.

Minzter is complacent about the safety of the effects of opioids on the nursing mother, which contrasts sharply with concerns expressed by Freeborn and colleagues (1980; Chapter 9, 'Breastfeeding'). The importance of maternal–newborn interaction following caesarean section is correctly emphasised by Minzter, but such interaction is only effective if the woman's pain control is adequate, which should be assessed as objectively as possible.

While Minzter shows very clearly the potential for a high standard of care following caesarean section, the reality may fall short. This is associated with observations by Wraight (1992) and Rajan (1993) of the limitations inherent in anaesthetic services (Chapter 2, 'Pain intervention research'). Services are finite and operating theatre activities are, probably appropriately, prioritised. These researchers draw our attention to the problems of labouring women and the midwives caring for them in locating anaesthetic personnel to provide specialist interventions. Inevitably, lower priority is given to women who have given birth but are still using, for example, PCA. It is my experience that the needs of this woman fall a long way behind those of her sisters in theatre and labour. The ethical dilemma of offering care, without staff to provide it (Wraight, 1992; Audit Commission, 1997), emerges again.

Summary

These examples of pain that follows interventions to facilitate the birth vary in their intensity and causality. There is also huge variation in our knowledge of the link between intervention and pain. Such gaps need to be filled, if, for no other reason, to be able to help women to prepare for and cope with the experience. It is necessary to continue asking: 'If women were fully informed would so many still agree so willingly?' (Newson, 1984).

Musculoskeletal pain

Back pain is the puerperal musculoskeletal pain that attracts most attention, possibly because it is so common, but also because there are many important issues related to it. Back pain has been discussed elsewhere (Chapter 6 and above). While there is a variety of other pain of musculoskeletal origin, that associated with the symphysis pubis now seems to be attracting the research and clinical attention that it deserves. The incidence of symphysial pain is estimated at between 1 in 300–20 000 births (Shepherd & Fry, 1996). Pain over the symphysis pubis is not unique to the puerperium, but, because this joint may be damaged during childbirth, such pain may begin postnatally or pre-existing pain may be aggravated (Shepherd & Fry, 1996). Thus, symphysis pubis pain is considered here.

There are at least three causes of symphysis pubis pain and Cockshoot (1995), under the heading of *Diastasis symphysis pubis*, discusses two of them. Diastasis is defined as 'the forcible separation of two parts that are normally joined together' (Anderson, 1994). This definition clearly applies to the traumatic separation of the symphysis during childbirth and has been attributed to 'precipitous (*sic*) labour, difficult instrumental delivery, cephalo-pelvic disproportion, previous or existing pelvic abnormality and multiparity' (Shepherd & Fry, 1996: 200). The lithotomy position is also blamed (Cockshoot, 1995). In such situations, this cartilaginous joint is overstretched or torn (Lowery, 1995) and the pain manifests itself suddenly, within hours after the birth.

The second cause of diastasis (Shepherd & Fry, 1996) relates to the supposedly physiological changes in the symphysis in preparation for childbirth, which are hard to envisage as 'forcible separation'. Lowery describes the increased laxity of the symphysis, which is hormonally induced, permitting greater mobility of this joint and, presumably, facilitating childbirth. He describes the diameter of the joint as increasing from the non-pregnant measurement of 4.9 mm to 7.1 mm. This marked increase is further enhanced by enzymatic resorption of the pubic bones (Shepherd & Fry, 1996).

A third cause of puerperal symphysial pain is the non-infectious inflammation of the symphysis, pubic bones and nearby structures known as osteitis pubis (Lentz, 1995). This author cites periosteal trauma during childbirth as the cause.

Regardless of the timing or the aetiology, the pain is remarkably similar. It has been described as 'extreme pain in both groins and symphysis pubis ... walking [was] a nightmare and all weightbearing activities [were] excruciatingly painful' (Shepherd & Fry, 1996: 199). Others support these authors' contention that pain changes the gait into a waddle (Lentz, 1995).

Care in labour involves avoiding abduction of the hips as far as possible. Jones and Sturdy (1990) maintain that no active treatment is likely to be needed postnatally, but others advocate a support (e.g. tubigrip) bandage applied by a physiotherapist (Cockshoot, 1995; Shepherd & Fry, 1996). If the cause is osteitis pubis, anti-inflammatory medication is appropriate (Lentz, 1995). Emotional support is needed by this woman who experiences a little-recognised pain, and is available from a self-help group (Cockshoot, 1995).

Little attention has been given to the recurrence risk. That this needs researching became clear to me when caring for a woman who had experienced symphysial pain following her previous birth. Her anxiety was profound and, despite my best efforts, marred an otherwise satisfying birth experience. She was eventually convinced when, following the birth, she walked painlessly to the shower.

Pain control in the puerperium

The limited attention given to the postnatal period in general and to pain in particular is, not surprisingly, reflected in the scanty research on pain control at the time of writing (Dewan *et al.*, 1993).

Non-pharmacological methods

I have referred to various non-pharmacological methods of pain control in the specific sections, such as those on breast pain and perineal pain. With the exception of work such as that by Dale and Cornwell (1994) on using lavender oil to reduce perineal pain, the non-pharmacological methods are unresearched. Thus, midwives are not yet able to confidently recommend their use.

Pharmacological methods

The pharmacological methods have attracted marginally more interest than their non-pharmacological counterparts in controlling postnatal pain. In their study of health after childbirth, MacArthur and colleagues (1991) found that general practitioners were keen to treat some painful conditions, such as haemorrhoids, migraine and headaches. It may be assumed that treatment comprised analgesic drugs. The relative benefits of two widely used oral analgesic agents (mefenamic acid and paracetamol) are the focus of Dewan and colleagues' discussion of pain relief (1993); they conclude that the former is more effective, and that 'side effects and concentrations in breast milk are negligible' (p. 66). In her account of analgesia after caesarean section, Minzter (1993) considers only pharmacological methods, with a focus on PCA. Her criteria for recommending certain medications relate to the mother's ability to interact with her baby, rather than these drugs' transfer via breast milk.

Minzter draws attention to the mother's need to assume some degree of control after surgery and uses this argument to advocate PCA. Similar logic has been applied more widely by our nursing cousins, who have introduced and evaluated self-administration of medicine (SAM) programmes (Furlong, 1996). Although many of these programmes have been introduced in medical wards and areas where each patient is prescribed a multiplicity of drugs, other areas have also been studied. Jones and colleagues (1996) undertook part of their SAM study in a gynaecology ward, whose drug administration and client population may bear comparison with the maternity area. Having established that a majority of the women would be happy to self-administer, a system to test out the feasibility of SAM was operationalised. Most of the medications were analgesics, were initially dispensed in bottles containing one day's supply and were kept in the bedside locker. These researchers found that, as well as reducing anxiety by increasing their control, patients experienced less delay in medication administration and that time and confusion were reduced during medicine rounds. A larger controlled study endorsed these findings and reported patients' increased sense of independence and their impression of saving nurses' time (Furlong, 1996). Contrary to staff anxieties, Jones and colleagues (1996) found that 'mistakes, stealing and misuse' did not cause problems. The disadvantages of staff administration by drug rounds of postnatal analgesia is spelt out by Myrnick (1981), who introduced a SAM programme in the maternity area. Like the recent nurse researchers, Myrnick found that the women were satisfied and that staff time was utilised more efficiently.

Thus, it would appear that such an innovation might provide both woman and midwife with learning opportunities.

Summary

The limited interest in the postnatal period is a continuing source of concern. Researchers suggest that this lack of interest leads to services failing to meet consumers' needs (Glazener *et al.*, 1993). These researchers also draw attention to the increased risk of maternal morbidity and mortality associated with interventive techniques. In more general terms, responsibility for postnatal ill-health has been allocated to society at large (Garcia & Marchant, 1993). This claim is based on society fostering such high expectations among women of getting 'back to normal' (1993) that women are prevented from seeking help when they do not 'match up with the images in the popular media' (1993: 3). Thus, maternal ill-health remains unreported and untreated. Of particular significance, Garcia and Marchant maintain, is the lack of any systematic feedback to the maternity unit staff. For this reason, a potential stimulus to change practice is unutilised.

I have shown that the pain that a woman experiences postnatally may relate to her care of her child, or to pathophysiological changes during or since the birth, labour or pregnancy. The duration of the pain is even less certain. Even though knowledge is increasing, there remain huge gaps in our knowledge of the duration of painful postnatal problems. Whether these gaps are filled depends on the preparedness of researchers and funding agencies to invest time and money in research which may at first sight appear unexciting and pedestrian. As Glazener and colleagues observe: '... many of the problems are not major but diminish the quality of life' (1993: 136). These researchers do not elucidate *whose* quality of life is diminished, but the effects may extend beyond the woman herself. It is only through such basic research that the first weeks, months and perhaps years of motherhood may become less painful for all involved.

Chapter 11
Fetal/Neonatal Pain

It is relatively recently that the subject of pain experienced by the neonate has been opened up to debate, which is only now resulting in serious attention being given to the closely related topic of fetal pain. Thus, many complex issues are being brought to light. In this chapter, in the hope of teasing out the issues, I focus first on the pathophysiology and then approach the ethical quagmire in which fetal/neonatal pain is submerged; I end by summarising the issues in the form of the practical applications of this material. Because the mother does, I use the term 'baby' here to indicate the fetus as well as the neonate. Additionally, when considering fetal age, postmenstrual not postconceptual age is utilised.

Traditionally, health care workers have chosen to believe that the baby does not suffer or experience pain (Franck, 1986; Penticuff, 1989; Fletcher, 1993). This belief continued at least until 1986 (Rawlinson, 1996). Such beliefs, which constitute denial, are attributable to ignorance, insensitivity, personal bias or inability to cope with the alternatives (Fletcher, 1990). This denial may be compounded to some extent by the nature of pain, which is essentially subjective. Thus, the emotional component of pain may not be identified in the fetus/neonate, leading to the concept of nociception, that is the reception of harmful stimuli, being preferred by some writers (Anand & Hickey, 1987; Fitzgerald, 1994; Campbell & Glasper, 1995).

Pathophysiological issues

In purely anatomical terms these traditional beliefs do not stand up to scrutiny. An example is the incomplete myelination of the peripheral nervous system, which has been cited to refute the existence of fetal/neonatal pain. Incomplete myelination has also been said to indicate neurological immaturity. While poor myelination may reduce the speed of conduction, one must remember that, in such small beings, the distances involved are not great so the time taken for the passage of impulses is unlikely to be greatly affected (Anand & Hickey, 1987). Following animal studies, Fitzgerald (1994) suggests that any early deficiency in myelination is corrected by the third trimester of fetal life or, after preterm birth, its neonatal equivalent.

Another example of a questionable belief is the lack of structural integrity of the neonatal nervous system. Fitzgerald's suggestion that the component parts and their connections are functional by the time of birth is progressed by Walco and colleagues, who consider the pain perception pathways to be completely developed by 29 weeks' gestation (1994). In contrast, though, the organisation of the responses may be incomplete, giving rise to less easily recognisable manifestations of pain, especially for those more accustomed to adult responses.

Another belief supporting the denial of fetal/neonatal pain is the suggestion that absence of memory of any painful event negates the potential for harm. Marshall and colleagues (1980), however, have shown that disturbed feeding and sleeping behaviour may follow inflicted or iatrogenic pain. Fitzgerald and Anand (1993) have extended this argument to suggest that responses to subsequent pain may also be affected. The Rawlinson report (1996) explains this phenomenon in terms of noxious fetal/neonatal stimuli modifying gene expression in the spinal cord to reduce pain thresholds. Such a reduction means that throughout life this person would experience greater pain following minor injury than he or she would otherwise have done. Thus, the potential for pain experience has been established, but the existence of that pain is harder to prove. Prechtl warns against attributing intentionality to the fetus when behaviour that is later characteristic of emotional states is observed (1985). Despite this caution, skin stimulation to the fetus clearly produces responses, even if they are not clearly or easily recognisably organised.

Walco and colleagues (1994) suggest that the difficulty of assessing neonatal pain may have provided another rationale for denying its existence. This suggestion is contradicted by those caring intensively for the neonate, who claim to be able to describe accurately neonatal pain expression (Penticuff, 1989; Carter, 1990; Hamblett, 1990).

Apart from the anatomical and physiological data already mentioned, the evidence for fetal/neonatal pain experience rests largely on hormonal and metabolic measures of stress (Walco *et al.*, 1994). The first study to provide fetal evidence was undertaken on babies subjected to 'intrauterine needling' for the sampling or transfusion of blood (n=30; Giannakoupoulos *et al.*, 1994). In the control group the needle was introduced at the insertion of the cord into the placenta; when this site was unavailable, intra-abdominal injection was necessary, providing the experiment group. Babies who underwent intra-abdominal injection showed increased cortisol and beta-endorphin levels, which correlated positively and significantly with the duration of the procedure. These authors interpret their data as evidence of fetal pain and recommend pain control medication prior to such interventions.

In response to this interpretation of Giannakoupoulos and colleagues' findings, Clark (1994) argues that the fetal stress response to this intervention was simply that. He states that the stress response manifests itself even in the presence of adequate analgesia and that it is an invalid proxy for pain measurement. Clark goes on to draw ludicrous comparisons, such as administering diamorphine prior to dental work or venepuncture, and questions the benefits of intrauterine analgesia. Thus, Giannakoupoulos and colleagues' attempt to open fetal pain to serious debate is effectively trivialised, just as neonatal pain has traditionally been denied and perhaps for the same reasons.

Ethical issues

Discussion of fetal and, to a lesser extent, neonatal pain inevitably raises a number of ethical issues. These relate initially to the status of the fetus, but may be broadened to the ethics of pain control more generally. While debates about fetal status are based on religious or secular principles, I consider here only secular arguments. The 'personhood' of the fetus has been used to justify his or her privileged position (Gillon, 1994). A more convincing argument in defence of the fetus's moral status may, however, be found in Gillon's 'consequentialist' argument. This view depends on the consideration extended to the fetus having the potential to benefit the person into whom the fetus develops (Benn, 1984). This argument requires the identification of the fetus with the person he or she will eventually become. Thus, fetal appearance is crucial, so that the more mature fetus is more likely to benefit (Engelhardt, 1986). While arguments about the moral status of the fetus tend to focus on the conflict between maternal and fetal rights associated with termination of pregnancy and other aspects of maternal choice, the consequentialist view clearly facilitates the serious consideration of fetal pain.

The work of Fan and colleagues (1994), who used muscle relaxants to facilitate intrauterine intervention, demonstrated the feasibility of fetal medication. It may be assumed therefore, as suggested by Giannakoupoulos and colleagues (1994), that the control of fetal pain is also feasible. The question that arises in this context, and which may also be relevant in others, is 'Because we can, must we?' In other words, is there any ethical requirement, obligation or compulsion for those who are able to control pain to do so?

Any attempt to answer this question must begin with the twin principles that underpin bioethics, that is beneficence and non-maleficence. These principles may be summarised in terms of '*primum non nocere*', which is translated as 'Above all do no harm' (Gillon, 1994). Within these safeguards the obligation to treat permits limited flexibility. Beauchamp and Childress discuss the conditions for overriding the general obligation to treat; these include pointless treatment and situations where the costs outweigh the benefits (1994). Gillon's conclusion is similar (1994), when he maintains that the practitioner is morally allowed not to obey a 'perfect duty' only when there is adequate justification for disobedience. Again, the balance of costs and benefits determines the decision of whether to treat. Unfortunately, the participant to whom the costs and benefits accrue is not always as clear. In clinical neonatal care, these principles are applied by Walco and colleagues; they argue that 'Denial of relief from pain . . . must be judged an ethically unjustified harm, unless such deprivation serves a substantially greater good' (1994: 542). This 'greater good' must be in terms of 'defined therapeutic benefits' (p. 543) and not the traditional and largely unsubstantiated beliefs with which I opened this section.

Clinical applications and the debates

Our increasing ability to observe the fetal condition, and particularly potentially life-threatening states, has led inevitably and inexorably to more and more complex intrauterine interventions (Whelton, 1993). Fetal haematological investigations and treatment have made way for fetal surgery such as vesico-amniotic shunt, to prevent pathological sequelae associated with obstructive uropathy. Intrauterine interventions will only be facilitated by fetal medication, such as that recounted by Fan and colleagues (1994; see above).

A more routine yet potentially painful intervention, whose effects have yet to be systematically investigated, is ultrasound (Beech & Robinson, 1994). The not infrequent reports of maternal recognition of changes in the pattern of fetal behaviour during ultrasound exposure remain anecdotal. The mother may attribute such a change in behaviour to unpleasant sensations:

'The scan upset the baby.'
'The baby jumped away every time the ultrasound probe was positioned.' (Beech & Robinson, 1994: 16)

More objective evidence emerged in a blind study by David and colleagues (1975), whose data showed a mean increase in fetal activity of 90% during ultrasound exposure, as assessed by fetal movement counting. The conclusion was that 'ultrasound increases fetal activity' (p. 63), but no explanation was forthcoming as to the reason. This research has not been pursued, possibly due to the huge potential of ultrasound to facilitate medical intervention.

Our increasing awareness of the likelihood of fetal pain may lead us to reassess some of the interventions which may be undertaken with little regard for the fetal effects. An example is the ubiquitous abdominal palpation which, as those of us who work in centres where fetal breathing observations are used know only too well, are associated with adverse changes in the pattern of fetal breathing. Similarly, although undertaken less frequently, any fetal effects of fetal blood sampling in labour tend to be disregarded.

Questions about neonatal pain have focused mainly on interventions such as circumcision in the North American literature and heelprick in the UK (Rushforth & Levene, 1993; Taddio *et al.*, 1997). Pharmacological remedies have been subjected to medical research (Levene, 1995), while more low-tech remedies have been studied by nursing personnel (Corff *et al.*, 1995). Penticuff (1989) extends these questions to include the cumulative effects of months of interventive activity on the vulnerable and ineffectually protesting sick neonate. The behaviourally immature pain responses associated with prolonged neonatal unit (NNU) care have been clearly demonstrated (Johnston & Stevens, 1996).

The observation and assessment of neonatal pain have shown huge strides forward recently, but their use clinically has not kept pace (McGrath & Unruh, 1994). Perhaps the multiplicity of neonatal pain scoring systems is indicative of the difficulty of devising one that is reliable and acceptable to practitioners. The neonatal infant pain score (NIPS) may be used to assess the response of preterm and term babies to needle puncture (Lawrence *et al.*, 1993). It utilises facial expression, limb movement and state of arousal, but the fact that cry and breathing pattern also feature makes it unsuitable for ventilated babies. Thus, the Distress Scale for Ventilated Newborn Infants (DSVNI) was developed for use during any invasive procedure. A pain score for the ventilated neonate should assume, as the DSVNI does, that the baby has experienced many invasive procedures and may have given up reacting to them healthily (Sparshott, 1997). When using the DSVNI, observations of facial expression and body movement, as well as recordings of heart rate, blood pressure, oxygen saturation and temperature are made before, during and after the intervention. The DSVNI demonstrates to the carer the extent to which the baby has been disquieted by the intervention as well as whether the baby has returned to a steady state subsequently. An assessment tool using only facial expression has been introduced to evaluate behavioural responses of healthy babies to acute pain such as heelprick (Rushforth & Levene, 1993). The four expressions (brow bulge, eye squeeze, nasolabial furrow and open mouth) were found significantly more frequently in babies experiencing a heelprick.

Stevens (1996) reminds us that such scoring systems were devised for and have been used to advantage in research situations. Despite this and in spite of evidence of their clinical reliability, these techniques are infrequently used in the NNU because they are time-consuming and require experienced coders.

As well as needing to assess the effect of painful invasive stimuli on a baby, it is necessary to consider the extent to which other aspects of the neonatal environment may be disturbing or discomforting. Sparshott (1997) categorises many features of the NNU environment as 'disturbing', such as light, noise, heat and nakedness. She continues by considering the 'discomforting' features of neonatal life, such as physical examination, hunger and rectal temperature taking. Clearly many of these disturbing and discomforting aspects, as well as the painful interventions, feature in the conventional care of the newborn; should we regard the responses, including pain, that they engender as iatrogenic? An example which Sparshott omits is the methods employed to elicit the Moro or startle reflex, which is part of the 'routine' physical examination. Striking the sides of the plastic cot is a fairly standard and probably anodyne method, but allowing the baby's head to drop or even smacking the baby's head are not unknown.

In the light of our knowledge of neonatal pain there are a number of possibilities for relatively straightforward changes in practice. The contribution of quality assessment should not be underestimated in such change, and this may be facilitated by parental pressure and even the 'legal community' (Walco *et al.*, 1994). Als and colleagues (1994) advocate developmentally sensitive neonatal care which minimises environmental stress and, although no claims are made to reduce pain, they may facilitate coping (Stevens, 1996). Sparshott (1997) lists the therapeutic interventions used to prevent or treat pain by pharmacological methods. She also lists the 'consolation' and 'cherishment' activities which are becoming standard, including variation in day/night lighting, noise reduction and facilitating skin-to-skin contact.

The more innovative consolation activities have been researched, such as music therapy for colicky babies (Larson & Ayllon, 1990). The mothers in the experiment group used behavioural therapy, involving rewarding non-crying with music and loving attention. Excessive crying was found to have decreased by 75% within 7 weeks. Music, however, was found to exert negligible effect on the intensely acute circumcision pain (Marchette *et al.*, 1989).

A consolation activity comprising 'nesting' in a containing and supported position during retinopathy screening was investigated by Slevin and Murphy (1996), who collected neurobehavioural and physiological data. Both groups of babies, nested and unnested, showed distressed behaviour, including defensive posture and 'swiping' movements, as well as self-consoling activity. Although the babies who were nested coped better with this invasive procedure, the findings were not statistically significant.

Perhaps because it is so frequently used, the treatment of pain caused by heelprick has been well-researched. Thirty preterm babies having 'heelsticks' were involved in a randomised trial to assess the effects of 'facilitated tucking' as a consolation activity following this procedure (Corff *et al.*, 1995). Physiological and neurobehavioural states were measured before, during and after the procedure. Facilitated tucking comprises 'gentle motoric containment of an infant's arms and legs in flexed, midline position close to the infant's trunk with the infant in a side-lying or supine position'. Facilitated tucking was associated with significantly lower heart rate change and significantly shorter periods of distress. On the basis of this study this intervention is recommended as an effective low-tech comfort measure. A similarly low-tech intervention is one that may have encountered adverse publicity. Now termed 'non-nutritive sucking', it was associated with 'dummies' or 'pacifiers' but holds out 'most promising' possibilities (Stevens, 1996: 232).

In a marginally more interventive study which raises other issues, 60 babies were randomly allocated to be given orally one of four solutions prior to heelprick (Ramenghi *et al.*, 1996). The solutions comprised sterile water, two different concentrations of sucrose and a sweet-tasting substance commercially described as sugar-free. The crying time and 3 minute pain scores were significantly reduced in those babies given the sweet-tasting substances, leading the researchers to suggest that some analgesic benefit was operating.

Clearly the major barrier to alleviating neonatal pain is in carers' attitudes, as simple yet effective non-pharmacological remedies have been identified. More interventive forms of pain control include the pharmacological approaches, which may be indicated postoperatively or during invasive diagnostic/therapeutic procedures. Their administration may be hampered by pharmacokinetic (movement within the body) and pharmacodynamic (dose-response) complexity in neonates and preterm infants; these phenomena differ markedly between babies and even more from adults (Stevens, 1996). Opioids' benefits are hindered by their lesser analgesic effects, especially when compared with the relative increase in the risk of respiratory depression. The non-opioid analgesics have little role in neonatal care because of problems such as uncertain efficacy and safety and their binding properties aggravating jaundice (Stevens, 1996).

Variability in the application of our knowledge of neonatal pain control was brought home to me after I was asked by a concerned mother whether her newborn daughter would be given 'pain killers' after her forthcoming surgery. On the basis of my reading about changing attitudes to neonatal pain, I reassured her. Discussing this with a neonatal nurse colleague later, I learned that my confidence had been misplaced. Apparently, the surgical unit to which the baby was transferred still clung to the outdated attitudes to neonatal pain with which I began this chapter.

Summary

I have established the importance of fetal/neonatal pain and I have considered the reasons for the variable impact of this knowledge on practice. The issue of fetal pain is so closely linked to the abortion debate that it has effectively been hijacked by the anti-choice lobby. This has resulted in it being a 'no go' area in relation to other areas of concern, such as ultrasound and fetal investigations (Peacock & Furedi, 1996). Unfortunately, this link in no way explains the limited application of this knowledge in neonatal care. These questions become more urgent when we recall that local anaesthetic is being recommended to be administered routinely prior to intravenous cannulation in adults.

Chapter 12
Conclusion

To summarise the argument that I have advanced in this book, I would like to focus on the significance of pain in childbearing. Having examined its individual or personal meanings already (Chapters 1 and 2), considering pain's meaning in more global terms may answer the question 'Why does pain in childbearing matter?' The answer may lie in the words that we use. As I mentioned in the Preface, pain tends to be addressed in terms of needing to be 'managed' at best, or more likely needing to be 'challenged', 'defeated' or 'conquered'. Are we really meant to believe, however, that these attacks on pain are intended only to relieve pain? Is it pure humanitarian altruism that underpins these attempts to resolve pain in childbearing? I suspect not.

My suspicion is supported by changing attitudes to pain memories. It was the obliteration of the memory of pain, rather than the pain itself, that was for the first half of this century the remedy for childbearing pain (Chamberlain, 1993). However, although having spent so long seeking obliteration of the memory of labour pain, our medical colleagues now argue that it 'is soon forgotten' (Reynolds, 1997b). This *volte-face* endorses my belief that other agendas are operating.

What are these agendas? It may be that extending the boundaries of knowledge through research encourages interest in remedying child-bearing pain. Alternatively, it has been suggested that increasing certain occupational groups' power base may be a factor (Mander, 1993b). A third possibility is even less acceptable. This is the reason suggested by Hardy (1991: 62) that staff encounter difficulty coping with a woman who is 'awake', 'moaning' or frequently 'moving position'. The quiet, smoothly functioning labour ward may, according to Schott and Henley (1996: 167), be interpreted as a sign of 'professional competence'. This quietness may be elevated to an art form, as recounted by an NCT teacher:

'Some years ago I was taken round a labour ward by the sister in charge. She stopped in the corridor and said "Listen". I could hear nothing and said so. "I know", she said, "aren't epidurals wonderful things?"' (Schott & Henley, 1996: 167)

Our medical colleagues' impotence may be influencing these attitudes as they write:

> 'My discomfort in the labour ward has been due to a feeling of barbarism when standing over someone in obvious pain which could easily be avoided or relieved.... "Shouldn't we be doing something?"' (Wilson, 1994: 447)

Thus, the rationale for attempting to control childbearing pain may be less than transparent. The intervention by which pain is controlled, though, may correlate with other interventions in childbearing in a number of ways. First, the prevention of pain may be presented as the rationale for intervention. Next, those interventions may, perhaps inadvertently, engender or aggravate the woman's pain. Additionally, the cultural environment in which the pain occurs may have been subjected to interventions that reduce the individual's ability to cope with pain. I will now examine more closely these associations.

Preventing pain as a rationale for intervention

The amelioration of the woman's pain, in terms of its intensity and/or its duration, may provide a rationale for interventions which directly aim to avoid the pain or indirectly aim to shorten the labour. The ultimate example of such an intervention is the Dublin protocol (O'Driscoll & Meagher, 1986). Its initiators cited humane altruism as the reason for the introduction of this battery of interventions, by reducing the duration of the woman's suffering. This claim contradicts the reports of women having labour augmented, who tell me that amniotomy or oxytocic administration brings an abrupt and unforeseen increase in their pain intensity. Thus, although pain is an inevitable aspect of physiological childbearing, it may, because of medicalisation, constitute a challenge. In this way pain, which in other contexts is inextricably associated with disease, is perceived, like disease, as presenting a challenge to be overcome. This view contrasts with regarding childbearing pain as an integral component of a physiological process which the woman is able to employ constructively.

Pain as a consequence of intervention

As well as happening spontaneously and usually physiologically in childbearing, pain is further significant because it may be caused in the course of treatment, that is following interventions in childbearing which are intended to be beneficial. These are the forms of pain that could appropriately be described as iatrogenic (Penn, 1986: 14; Melzack & Wall, 1991). The augmentation of labour mentioned above may serve as one example, but other examples are better documented.

One example of iatrogenic pain is our use of vaginal examination (VE) in labour, which has been shown to be both distasteful and painful for the woman (Bergstrom *et al.*, 1992; Clement, 1994) as well as carrying long-term consequences (Menage, 1993). Uncertainty about the need for this intervention has been aggravated by the serious doubts which have been cast on the value of the information thus obtained (Tuffnell *et al.*, 1989; Robson, 1992). The contribution of this 'invasive intervention of as yet unproved value' (Enkin, 1992: 20) needs researching if its routine use is to continue.

A further example of iatrogenic pain is found in the literature on perineal suturing. That this intervention is painful for the woman is well-known (Wraight, 1993), but the need for it to be undertaken routinely is less clear (Chapter 10). The need for suturing is further called into question by the increasing body of evidence indicating the hazardous use of particular suture materials and techniques (Howard *et al.*, 1995b). Thus, the pain of suturing as well as the longer term perineal pain is iatrogenic.

My final and ultimate example of iatrogenic pain, in that it comprises an intervention in a physiological process which may actually engender pain, is postepidural back pain. Our obstetric anaesthetist colleagues, though, continue to 'protest too much' against its existence (Reynolds, 1997a).

Cultural iatrogenesis

Having considered examples of iatrogenic pain which are specific to childbearing, it is now necessary to look more broadly at the Western societal attitude to pain. As Illich suggests (1976), there is a movement to persuade individuals that they are unable to cope with or endure pain, which, he maintains, is largely medically driven and is summarised thus: 'Medical enterprise saps the will of people to suffer their reality' (Illich, 1976: 127).

As I have discussed (Chapter 1), culture lends meaning to pain, including childbearing pain, which in turn, Illich maintains, imbues the person with the ability to cope (1976). Traditional coping skills, which have grown up over centuries and generations of women, are 'trammeled' by medical progress. Thus, by depriving the person of the suffering, she is denied the opportunity to enjoy the success of coping (p. 128) and the sense of achievement which it brings with it (Flint, 1997). Women find themselves being encouraged not to cope by being told, 'You don't get a medal for being a martyr' (Langford, 1997: 6).

It may be that Illich's words are particularly apposite in the context of childbearing pain: 'Now an increasing portion of all pain is man-made.' (1976: 135)

References

Abboud, T.K., Sarkis, F., Hung, T.T. (1983) Effects of epidural anaesthesia during labour on maternal plasma beta-endorphin levels. *Anesthesiology* 59(1), 1–5.

Abboud, T.K., Yanage, T., Artal, R., Costandi, J., Henriksen, E. (1985) Effects of epidural analgesia during labour on fetal plasma catecholamine release. *Regional Anesthesia* 10(4), 170–174.

Abouleish, E., Depp, R. (1975) Acupuncture in obstetrics. *Anesthetic Analgesia* 54, 83–8.

Abu-Saed, H., Tesler, M. (1986) Pain. In: *Pathophysiologic Phenomenon in Nursing* (eds V. Carrier & A. West), pp. 235–69. W.B. Saunders, Philadelphia.

Achterberg, J. (1990). *Woman as Healer*. Rider, London.

Adams, J.Q., Alexander, A.M., Jr (1958) Alterations in cardiovascular physiology during labour. *Obstetrics and Gynaecology* 12 (whole volume), 542–9

Ader, L., Hansson, B., Wallin, G. (1990) Parturition pain treated by intracutaneous injections of sterile water. *Pain* 41(2), 133–8.

Adoni, A., Anteby, E. (1991) The use of histoacryl for episiotomy repair. *British Journal of Obstetrics and Gynaecology*, 98(5), 476–8

Ahlborg, G., Axelsson, J., Bodin, L. (1996) Shift work nitrous oxide exposure and subfertility among Swedish midwives. *International Journal of Epidemiology* 25(4), 783–90.

Ahmad, W.I.V. (1993) *The Politics of 'Race' and Health*. University of Bradford.

Albe-Fessard, D., Levante, A., Lamour, Y. (1974) Origins of spinothalamic and spinoreticular pathways in cats and monkeys. In: *Advances in Neurology 4* (ed J. Bonica), pp. 157–68. Raven Press, New York.

Alderdice, F., Renfrew, M., Marchant, S., *et al.* (1995) Labour and birth in water in England and Wales: survey report. *British Journal of Midwifery* 3(7), 375–82.

Allbright, G.A., Joyce, T.H., Stevenson, D.K. (1986) Systemic analgesia. In: *Anaesthesia in Obstetrics* (eds G.A. Allbright, J.E. Ferguson, T.H. Joyce, D.K. Stevenson). Butterworths, London.

Allcock, N. (1996a) The use of different research methodologies to evaluate effectiveness of programmes to improve the care of patients in postoperative pain. *Journal of Advanced Nursing* 23(1), 32–8.

Allcock, N. (1996b). Factors affecting the assessment of postoperative pain. *Journal of Advanced Nursing* 24:6, 1144–51.

Allotey, J.C., Louca, O. (1997). Thromboembolic disorders: treatment and diagnosis. *British Journal of Midwifery* 5(2), 75–9.

Als, H., Lawhon, G., Duffy, F., McAnulty, G.B., Gibes-Grossman, R., Blickman, J.G. (1994) Individualised development care for the very low birth weight preterm infant. *Journal of the American Medical Association* 272(11), 853–8.

Amir, L.H., Dennerstein, L., Garland, S.N., Farish, S.J. (1996) Psychological aspects of nipple pain in lactating women. *Journal of Psychosomatic Obstetrics and Gynaecology*, 17(1), 53–8.

Anand, K.J.S., Hickey, P.R. (1987) Pain and its effects in the human neonate and fetus. *New England Journal of Medicine* 317(21), 1321–9

Ananth, C.V., Wilcox, A.J., Savitzda, D.A., Bowes, W.A., Luther, E.R. (1996) Effect of maternal age and parity on the risk of uteroplacental bleeding disorders in pregnancy. *Obstetrics and Gynaecology* 88 (4Pt1), 511–16

Anderson, K.N. (ed) (1994) *Mosby's Medical Nursing and Allied Health Dictionary*. Mosby, St Louis.

Andrews, C.M., Chrzanowski, M. (1990) Maternal position, labour, and comfort. *Applied Nursing Research* 3, 7.

Andrews, C.M., O'Neill, L.M. (1994) Use of pelvic tilt exercise for ligament pain relief. *Journal of Nurse-Midwifery* 39(6), 370–374.

Anionwu, E.N. (1996) Sickle cell and thalassaemia: some priorities for nursing research. *Journal of Advanced Nursing* 23(5), 853–5.

APA & NPSP (1982) *Handbook of Non-prescription Drugs, 7th edn. Drug Information for the Health Care Professional*. American Pharmaceutical Society and National Professional Society of Pharmacists, Washington.

Argyle, M. (1989) *The Social Psychology of Work*. Penguin, Harmondsworth.

Arndt, M. (1994) Nurses' medication errors. *Journal of Advanced Nursing* 19(3), 19–26.

Arney, W.R. (1982) *Power and the Profession of Obstetrics*. University of Chicago Press, Chicago.

Arney, W., Neill, J. (1982) The location of pain in natural childbirth: natural childbirth and the transformation of obstetrics. *Sociology of Health and Illness* 7(1), 375–400.

Arthurs, G. (1994) Hypnosis and acupuncture in pregnancy. *British Journal of Midwifery*, 2(10), 495–8.

Astley, A. (1990) A history of pain. *Nursing* 4(17), 33–5.

Atkinson, F.I. (1988) Non-response rates in nursing research. *Senior Nurse* 8(5), 23.

Atlay, R.D., Gillison, E.W., Horton, A.L. (1973) A fresh look at pregnancy heartburn. *Journal of Obstetrics and Gynaecology of the British Commonwealth* 80, 63–6.

Audit Commission (1997). *First Class Delivery: improving Maternity Services in England and Wales*. HMSO, London.

Baines, M. (1990) *Living With Dying: The Management of Terminal Disease*. Oxford University Press, Oxford.

Balaskas, J., Gordon, Y. (1990) *Waterbirth*. Unwin, London.

Ball, J.A. (1991) Foreword. In: *Postnatal Care: A Research-Based Approach* (eds J. Alexander, V. Levy, R.S. Roch). Macmillan, London.

Ball, J.A. (1993) Complications of the puerperium. In: *Myles Textbook for*

Midwives (eds V.R. Bennett & L.K. Brown), pp. 477–88. Churchill Livingstone, Edinburgh.

Bancroft, J. (1994) *Human Sexuality and Its Problems*, 2nd edn. Churchill Livingstone, Edinburgh.

Banks, E. (1992) Labouring in comfort. *Nursing Times* 88(31), 40–41.

Bansen, S.S. Stevens, H.A. (1992) Women's experiences of miscarriage in early pregnancy. *Journal of Nurse-Midwifery* 37(2), 84–90.

Banta, D., Thacker, S.B. (1982) Benefits and risks of episiotomy. *Birth* 9(1), 25–30.

Baram, D.A. (1995) Hypnosis in reproductive health care: a review and case reports. *Birth*, 22(1), 37–42.

Barclay, L.M. Everitt, L., Rogan, F., Schmied, V., Wyllie, A. (1997) Becoming a mother – an analysis of women's experience of early motherhood. *Journal of Advanced Nursing* 25(4), 719–28.

Barclay, L.M., Lloyd, B. (1996) The misery of motherhood: alternative approaches to maternal distress. *Midwifery* 12(3), 136–9.

Barker, P.J. (1991) Interview. In: *The Research Process in Nursing* (ed D.F.S. Cormack). Blackwell Science, Oxford.

Barry, C, Fox, R., Stirrat, G. (1994) Upper abdominal pain in pregnancy may indicate pre-eclampsia. *British Medical Journal* 308(6943), 1562–3.

Basbaum, A.I., Clanton, C.H., Fields, H.L. (1976) Opiate and stimulus-produced analgesia: functional anatomy of a medullospinal pathway. *Proceedings of the National Academy of Sciences of the United States of America* 73(12), 4685–8.

Basbaum, A.I., Fields, H.L. (1978) Endogenous pain control mechanisms: review and hypothesis. *Annals of Neurology* 4(5), 451–62.

Baskett, T.F. (1985) *Essential Management of Obstetric Emergencies*, pp. 43–52. John Wiley, Chichester.

Baylis, C., Davison, J. (1991) The urinary system. In: *Clinical Physiology of Obstetrics* (F.E. Hytten & G. Chamberlain), pp. 245–302. Blackwell Science, Oxford.

Bayliss, P.F.C. (1980) *Law on Poisons, Medicines and Related Substances*. Ravenswood, Beckenham.

Beard, R.W. (1978) Future developments in obstetrics. *Midwife, Health Visitor and Community Nurse* August.

Beauchamp, T.L., Childress, J.F. (1994) *Principles of Biomedical Ethics*, 4th edn. Oxford University Press, Oxford.

Beech, B.L. (1995a) Conscious during a general anaesthetic caesarean operation. *AIMS Journal* 7(3), 8–10.

Beech, B.L. (1995b) Water labour water birth. *AIMS Journal* 7(1), 1–3.

Beech, B.L., Robinson, J. (1994) *Ultrasound – Unsound*. Association for the Improvement in Maternity Services, London.

Beinart, J. (1990) Obstetric analgesia and the control of childbirth in twentieth-century Britain. In: *The Politics of Maternity Care: Services for Child-bearing Women in Twentieth-Century Britain* (J. Garcia, R. Kilpatrick & M.P.M. Richards), pp. 116–32. Clarendon, Oxford.

Bendelow, G.A., Williams, S.J. (1995) Transcending the dualisms: towards a sociology of pain. *Sociology of Health and Illness* 17(2), 139–65.

Benn, S.J. (1984) Abortion infanticide and respect for persons. In: *The*

Problem of Abortion (ed J. Feinberg), pp. 135–44. Wadsworth, Belmont.

Bennett, R.L., Batenhorst, R.L., Bivens, B.A., Bell, R.M., Graves, D.A., Foster, T.S. (1992) Patient controlled analgesia: a new concept of pain relief. *Annals of Surgery* 195(6), 700–704.

Bennett, V.R., Brown, L.K. (eds) (1993) *Myles Textbook for Midwives*. Churchill Livingstone, Edinburgh.

Benson, H., Beary, J.F., Carol, M.P. (1974) The relaxation response. *Psychiatry* 37, 37.

Benson, H., Kotch, J.B., Crassweiler, K.D., Greenwood, M.M. (1977) Historical and clinical considerations of the relaxation response. *American Scientist* 65, 441–5.

Bensoussan, A. (1991) *The Vital Meridian: A Modern Exploration of Acupuncture*. Churchill Livingstone, Edinburgh.

Bergstrom, L., Roberts, J., Skillman L., Seidel, J. (1992) 'You'll feel me touching you, sweetie . . .'. *Birth* 19(1), 10–18.

Bergum, V. (1989) *Woman to Mother: A Transformation*. Bergin and Harvey Publishers, Massachusetts.

Bernat, S., Woolridge, J.P., Snell, L. (1992) Biofeedback assisted relaxation to reduce stress in labour. *Journal of Obstetric Gynaecological and Neonatal Nursing* 21(4), 295–303.

Beutel, M., Deckhardt, R., von Rad, M., Wiener, H. (1995) Grief and depression after miscarriage. *Psychosomatic Medicine* 57(6), 517–26.

Bishop, B. (1980) Pain: its physiology and rationale for management: analgesic systems of the CNS. *Physical Therapy* 60(1), 21–3.

Blackburn, S.T., Loper, D.L. (1992) *Maternal, Fetal and Neonatal Physiology: A Clinical Perspective*. W.B. Saunders, Philadelphia.

Blair, R.W., Ammons, W.S., Foreman, R.D. (1984) Responses of thoracic spinothalamic and spinoreticular cells to coronary artery occlusion. *Journal of Neurophysiology* 51(4), 636–48.

Blanchard, E.B., Ahles, T.A. (1990) Biofeedback therapy. In: *The Management of Pain*, 2nd edn. (eds J.J. Bonica, J.D. Loesser, C.R. Chapman & W.E. Fordyce). Lea & Febiger, Philadelphia.

Blanchard, E.B., Epstein, L.H. (1978). *A Biofeedback Primer*. M.A. Addison-Wesley, Reading.

Blendis, L.A. (1994) Abdominal pain. In: *Textbook of Pain*, 3rd edn. (eds P.D. Wall & R. Melzack). Churchill Livingstone, Edinburgh.

Bloomfield, S.S., Mitchell, J., Cissel, G., Barden, T.P. (1986) Flurbiprofen aspirin codeine and placebo for postpartum uterine pain. *American Journal of Medicine* 24(80)(a), 65–70.

Bobak, I.M. (1993) Second trimester. In: *Maternity and Gynecologic Care: The Nurse and the Family*, 5th edn. (I.M. Bobak & M.D. Jensen), pp. 299–319. Mosby, St Louis.

Bobak, I.M., Jensen, M.D. (1993) *Maternity and Gynecologic Care: The Nurse and the Family*, 5th edn. Mosby, St Louis.

Bobak, I.M., Starn, J.R. (1993) Third trimester. *Maternity and Gynecologic Care: The Nurse and the Family*, 5th edn. (I.M. Bobak & M.D. Jensen), pp. 321–47. Mosby, St Louis.

Bogod, D. (1995) Advances in epidural analgesia for labour: progress versus prudence. *Lancet*, 345, 1129–30.

Bond, M.R. (1984) *Pain: Its Nature, Analysis and Treatment.* Churchill Livingstone, Edinburgh.

Bonica, J.J. (1973) Maternal respiratory changes during pregnancy and parturition. In: *Parturition and Perinatology* (ed G.F. Marx), pp. 1–19. F.A. Davis, Philadelphia.

Bonica, J.J. (1975) The nature of pain of parturition. In: *Obstetric Analgesia–Anaesthesia: Recent Advances and Current Status* (J.J. Bonica). W.B. Saunders, Philadelphia.

Bonica, J.J. (1980) Labour pain: mechanisms and pathways. In: (eds G.F. Marx & G.M. Bassell), *Obstetric Analgesia and Anesthesia*, pp. 173–95. Elsevier/North-Holland Biomedical Press, Amsterdam.

Bonica, J.J. (1990a) History of pain concepts and therapies. In: *The Management of Pain*, 2nd edn. (J.J. Bonica, J.D. Loeser, C.R. Chapman & W.E. Fordyce), Chapter 1. Lea & Febiger, Philadelphia.

Bonica, J.J. (1990b) Painful disorders of the respiratory system. In: *The Management of Pain*, 2nd edn. (J.J. Bonica, J.D. Loeser, C.R. Chapman & W.E. Fordyce), pp. 1043–61) Lea & Febiger, Philadelphia.

Bonica, J.J. (1994) Labour pain. In: *Textbook of Pain*, 3rd edn. (eds P.D. Wall & R. Melzack), pp. 615–41. Churchill Livingstone, Edinburgh.

Bonica, J.J. Albe-Fessard, D. (1976) *Advances in Pain Research and Therapy* 1. Raven Press, New York.

Bonica, J.J., Chadwick, H.S. (1989) Labour pain. In: *Textbook of Pain* (eds P.D. Wall & R. Melzack), pp. 482–99. Churchill Livingstone, New York.

Bonica, J.J., McDonald, J.S. (1990) The pain of childbirth. In: *The Management of Pain*, 2nd edn. (J.J. Bonica, J.D. Loeser, C.R. Chapman & W.E. Fordyce), pp. 1313–43. Lea & Febiger, Philadelphia.

Bonica, J.J. Ueland, K. (1969) Heart disease. In: *Principles and Practice of Obstetric Analgesia and Anesthesia* 2nd edn. (ed. J.J. Bonica), pp. 941–77. F.A. Davis, Philadelphia.

Bonnel, A.M., Boureau, F. (1985) Labour pain assessment: validity of a behavioural index. *Pain* 22(1), 81–90.

Booth, B. (1993a) Hypnotherapy. *Nursing Times*, 89(40), 42–5.

Booth, B. (1993b) Shiatsu. *Nursing Times* 89(46), 38–40.

Booth, B. (1993c) Therapeutic Touch. *Nursing Times* 89(31), 48–50.

Booth, B. (1994) Reflexology. *Nursing Times* 90(1), 38–40.

Boswell, M.V., Hameroff, S.R. (1996) Theoretical mechanisms of general anesthesia. In: *Physiologic and Pharmacologic Bases of Anesthesia* (ed V.J. Collins), Chapter 25. Williams Wilkins, Baltimore.

Bourbonnais, F. (1981) Pain assessment: development of a tool for the nurse and the patient. *Journal of Advanced Nursing* 6(4), 277–82.

Bowlby, J. (1969) *Attachment and Loss. Volume 1: Attachment.* Hogarth, London.

Bowler, I.M.W. (1993) Stereotypes of women of Asian descent in midwifery: some evidence. *Midwifery* 9(1), 7–16.

Bracken, M., Enkin, M., Campbell, H., Chalmers, I. (1989) Symptoms in pregnancy: nausea and vomiting, heartburn, constipation and leg cramps. In: *Effective Care in Pregnancy and Childbirth* (eds I. Chalmers, M. Enkin & M.J.N.C. Keirse), pp. 501–511. Oxford University Press, Oxford.

Brayshaw, E. (1993) Special exercises for pregnancy, labour and the puerperium. In: *Myles Textbook for Midwives* (eds V.R. Bennett & L.K. Brown), pp. 633–47. Churchill Livingstone, Edinburgh.

Breen, T.W., Ransil, B.J., Groves, P.A., Oriol, N.E. (1994) Factors associated with back pain after childbirth. *Anesthesiology*, 81(1), 29–34.

Brettle, R.P., MacCallum, C.J. Murdoch, J.McC., Gray, J.A. (1986) The adult female – a 20-year study of bacteriuria in female patients. In: *Microbial Diseases in Nephrology* (W.W. Asscher & W. Brumfitt), pp. 257–72. Wiley, Chichester.

Brodwin, P.E., Kleinman, A. (1987) The social meanings of chronic pain. In: *Handbook of Chronic Pain Management* (G.D. Burrows, D. Elton & G.V. Stanley) Elsevier, Amsterdam.

Brooten, D.A., Brown, L.P., Hollingsworth, A.O., Tanis, J.L., Donlen, J. (1983) A comparison of four treatments to prevent and control breast pain and engorgement in nursing mothers. *Nursing Research* 32(4), 225–9.

Brown, A.G., Fyffe, R.E.W. (1981) Form and function of dorsal horn neurones with axons ascending the dorsal column in cat. *Journal of Physiology*, 321 (whole volume), 31–47.

Brown, A.G., Hamann, W.C., Martin, H.G. (1975) Effects of activity in non-myelinated afferent fibres on the spinocervical tract. *Brain Research* 98(2), 243–59.

Brown, C. (1982) Therapeutic effects of bathing during labor. *Journal of Nurse-Midwifery* 27, 13–6.

Brownridge, P. (1995) The nature and consequences of childbirth. *European Journal of Obstetrics and Gynecology*, 59 (Suppl.), S9–S15.

Brozovic, M., Davies, S.C., Brownell, A.I. (1987) Acute admissions of patients with sickle cell disease who live in Britain. *British Medical Journal* 294, 1206–1208.

Brucker, M.C. (1988) Managing gastrointestinal problems in pregnancy. *Journal of Nurse-Midwifery* 33(2), 67–73.

Brunner, L.S., Suddarth, D.S. (1992) *The Textbook of Adult Nursing.* Chapman Hall, London.

Bundsen, P., Ericson, K. (1982) Pain relief in labour by transcutaneous electrical nerve stimulation: safety aspects. *Acta Obstetrica Gynecologica Scandinavica* 61, 1–5.

Burgess, P.R. (1974) Patterns of discharge evoked in cutaneous nerves and their significance for sensation. In: *Advances in Neurology*, 4th edn. (ed J.J. Bonica), pp. 11–18. Raven Press, New York.

Butler, M. (1995) Use of anticoagulants in hospital and community. *Nursing Times* 91(29), 36–7.

Caldeyro-Barcia, R.S., Poseiro, J.J. (1960) Physiology of the uterine contraction. *Clinical Obstetrics and Gynaecology* 3(2), 386–408.

Calguneri, M., Bird, H.A. Wright, V. (1982) Changes in joint laxity occurring during pregnancy. *Annals of the Rheumatic Diseases* 41, 126–8.

Callam, M.J. (1994) Epidemiology of varicose veins. *British Journal of Surgery*, 81(2), 167–73.

Cammu, H., Clasen, K., van Wettere, L., Derde, M.P. (1994) 'To bathe or not to bathe' during the first stage. *Acta Obstetrica Gynecologica Scandinavica* 73(6), 468–72.

Campbell, S., Glasper, E.A. (1995) *Whaley and Wong's Children's Nursing.* Mosby, St Louis.

Campion, M.J. (1990) *The Baby Challenge: A Handbook on Pregnancy for Women with a Physical Disability.* Routledge, London.

Cannon, W.B. (1932) *The Wisdom of the Body.* Appleton, New York.

Carlisle, D. (1996) An injection of danger. *Nursing Times* 92(34), 26–8.

Carter, B. (1990) A universal experience. *Paediatric Nursing,* 2(7), 8–10.

Carter, J., Duriez, T. (1986) *With Child: Birth Through the Ages.* Mainstream Publishing, Edinburgh.

Cartwright, D. (1979) Contemporary social psychology in historical perspective. *Social Psychology Quarterly* 42(1), 82–93.

Carty, E.A., Conine, T.A. (1983) *Childbirth Education for Women with Arthritis.* British Columbia Health Care Research Foundation, University of British Columbia.

Carty, E.A., Conine, T.A., Wood-Johnson, F. (1986) Rheumatoid arthritis pregnancy: helping women to meet their needs. *Midwives Chronicle* 99(1186), 254–6.

Cassell, E.J. (1982) The nature of suffering and the goals of medicine. *New England Journal of Medicine* 206, 639–42.

Castro, M. (1992) *Homeopathy for Mother and Baby.* Macmillan, London.

Caton, D. (1985) The secularisation of pain. *Anaesthesiology* 62, 493–501.

Cawthra, A.M. (1986) The use of pethidine in labour. *Midwives Chronicle* 99 (1183), 178–81.

Cerveno, F., Iggo, A., Molony, V. (1977) Responses of spinocervical tract neurones to noxious stimulation to the skin. *Journal of Physiology,* 267 (2), 537–58.

Chalmers, I. (1993) Effective care in midwifery: research, the professions and the public. *Midwives Chronicle,* 106 (1260), 3–12.

Chalmers, I., Enkin, M., Keirse, M.J.N.C. (1989) *Effective Care in Pregnancy and Childbirth.* Oxford University Press, Oxford.

Chalmers, I., Grant, A. (1996) Salutary lessons from the collaborative eclampsia trial. *Evidence-based Medicine* 1(2), 39–40.

Chamberlain, G. (1993) The history of pain relief in labour. In: *Pain and its Relief in Childbirth* (G. Chamberlain, A. Wraight & P. Steer), Chapter 1. Churchill Livingstone, Edinburgh.

Chamberlain, G., Wraight, A., Steer, P. (1993) *Pain and its Relief in Childbirth.* Churchill Livingstone, Edinburgh.

Chapman, C.R. (1984) New directions in the understanding and management of pain. *Social Science & Medicine* 19, 1261–77.

Chapman, C.R., Gunn, C.C. (1990) Acupuncture. In: *The Management of Pain,* 2nd edn. (eds J.J. Bonica, J.D. Loeser, C.R. Chapman & W.E. Fordyce), pp. 1805–1821. Lea & Febiger, Philadelphia.

Chapman, R. (1985) Psychological factors in post-operative pain. In: *Acute Pain* (eds G. Smith & B. Corino), pp. 22–41. Butterworths, London.

Cherny, N.I., Portenoy, R.K. (1994) The management of cancer pain. *Cancer: Journal of Clinical Care* 44(5), 263–303.

Chesley, L.C. (1978) *Hypertensive Disorders in Pregnancy.* Appleton Century Crofts, New York.

Chestnut, D.H., McGrath, J.M., Vincent, R.D. *et al.* (1994) Does early administration of epidural analgesia affect obstetric outcome in nulliparous women who are in spontaneous labour? *Anaesthesiology* 80, 1201–1208.

Chestnut, D.H., Vandewalker, G.E., Owen, O.L., Bates., J.N., Choi, W.W. (1987) The influence of continuous epidural bupivicaine analgesia on the second stage of labour and method of delivery on the nulliparous woman. *Anaesthesiology* 66, 774–80.

Cheung, N.F. (1994) Pain in normal labour. *Midwives Chronicle* 107 (1277), 212–16.

Church, S., Lyne, P. (1994) Research-based practice: some problems illustrated by the discussion of evidence concerning the use of pressure-relieving devices in nursing and midwifery. *Journal of Advanced Nursing* 19(3), 513–18.

Clark, D.A. (1994) Stress without distress: the intrauterine perspective. *Lancet* 344 (8915), 73–4.

Claye, A.M. (1954) Obstetric anaesthesia and analgesia. In: *Historical Review of British Obstetrics and Gynaecology 1800–1950* (eds J.M. Munro-Kerr, R.W. Johnstone & M.H. Phillips), Chapter 27. Churchill Livingstone, Edinburgh.

Clement, S. (1994) Unwanted vaginal examinations. *British Journal of Midwifery* 2(8), 368–70.

Cloake, M. (1991) Report on Confidential Enquiries into maternal deaths in the UK 1985–7: a summary of the main points. *Health Trends* 23(1), 4–5.

Cluett, E. (1994) Analgesia in labour: a review of the TENS method. *Professional Care of Mother and Child* 4(2), 50–52.

Cochrane, S. (1992) Perineal trauma. *Nursing Times* 88(21), 64.

Cockshoot, A. (1995) Diastasis symphysis pubis – a painful problem. *Changing Childbirth Update* 4, 10.

Cohen, A. (1974) Introduction. In: *Urban Ethnicity* (ed A. Cohen) Tavistock ASA Monographs: 12, London.

Cohen, M. (1961) *Nature: The Philosophy of John Stuart Mill*. Modern Library, New York.

Cole, P.V., Nainby-Luxmoore, R.C. (1962) Respiratory volumes in labour. *British Medical Journal* 1(5285), 1118.

Combes, G., Schonveld, A. (1992) *Life Will Never be the Same Again: Learning to be a First-Time Parent*. Health Education Authority, London.

Conduit, E. (1995) *The Body Under Stress: Developing Skills for Keeping Healthy*. Erlbaum Associates, Hove.

Cooper, P.J. Murray, L., Hooper, R., West, A. (1995) The development and validation of a predictive index for postpartum depression. *Psychological Medicine* 26(3), 627–34.

Copp, L.A. (1974) The spectrum of suffering. *American Journal of Nursing* 74, 491.

Copp, L.A. (1985) *Recent Advances in Nursing: Perspectives on Pain*. Churchill Livingstone, Edinburgh.

Copp, L.A. (1994) Illness and the human spirit. *Quality of Life* 2(3), 50–55.

Copstick, S., Hayes, R.W., Taylor, K.E., Morris, N.F. (1985) A test of a common assumption regarding the use of antenatal training during labour. *Journal of Psychosomatic Research* 20, 215–18.

Corff, K.E., Seiderman, R., Venkaraman, P.S., Lutes, P., Yates, B. (1995) Facilitated tucking: a non-pharmacologic comfort measure for pain in preterm neonates. *Journal of Obstetric, Gynecological and Neonatal Nursing* 24(2), 143–7.

Cottrell, B.H., Shannahan, M.D. (1986) Effect of the birth chair on duration of second stage labor and maternal outcome. *Nursing Research* 35(6), 364–7.

Covino, B. (1993) Local anesthetics. In: *Postoperative Pain Management* (eds F.M. Ferrante & T.R. Vadebonoueur), pp. 211–53. Churchill Livingstone, New York.

Cox, B.M. (1990) Drug tolerance and physical dependence. In: *Principles of Drug Action: The Basis of Pharmacology*, 3rd edn. (W.B. Pratt & P. Taylor), pp. 639–90. Churchill Livingstone, Edinburgh.

Cox, J.L. (1986) *Postnatal Depression: A Guide for Health Professionals.* Churchill Livingstone, Edinburgh.

Craig, K.D., Wyckoff, M.G. (1987) Cultural factors in chronic pain management. In: *Handbook of Chronic Pain Management* (G.D. Burrows, D. Elton & G.V. Stanley), p. 99. Elsevier, Amsterdam.

Craigin, E. (1916) Conservatism in obstetrics. *New York State Journal of Medicine*, 104, 1.

Crasilneck, H.B., Hall, J.A. (1985) *Clinical Hypnosis: Principles and Applications*, 2nd edn. Grune Stratton, Orlando.

Crowe, K, von Bayer, C. (1989) Predictors of a positive childbirth experience. *Birth* 16(2), 59–63.

Crowell, M.K., Hill, P.D., Humenick, S.S. (1994) Relationship between obstetric analgesia and time of effective breast feeding. *Journal of Nurse-Midwifery* 39(3), 150–156.

Crown, J. (1989) *Report of the Advisory Group on Nurse Prescribing.* Department of Health, London.

Culp, E., Osofsky, H.J. (1989) Effects of cesarean on parental depression, marital adjustment and mother–infant interaction. *Birth* 16(2), 53–8.

Cumberlege, J. (1986) *Neighbourhood Nursing: A Focus for Care.* Department of Health and Social Security, London.

Cunningham, F.G., Lucas, M.J. (1994) Urinary tract infections complicating pregnancy. *Baillière's Clinical Obstetrics and Gynaecology* 8(2), 353–73.

Cupit, G.C., Rotmensch, H.H. (1992) Principles of drug therapy. In: *Principles and Practice of Medical Therapy in Pregnancy* (ed N. Gleicher), pp. 68–79. Appleton & Lange, Norwalk.

Dahl, V. Aames, T. (1991) Sterile water papulae for analgesia during labour. *Tidsskr Nor Laegeforen* 111(12), 1484–7.

Dahle, L.O., Berg, G., Hammar, M., Hurtig, M., Larsson, L. (1995) The effect of oral magnesium substitution on pregnancy-induced leg cramps. *American Journal of Obstetrics and Gynecology* 173(1), 175–80.

Dale, A., Cornwell, S. (1994) The role of lavender oil in relieving perineal discomfort following childbirth: a blind randomised controlled trial. *Journal of Advanced Nursing* 19(1), 89–96.

Daley, B. (1997) Therapeutic touch, nursing practice and contemporary cutaneous wound healing research. *Journal of Advanced Nursing* 25(6), 1123–32.

216   *Pain in Childbearing and its Control*

David, H., Weaver, J.B., Pearson, J.F. (1975) Doppler ultrasound and fetal activity. *British Medical Journal* 2, 62–4.

Davies, J. (1993) Mothers at risk. *Modern Midwife* 3(4), 31–3.

Davies, S.C. (1994) Foreword. In: *Sickle Cell Disease: A Psychosocial Approach* (K. Midence & J. Elander). Radcliffe Medical Press, Oxford.

Davitz, L.J., Sameshima, Y., Davitz, J. (1976) Suffering as viewed in six different cultures. *American Journal of Nursing* 76(8), 1296–7.

Davitz, L.L., Davitz, J.R. (1985) Culture and nurses' inferences of suffering. In: *Recent Advances in Nursing: Perspectives on Pain* (L.A. Copp), Chapter 2. Churchill Livingstone, Edinburgh.

Dening, F. (1982) The woman's stoole or the parturition chair. *Midwives Chronicle* 95(1139), 440–442.

Department of Health (1996) *Report on Confidential Enquiries into Maternal Deaths in the UK*. HMSO, London.

De Voe, S.T., De Voe, K., Jr, Rigsby, W.V.C., McDaniels, B.A. (1969) Effect of meperidine on uterine contractility. *American Journal of Obstetrics and Gynecology* 105, 1004–1007.

Dewan, G., Glazener, C., Tunstall, M. (1993) Postnatal pain: a neglected area. *British Journal of Midwifery* 1(2), 63–6.

Dickersin, K. (1989) Pharmacological pain control during labour. In: *Effective Care in Pregnancy and Childbirth* (eds I. Chalmers, M. Enkin & M.J.N.C. Keirse). Oxford University Press, Oxford.

Dick-Read, G. (1933) *Natural Childbirth*. W. Heinemann, London.

Dick-Read, G. (1962) *Childbirth Without Fear*. Dell, New York.

Di Franco, J. (1988) Relaxation: biofeedback. In: *Childbirth Education: Practice, Research and Theory* (F.H. Nichols & S.S. Humenick), Chapter 9. W.B. Saunders, Philadelphia.

Disaia, P., Creasman, J. (1984) *Clinical Gynaecologic Oncology*, 2nd edn. Mosby, St Louis.

Dobson, S.M. (1991) *Transcultural Nursing*. Scutari Press, London.

Dominian, J. (1981) *Depression*. Fontana, London.

Donaldson, J.O. (1995) Neurological disorders. In: *Medical Disorders in Obstetric Practice*, 3rd edn. (ed. M de Swiet), pp. 535–51. Blackwell Science, Oxford.

Doughty, A. (1987) Landmarks in the development of regional anaesthesia in obstetrics. In: *Foundations of Obstetric Anaesthesia* (ed. B.M. Morgan), pp. 1–18. Farrand Press, London.

Douglas, C.P. (1968) Thromboembolic disease in pregnancy and the puerperium. *Midwife, Health Visitor and Community Nurse*, 4, 413–15.

Doyle, P.M., Johanson, R., Geetha, T., Wilkinson, P. (1993) A prospective randomised controlled trial of perineal repair after childbirth. *British Journal of Obstetrics and Gynaecology* 100(1), 93–4.

Drew, J. (1992) Pain. *International Journal of Childbirth Education* 7(1), 35–6.

Drewett, R.F., Kahn, H., Parkhurst, S., Whiteley, S. (1987) Pain during breastfeeding: the first three months postpartum. *Journal of Reproductive and Infant Psychology* 5(3), 183–6.

Duchene, P. (1989) Effects of biofeedback on childbirth pain. *Journal of Pain and Symptom Management*, 4, 117–123.

Duley, L. (1994) Maternal mortality and eclampsia: the eclampsia trial. *MIDRS. Midwifery Digest* 4(2), 176–8.

Durham, C.F., McCain, C.F. (1993) Medical–surgical problems and trauma. In: *Maternity and Gynecologic Care: The Nurse and the Family*, 5th edn. (I.M. Bobak & M.D. Jensen), pp. 960–991. Mosby, St Louis.

Durham, L., Collins, M. (1986) The effect of music as a conditioning aid in prepared childbirth education. *Journal of Obstetric, Gynaecological and Neonatal Nursing* 15(3), 268–70.

Dutro, S., Wheeler, L. (1991) Pregnancy and exercise. In: *Conservative Care of Low Back Pain* (eds A.H. White & R. Anderson). Williams & Wilkins, Baltimore.

Dyson, S., Fielder, A., Kirkham, M. (1996a) Haemoglobinopathies, antenatal screening and the midwife. *British Journal of Midwifery* 4(6), 319–322.

Dyson, S., Fielder, A., Kirkham, M. (1996b) Midwives' knowledge of haemoglobinopathies. *Modern Midwife* 6(7), 22–5.

Eboh, W., van der Akker, O. (1994) Antenatal care of women with sickle cell disease. *British Journal of Midwifery* 2(1), 6–11.

Edgar, L., Smith-Hanrahan, C.M. (1992) Nonpharmacological pain management. In: *Pain Management: Nursing Perspective* (eds J. Watt-Watson & M.I. Donovan). Mosby, St Louis.

Editorial (1991) Catheter-acquired urinary infection. *Lancet* 338, 857–8.

Edwards, M.R., Nichols, F.H. (1988) Group process. In: *Childbirth Education: Practice, Research and Theory* (F.H. Nichols & S.S. Humenick), Chapter 24. W.B. Saunders, Philadelphia.

Egley, C., Cefalo, R.C. (1985) Abruptio placentae. In: *Progress in Obstetric and Gynaecology 5* (ed. J. Studd), pp. 108–120. Churchill Livingstone, Edinburgh.

Eisenach, J.C., Dobson, E.C., Inturrisi, C., Hood, D.D., Agner, P.B. (1990) Effect of pregnancy and pain on cerebrospinal fluid immunoreactive encephalins and norepinephrine in healthy humans. *Pain* 43, 149–54.

Ekman-Ordeberg, G., Salgeback, S., Ordeberg, G. (1987) Carpal tunnel syndrome in pregnancy: a prospective study. *Acta Obstetrica Gynecologica Scandinavica* 66(3), 233–5.

Elbourne, D. (1987) Subjects' views about participation in a randomised controlled trial. *Journal of Reproductive and Infant Psychology* 5:1, 3–8.

El Halta, V. (1996) Posterior labor – a pain in the back! Its prevention and cure. *Clarion* 11(1), 6–7, 12–13.

Engelhardt, H.T., Jr (1986) *The Foundations of Bioethics*. Oxford University Press, New York.

Enkin, M., Smith, S.L., Dermer, S.W., Emmett, J.O. (1972) An adequately controlled study of the effectiveness of P.P.M. training. In: *Psychosomatic Medicine in Obstetrics and Gynaecology* (N. Morris). Kargar, Basel.

Enkin, M.W. (1992) Commentary. *Birth* 19(1), 19–20.

L'Esperance, C.M. (1980) Pain or pleasure: the dilemma of early breastfeeding. *Birth and the Family Journal*, 7, 21–6.

Evans, S. (1992) The value of cardiotocograph monitoring in midwifery. *Midwives Chronicle* 105(1248), 4–11.

Eriksson, M., Ladfors, L., Mattsson, L.A., Fall, O. (1996) Warm tub bath during labour. *Acta Obstetrica Gynecologica Scandinavica* 75(7), 642–4.

Everett, C., Ashurst, H., Chalmers, I. (1987) Reported management of threatened miscarriage by general practitioners in Wessex. *British Medical Journal* 295, 583–6.

Ewen, A., McLeod, D.D., McLeod, D.M., Campbell, A., Tunstall, M.E. (1986) Continuous infusion epidural anagesia in obstetrics: a comparison of 0.08% and 0.25% bupivicaine. *Anaesthesia* 41, 143–7.

Fagerhaugh, S.Y., Strauss, A. (1977) *Politics of Pain Management: Staff-Patient Interaction.* Addison-Wesley, Menlo Park.

Fairley, P. (1978) *The Conquest of Pain.* Michael Joseph, London.

Fan, S.Z., Susetio, L., Tsai, M.C. (1994) Neuromuscular blockade of the fetus with pancuronium and pipecuronium for intrauterine procedures. *British Journal of Anaesthesia* 49(4), 284–6.

Feeney, J.G. (1982) Heartburn in pregnancy. *British Medical Journal* 284, 1138–9.

Ferrante, F.M., Ostheimer, G.W., Covino, B.G. (eds) (1990) *Patient Controlled Analgesia,* 2nd edn. Blackwell Science, Oxford.

Ferrell-Torry, A., Glick, O.J. (1993) The use of therapeutic massage as a nursing intervention to modify anxiety and the perception of cancer pain. *Cancer Nursing* 16(2), 93–101.

Fields, H.L. Basbaum, A.I. (1989) endogenous pain control mechanisms. In: *Textbook of Pain* (eds P.D. Wall & R. Melzack), pp. 206–217. Churchill Livingstone, Edinburgh.

Fishel, A. (1981) Mental health. In: *Health Care of Women: A Nursing Perspective* (eds C.I. Fogel & N.F. Woods). Mosby, St Louis.

Fisher, A, Prys-Roberts, C. (1968) Maternal pulmonary gas exchange. A study during normal labour and extradermal blockage. *Anaesthesia* 23(3), 350–355.

Fitzgerald, M. (1994) Neurobiology of fetal and neonatal pain. In: *Textbook of Pain,* 3rd edn. (eds P.D. Wall & R. Melzack), pp. 153–64. Churchill Livingstone, Edinburgh.

Fitzgerald, M., Anand, K.J.S. (1993) Developmental neuroanatomy and neurophysiology of pain. In: *Pain in Infants, Children and Adolescents* (eds N.L. Schechter, C.B. Berde & M. Yaster). Williams & Wilkins, Baltimore.

Fleming, N., Schafer, A.W. (1989) Postpartum perineal pain and sexual function in women with and without episiotomies. In: *The Free Woman* (eds E.V. van Hall & W. Everaerd). Parthenon, Carnforth.

Fleming, V.E.M. (1992) Client education: a futuristic outlook. *Journal of Advanced Nursing* 17(2), 158–63.

Fletcher, D.V. (1990) *A Study of Neonatal Nurses' and Midwives' Perceptions of Pain and Discomfort in the Neonate.* Internal Report, March, Glasgow Royal Maternity Hospital, Glasgow.

Fletcher, V. (1993) Pain and the neonate. In: *Midwifery Practice: A Research-Based Approach* (J. Alexander, V. Levy & S. Roch), Chapter 8. Macmillan, London.

Fleuren, M., Grol, R., De Haan, M., Wijkel, D. (1994) Care for the imminent miscarriage by midwives and G.P.s. *Family Practice* 11 (3), 275–81.

Flint, C. (1989) *The 'Know Your Midwife' Report.* South West Thames Regional Health Authority.

Flint, C. (1997) Do you want an epidural? *MIDIRS Midwifery Digest* 7(1), 60–61.

Flynn, A.M., Kelly, J., Hollins, G., Lynch, P.F. (1978) Ambulation in labour. *British Medical Journal*, 2, 591–3.

Fordham, M., Dunn, V. (1994) *Alongside the Person in Pain*. Baillière Tindall, London.

Formato, L-S (1985) Routine prophylactic episiotomy. *Journal of Nurse-Midwifery* 30(3), 144–8.

Fox, H. (1978) *Pathology of the Placenta*. W.B. Saunders, London.

Foxman, B., Schwartz, K., Looman, S.J. (1994) Breastfeeding practices and lactation mastitis. *Social Science and Medicine* 38(5), 755–61.

Franck, L.S. (1986) A new method to quantitatively describe pain behaviour in infants. *Nursing Research*, 35(1), 28–31.

Fraser, R., Watson, R. (1989) Bleeding during the latter half of pregnancy. In: *Effective Care in Pregnancy and Childbirth* (eds I. Chalmers, M. Enkin & M.J.N.C. Keirse), pp. 594–611. Oxford University Press, Oxford.

Freeborn, S.F., Calvert, R.T., Black, P. (1980) Saliva and blood pethidine concentrations in the mother and newborn baby. *British Journal of Obstetrics and Gynaecology* 87, 966–9.

Freeman, R.M., Macaulay, A.J., Eve, L., Chamberlain, C.V.P., Bhat, A.V. (1986) Randomised trial of self-hypnosis for analgesia in labour. *British Medical Journal*, 292, 657–8.

Freire, P., Shor, I. (1987) *A Pedagogy for Liberation; Dialogues on Transforming Education*. Macmillan Education, Basingstoke.

Fridh, G., Kopare, T., Gaston-Johansson, F., Norvell, K.T. (1988) Factors associated with more intense labor pain. *Research in Nursing and Health* 11, 117–24.

Furlong, S. (1996) Do programmes of medicine self-administration enhance patient knowledge, compliance and satisfaction? *Journal of Advanced Nursing* 23(6), 1254–62.

Fusi, L., Maresh, J.A., Steer, P.J. (1989) Maternal pyrexia associated with the use of epidural analgesia in labour. *Lancet* i, 1250–1252.

Gamsu, H.R. (1993) Neonatal effects. In: *Pain and its Relief in Childbirth* (eds. G. Chamberlain, A. Wraight & P. Steer). Churchill Livingstone, Edinburgh.

Garcia, J. (1987). Sharing research results with patients: the views of care-givers involved in a randomised controlled trial. *Journal of Reproductive and Infant Psychology* 5(1), 9–14.

Garcia, J, Marchant, S. (1993) Back to normal? Postpartum health and illness 1992. *Research and the Midwife Conference Proceedings*, 1990, University of Manchester.

Garland, D., Jones, K. (1994) Waterbirth, first stage immersion or non-immersion? *British Journal of Midwifery* 2(3), 113–20.

Gaston-Johansson, F., Fall-Dickson, J.M. (1995) The importance of nursing research design and methods in cancer pain management. *Nursing Clinics of North America* 30, 4.

Gaylard, D (1990) Epidural analgesia by continuous infusion. In: *Epidural and Spinal Blockade in Obstetrics* (ed F. Reynolds). Baillière Tindall, London.

Gélis, J. (translated by Morris, R.) (1991) *History of Childbirth*. Polity Press, Cambridge.

Giannakoupoulos, X., Sepulveda, W., Kourtis, N.M. (1994) Fetal plasma cortisol and beta-endorphin response to intrauterine needling. *Lancet*, 344(8915), 77–8.

Gibson, R.G., Gibson, S.L., McNeill, A.D., Buchanan, W.W. (1980) Homeopathic therapy in rheumatoid arthritis. *British Journal of Clinical Pharmacology.* 9(5), 453–9.

Gillies, H.C., Rogers, H.J., Spector, R.G., Trounce, J.R. (1986) *A Textbook of Clinical Pharmacology.* Hodder Stoughton, London.

Gillon, R. (1994) *Principles of Health Care Ethics.* Wiley, Chichester.

Gintzler, A.R. (1980) Endorphin-mediated increases in pain threshold during pregnancy. *Science* 210 (4466), 193–5.

Glazener, C.M.A., MacArthur, C., Garcia, J. (1993) Postnatal care: time for a change. *Contemporary Reviews in Obstetrics and Gynaecology* 5(3), 130–136.

Gould, D. (1990) *Nursing Care of Women.* Prentice Hall, London.

Grant, A. (1989a) Repair of perineal damage after childbirth. In: *Effective Care in Pregnancy and Childbirth* (eds I. Chalmers, M. Enkin & M.J.N.C. Keirse), pp. 1170–81. Oxford University Press, Oxford.

Grant, A. (1989b) The choice of suture materials and techniques for repair of perineal trauma: an overview of the evidence from controlled trials. *British Journal of Obstetrics and Gynaecology* 96(11), 1281–9.

Grant, A., Sleep, J. (1989) Relief of perineal pain and discomfort after childbirth. *Effective Care in Pregnancy and Childbirth* (eds I. Chalmers, M. Enkin & M.J.N.C. Keirse), pp. 1347–58. Oxford University Press, Oxford.

Grant, A., Sleep, J., McIntosh, J., Ashurst, H. (1989) Ultrasound and pulsed electromagnetic treatment for perineal trauma. A randomised placebo controlled trial. *British Journal of Obstetrics and Gynaecology* 96, 434–9.

Green, J, Coupland, V.A., Kitzinger, J.V. (1988) *Great Expectations: A Prospective Study of Women's Expectations and Experiences of Childbirth.* Child Care and Development Group, University of Cambridge, Cambridge.

Green, J.M. Kitzinger, J.V. Coupland, V.A. (1990) Stereotypes of childbearing women: a look at some evidence. *Midwifery* 6(3), 125–32.

Gregg, R.H. (1978) Biofeedback relaxation training effects in childbirth. *Behavioural Engineering* 4, 57–61.

Gregor, M., Zimmerman, M. (1973) Dorsal root potentials produced by afferent volleys in cutaneous group three fibres. *Journal of Physiology* 232(3), 413–25.

Grieff, J.M.C., Tordoff, S.G., Griffiths, R., May, A.E. (1994) Acid aspiration prophylaxis in 202 obstetric anaesthetic units in the UK. *International Journal of Obstetric Anaesthesia* 3(3), 137–42.

Guilbaud, G., Besson, M.J., Oliveras, J.L. Liebeskind, J.C. (1973) Suppression by LSD of the inhibitory effect exerted by dorsal raphe stimulation on certain spinal cord interneurons in the cat. *Brain Research* 61 (whole volume), 417–22.

Gunther, M. (1945) Sore nipples: causes and prevention. *Lancet* 2, 590–593.

Gunther, M. (1958) Discussion on the breast in pregnancy and lactation. *Proceedings of the Royal Society of Medicine* 51, 506–509.

Guzinski, G.M. (1990) Gynecologic pain. (eds J.J. Bonica, J.D. Loeser, C.R. Chapman & W.E. Fordyce), pp. 1344–67. *The Management of Pain*, 2nd edn. Lea & Febiger, Philadelphia.

Haber, L.H., Moore, B.D., Willis, W.D. (1982) Electrophysiological response properties of spinoreticular neurons in monkey. *Journal of Comparative Neurology* 207(1), 75–84

Hacker, N.F., Jochimsen, P.R. (1986) Common malignancies among women: sites and treatment. In: *Women with Cancer: Psychological Perspectives* (ed. B.L. Andersen), pp. 3–58. Springer-Verlag, New York.

Hagbarth, K.E., Kerr, D.B. (1954) Central influences on spinal afferent conduction. *Journal of Neurophysiology*, 17(3), 295–307.

Hagerdal, M., Morgan, C.W., Sumner, A.E., Gutsche, B.D. (1983) Minute ventilation and oxygen consumption during labour with epidural analgesia. *Anesthesiology* 59(5), 425–7.

Haldeman, S. (1989) Manipulation and massage for the relief of pain. In: *Textbook of Pain* (eds P.D. Wall & R. Melzack), pp. 942–51. Churchill Livingstone, Edinburgh.

Haldeman, S. (1994) Manipulation and massage for the relief of back pain. In: *Textbook of Pain* (eds P.D. Wall & R. Melzack), 3rd edn. pp. 1251–62. Churchill Livingstone, Edinburgh.

Halksworth, G. (1993) Exercise and pregnancy. In: *Midwifery Practice – A Research-Based Approach* (eds J. Alexander & V. Roch), Chapter 3. Macmillan, London.

Halldorsdottir, S., Karlsdottir, S.I. (1996) Journeying through labour and delivery: perceptions of women who have given birth. *Midwifery* 12(2), 48–61.

Hallgren, A., Kihlgren, M., Norberg, A. (1994) A descriptive study of childbirth education provided by midwives in Sweden. *Midwifery* 10(4), 215–24.

Hallgren, A., Kihlgren, M., Norberg, A., Forslin, L. (1995) Women's perceptions of childbirth and childbirth education before and after education and birth. *Midwifery* 11(3), 130–137.

Hallin, R.G., Torebjork, H.E. (1974) Activity in unmyelinated nerve fibres in man. In: *Advances in Neurology*, 4th edn. (ed J.J. Bonica), pp. 19–27. Raven Press, New York.

Hamblett, D. (1990) Pain in the neonate. *Paediatric Nursing* 2(1), 14–15.

Handfield, B., Bell, R. (1995) Do childbirth classes influence decision making about labour and postpartum issues? *Birth* 22(3) 153–60.

Hanser, S.B., Larson, S.C., O'Connell, A.S. (1983) The effect of music on relaxation of expectant mothers during labour. *Journal of Music Therapy* 20, 50–58.

Hanser, S.B., Thompson, L.W. (1994) Effects of music therapy strategy on depressed older adults. *Journal of Gerontology*, 49(6), 265–9.

Hardy, J. (1991). A randomised controlled trial into the use of TENS in labour. *Research and the Midwife Conference Proceedings*, 1990, University of Manchester.

Harris, B.G. (1990) Issues in nursing care of pregnant patients with cancer. *NAACOGS Clinical Issues in Perinatal Women's Health* 1(4), 423–36.

Harris, M. (1992) The impact of research findings on current practice in relieving postpartum perineal pain in a large district general hospital. *Midwifery* 8(3), 125–31.

Harrison, R.F., Woods, T., Shore, M., Mathews, G., Unwin, A. (1986) Pain relief in labour using transcutaneous electrical nerve stimulation (TENS): a TENS/TENS placebo controlled study in 2 parity groups. *British Journal of Obstetrics and Gynaecology*, 93(7), 739–46.

Hawkins, J. (1994) Use of TENS for pain relief in labour. *British Journal of Midwifery* 2(10), 487–90.

Hawkins, S. (1995). Water vs. conventional births: infection rates compared. *Nursing Times*, 91(11), 38–40.

Hay-Smith, A.J., Mantle, J.W. (1996) Surveys of the experience and perceptions of postnatal superficial dyspareunia. *Physiotherapy* 82(2), 91–7.

Hayward, J. (1975) *Information: a Prescription Against Pain*. Royal College of Nursing, London.

Head, M. (1993) Dropping stitches. *Nursing Times* 89(33), 64–5.

Helman, C. (1984) Pain and culture. In: *Culture, Health and Illness* (C. Helman), Chapter 6. Wright, Bristol.

Hendricks, C.H. Quilligan, E.J. (1956) Cardiac output during labour. *American Journal of Obstetrics and Gynecology* 71(5), 953–72.

Henschel, D., Inch, S. (1996) *Breastfeeding: A Guide for Midwives*. Hale Books for Midwives Press, Manchester, and the Royal College of Midwives, London.

Herbert, P. (1994) Support of first time mothers in the first three months after birth. *Nursing Times* 90(24), 36–7.

Heywood, A.M., Ho, E. (1990) Pain relief in labour. In: *Intrapartum Care: A Research-Based Approach* (J. Alexander, V. Levy & S. Roch), pp. 70–121. Macmillan, London.

Hibbard, B.M., Scott, D.B. (1990) The availability of epidural anaesthesia and analgesia in obstetrics. *British Journal of Obstetrics and Gynaecology* 97, 402–405.

Hicks, C. (1992). Research in midwifery: are midwives their own worst enemies? *Midwifery* 8(1), 12–18.

Higgins, C. (1995) Microbiological examination of urine in urinary tract infection. *Nursing Times* 91(11), 33–5.

Hignett, S. (1996) Work related back pain in nurses. *Journal of Advanced Nursing* 23(6), 1238–46.

Hilgard, E.R. (1973) A neodissociation theory of pain reduction in hypnosis. *Psychological Review* 80, 396–411.

Hilgard, E.R. Hilgard, J.R. (1986) *Hypnosis in the Relief of Pain*, 2nd edn. Kaufmann, Los Altos.

Hillan, E.M. (1992a) Research and audit: women's views of caesarean section. In: *Women's Health Matters* (ed H. Roberts), pp. 157–75. Routledge, London.

Hillan, E.M. (1992b) Short term morbidity associated with caesarean delivery. *Birth* 19(4), 190–194.

Hillman, P, Wall, P.D. (1969) Inhibitory and excitatory factors influencing the receptor fields of lamina five spinal cord cells. *Experimental Brain Research* 9(4), 284–306.

Hinchliff, S., Montague, S. (1988) *Physiology for Nursing Practice*. Baillière Tindall, London.

HMSO (1991) *Health after Childbirth.* University of Birmingham and HMSO, London.

HMSO (1996) *Report on Confidential Enquiries into Maternal Deaths in the UK 1991–93.* HMSO, London.

Hodnett, E.D. (1994) Support from caregivers during childbirth. In: *Pregnancy and Childbirth Module* (eds J.P. Neilson, C.A. Crowther, E.D. Hodnett, G.J. Hofmer, M.J.N.C. Keirse & M.J. Renfrew), *The Cochrane Database of Systematic Reviews* (updated 6 June 1996), available in The Cochrane Library. The Cochrane Collaboration, Issue 2, Oxford Update Software, 1996.

Hodnett, E.D. Osborn, R.W. (1989) A randomised trial of the effects of monitrice support during labour: mothers' views two to four weeks postpartum. *Birth* 16(4), 177–83.

Hofmeyr, G.J., Nikodem, V.C. (1996) Achieving mother and baby friendliness – the evidence for labour companions. In: *Baby Friendly Mother Friendly* (ed S.F. Murray), p. 89. UNICEF and Mosby, London.

Hollister, L.E. (1992) Drugs of abuse. In: *Basic and Clinical Pharmacology* (B.G. Katzung), pp. 437–51. Lange, Connecticut.

Hollman, A., Jouppila, R., Jouppila, P., Koivula, A., Vierrola, H. (1982) Effect of extradural analgesia using bupivicaine and 2-chloroprocaine on intervillous blood flow during labour. *British Journal of Anaesthesia* 54(8), 837–42.

Holwell, D.L. (1994) A double blind randomised controlled trial evaluating the homeopathic remedy Arnica Montana. In: *MIRIAD: a Sourcebook of Information about Research in Midwifery.* Hale Books for Midwives Press, Manchester.

Horan, J.J., Layng, F.C., Pursell, C.H. (1976) Preliminary study of effects of 'in vivo' emotive imagery on dental discomfort. *Perception and Motor Skills* 42, 105–106.

House of Commons (1992) *Health Committee Second Report.* Maternity Services, HMSO, London.

Howard, R.J. Tuck, S.M., Pearson, T.C. (1995a) Pregnancy and sickle cell disease in the UK. *British Journal of Obstetrics and Gynaecology* 102(12), 947–51.

Howard, S., McKell, D., Mugford, M., Grant, A. (1995b) Cost-effectiveness of different approaches to perineal suturing. *British Journal of Midwifery* 3(11), 587–90, 603–605.

Howell, C.J. Chalmers, I. (1992) A review of prospectively controlled comparisons of epidural with non-epidural forms of pain relief during labour. *International Journal of Obstetrical Anaesthesia* 1, 93–110.

Huch, A., Huch, R., Schneider, R., Rooth, G. (1977) Continuous transcutaneous monitoring of foetal oxygen tension during labour. *British Journal of Obstetrics and Gynaecology* 84 (Suppl.), S1–S39.

Hunt, S., Symonds, A. (1995) *The Social Meaning of Midwifery.* Macmillan, London.

Hytten, F.E. (1991) The alimentary system. In: *Clinical Physiology in Obstetrics* (F.E. Hytten & G. Chamberlain), Chapter 5. Blackwell Science, Oxford.

International Association for the Study of Pain (1979) Pain terms: a list with definitions and notes on usage. *Pain* 6, 249–52.

Ignelzi, R.J., Atkinson, J.H. (1980) Pain and its modulation. *Neurology* 6(5), 577–90.

Iles, S. (1989) The loss of early pregnancy. In: *Psychological Aspects of Obstetrics and Gynaecology* (ed M. Oates), pp. 769–90. Baillière Tindall, London.

Illich, I. (1976) *Medical Nemesis: The Expropriation of Health*. Pantheon Books, New York.

Impey, L., Hughes, J. (1995) Abdominal pain in pregnancy: who needs to be admitted? *Journal of Obstetrics and Gynaecology* 15(6), 263–5.

Inch, S. (1996) The importance of breastfeeding. *MIDIRS Midwifery Digest* 6(2), 208–211.

Inch, S., Fisher, C. (1996) Mastitis: infection or inflammation? *Practitioner* 239, 472-6.

Inch, S., Renfrew, M.J. (1989) Common breastfeeding problems. In: *Effective Care in Pregnancy and Childbirth* (eds I. Chalmers, M. Enkin & M.J.N.C. Keirse), pp. 1375–89. Oxford University Press, Oxford.

Jacobsen, E.J. (1938) *Progressive Relaxation*. University of Chicago, Illinois.

Jamieson, L. (1993) Preparing for parenthood: daily life in pregnancy. In: *Myles Textbook for Midwives* (eds V.R. Bennett & L.K. Brown), pp. 106–122. Churchill Livingstone, Edinburgh.

Jebali, C. (1993) A feminist perspective on postnatal depression. *Health Visitor*, 66(2), 59–60.

Jeffery, P. (1989) *Labour Pains and Labour Power: Women and Childbearing in India*. Zed Books, London.

Jessel, T.M., Iversen, L.L. (1977) Opiate analgesics inhibit substance P release from rat trigeminal nucleus. *Nature* 268(5620), 549–51.

Jessup, B.A., Gallegos, X. (1994) Relaxation and biofeedback. In: *Textbook of Pain*, 3rd edn. pp. 1321–36. Churchill Livingstone, Edinburgh.

Jimenez, S.L.M. (1988) Supportive pain management strategies. In: *Childbirth Education: Practice Research and Theory* (F.H. Nichols & S.S. Humenick), Chapter 6. W.B. Saunders, Philadelphia.

Johnston, C.C. Stevens, B.J. (1996) Experience in an NNICU affects pain response. *Pediatrics* 98(5), 925–30.

Johnston, J., Minchin, M. (1994) When there were no more cabbage leaves. *Australian Lactation Consultants Association News* 5(1), 8–10.

Johnson, M. (1977) Assessment of clinical pain. In: *Pain: A Source Book for Nurses and Other Health Professionals* (ed A.K. Jacox), pp. 107–138. Little Brown & Co, Boston.

Jones, D.G. Sturdy, D.E. (1990) Orthopaedic causes of pelvic pain. In: *Pelvic Pain in Women: Diagnosis and Management* (ed I. Rocker). Springer-Verlag, New York.

Jones, K. (1994) Alternative therapies in pregnancy. *British Journal of Midwifery* 2(10), 491–4.

Jones, L., Arthurs, G.J., Sturman, E., Bellis, L. (1996) Self-medication in acute surgical wards. *Journal of Clinical Nursing* 5(4), 229–32.

Jordan, B. (1978) *Birth in Four Cultures*. Monographs in Women's Studies. Eden Press, Vermont.

Jouppila, P., Jouppila, R., Hollman, A., Koivula, A. (1982) Lumbar epidural analgesia to improve intervillous blood flow during labour in severe pre-eclampsia. *Obstetrics and Gynecology* 59(2), 158–61.

Jouppila, R., Jouppila, P., Moilanen, K., Pakarinen, A. (1980) The effect of segmental epidural analgesia on maternal prolactin during labour. *British Journal of Obstetrics and Gynaecology* 31, 1–10.

Jungman, R. (1988) Relaxation: acupressure. In: *Childbirth Education: Practice Research and Theory* (F.H. Nichols & S.S. Humenick), Chapter 11. W.B. Saunders, Philadelphia.

Kaplan, B. (1994) Homeopathy: 2. In pregnancy and for the under fives. *Professional care of the mother and child* 4(6), 185–7.

Kass, E.H. (1978) Horatio at the orifice: the significance of bacteriuria. *Journal of Infectious Diseases* 138, 546–57.

Keele, K.D. Armstrong, D. (1964) *Substances Producing Pain and Itch.* Arnold, London.

Keep, N.B. (1995) Identifying pulmonary embolism. *American Journal of Nursing* 95(4), 52.

Keirse, M.J.N.C., Chalmers, I. (1989) Methods for inducing labour. In: *Effective Care in Pregnancy and Childbirth* (eds I. Chalmers, M. Enkin & M.J.N.C. Keirse), Chapter 62. Oxford University Press, Oxford.

Keirse, M.J.N.C., Enkin, M., Lumley, J. (1989) Social and professional support during childbirth. *Effective Care in Pregnancy and Childbirth* (eds I. Chalmers, M. Enkin & M.J.N.C. Keirse), Chapter 49. Oxford University Press, Oxford.

Kemp, T. (1996) The use of transcutaneous electrical nerve stimulation on acupuncture points in labour. *Midwives* 109 (1307), 13–20.

Keng, T.M., Bucknall, T.E. (1989) A clinical trial of tissue adhesive (histocryl) in skin closure of groin wounds. *Medical Journal of Malaysia* 44(2), 122–8.

Kennedy, D. (1978) DES and breast cancer. *Food and Drug Administration Drug Bulletin,* 8, 10.

Kennell, J.H., Klaus, M., McGrath, S., Robertson, S., Hinkley, C. (1988) Medical intervention: the effect of social support. *Paediatric Research* 23, 211A.

Kennell, J.H., Klaus, M., McGrath, S., Robertson, S., Hinkley, C. (1991) Continuous emotional support during labour in a US hospital: a randomised controlled trial. *Journal of the American Medical Association* 265(17), 2197–2201.

Kepes, E.R., Claudio-Santiago, M. (1996) Patient-controlled analgesia. In: *A Practical Approach to Pain Management* (eds M. Lefkowitz & A.H. Lebovitz), pp. 15–19. Little Brown & Co, Boston.

Kerr, F.W.L. (1975) Neuroanatomical substrates of nociception in the spinal cord. *Pain* 1(4), 325–56.

Khamashta, M.A., Hughes, G.R. (1996). Pregnancy in systemic lupus erythematosus. *Current Opinions in Rheumatology* 8(5), 424–9.

Kickbusch, I. (1989) Self-Care in Health Promotion. *Social Science and Medicine* 29(2), 125–30.

Kimmey, M.B., Silverstein, F.E. (1990) Diseases of the gastrointestinal tract. In: *The Management of Pain,* 2nd edn. (eds J.J. Bonica, J.D. Loeser, C.R. Chapman & W.E. Fordyce), pp. 1186–1213. Lea Febiger, Philadelphia.

King, H. (1988) The early anodynes: pain in the ancient world. In: *The History and Management of Pain* (R.D. Mann), Chapter 3. Parthenon, Carnforth.

Kingham, D.J. (1994) On the general theory of neural circuitry. *Medical Hypotheses* 42(5), 291–8.

Kirkham, M. (1989) Midwives and information giving during labour. In: *Midwives, Research and Childbirth 1* (S. Robinson & A.M. Thomson). Chapman & Hall, London.

Kitzinger, J. (1989) Strategies of the early childbirth movement: a case study of the National Childbirth Trust. *The Politics of Maternity Care: Services for Childbearing Women in Twentieth-Century Britain* (J. Garcia, R. Kilpatrick & M.P.M. Richards). Clarendon, Oxford.

Kitzinger, S. (1978) Pain in childbirth. *Journal of Medical Ethics* 4, 119–21.

Kitzinger, S. (1987a) *Giving Birth: How It Really Feels*. Gollancz, London.

Kitzinger, S. (1987b) *Some Women's Experiences of Epidurals: A Descriptive Study*. National Childbirth Trust, London.

Kitzinger, S. (1989) Perceptions of pain in home and hospital birth. In: *The Free Woman: Women's Health in the 1990s* (eds E.V. van Hall & W. Everaerd), pp. 90–100. Parthenon, Carnforth.

Kitzinger, S. (1992a) Birth plans. *Birth* 19(1), 36–7.

Kitzinger, S. (1992b) Reply to a letter. *Birth* 19(2), 110–111.

Kitzinger, S. (1995) Sexuality in the postpartum period: a review. *MIDIRS Midwifery Digest* 5(4), 451.

Kitzinger, S. (1996) Sentenced to hard labour. *The Independent* 8 July.

Klaus, M., Kennell, J.H., Robertson, S., Sosa, R. (1986) Effects of social support during parturition. *British Medical Journal* 29(3), 585–7.

Kleinman, A., Brodwin, P.E., Good, B.J., Good, M.-J.D.V. (1992) Pain as human experience: an Introduction. In: Good M-JDV, Brodwin P.E., Good B.J., Kleinman, A. *Pain as Human Experience: An Anthropological Perspective* (M-JDV Good, P.E. Brodwin, B.J. Good & A. Kleinman), Chapter 1. University of California Press, Berkeley.

Klopper, A. (1991) The ovary. In: *Clinical Physiology in Obstetrics* (F.E. Hytten & G. Chamberlain), pp. 337–92. Blackwell Science, Oxford.

Knights, J. (1986) Use of meptazinol in routine obstetric practice in a district general hospital. *Midwives Chronicle* 99(1183), 182–3.

Konotey-Ahulu, F.I.D. (1991) *The Sickle Cell Disease Patient*. Macmillan, London.

Koshy, M. (1995) Sickle cell disease and pregnancy. *Blood Reviews* 9(3), 157–64.

Krieger, D. (1979) *The Therapeutic Touch: How to Use Your Hands to Help or Heal*. Prentice Hall, New Jersey.

Kristiansson, P., Svardsudd, K., von Schoultz, B. (1996) Back pain during pregnancy: a prospective study. *Spine* 21(6), 702–709.

Kübler-Ross, E. (1970) *On Death and Dying*. Tavistock Publications, London.

Lamaze, F. (1956) *Painless Childbirth: Psychoprophylactic Method*. Regnery, Chicago.

Lamaze, F. (1970) *Painless Childbirth: Psychoprophylactic Method*. Regnery, Chicago.

Lambert, W.E., Libman, E., Poser, E.G. (1960) The effect of increased salience of membership group on pain tolerance. *Journal of Personality* 38, 350–57.

Lamotte, C., Perl, C.B., Snyder, S.H. (1976) Opiate receptor binding in primate spinal cord. Distribution and changes after dorsal root section. *Brain Research* 112(2), 407–412.

Langford, J. (1997) The legendary pain of labour. *New Generation* 16(1), 6–7.

Larson, K., Ayllon, T. (1990) The effects of contingent music. *Behaviour Research and Therapy* 28(2), 119–25.

Lasa, C.I., Kidd, R.R., Nunez, H.A., Drohan, W.N. (1993) Effect of fibrin glue and opsite on open wounds. *Journal of Surgical Research* 54(3), 202–206.

Lawrence, J., Alcock, D., McGrath, P., Kay, J., MacMurray, S.B., Dulberg, C. (1993) The development of a tool to assess neonatal pain. *Neonatal Network* 12(6), 59–65.

Lawrence, R.A. (1989) *Breastfeeding: A Guide for the Medical Profession*, 3rd edn. Mosby, St Louis.

Leap, N. (1997) Being with women in pain. *British Journal of Midwifery* 5(5), 263d,s.

Leder, D. (1986) Toward a phenomenology of pain. *Review Existential Psychologist and Psychiatry* 19(2), 255–66.

Lederman, E., Lederman, R.P., Work, B.A., McCann, D.S. (1981) Maternal psychological and physiological correlates of fetal–newborn health status. *American Journal of Obstetrics and Gynecology* 139(8), 956–8.

Lederman, R.P., Lederman, E., Work, B.A., Jr (1978). The relationship of maternal anxiety, plasma catecholamine and plasma cortisol to progress in labor. *American Journal of Obstetrics and Gynecology* 132(5), 495–500.

Lederman, R.P., McCann, D.S., Work, B.A., Huber, M.J. (1977) Endogenous plasma epinephrine and norepinephrine in last-trimester pregnancy and labor. *American Journal of Obstetrics and Gynecology* 129(1), 58.

Lee, M.H.M. Itoh, M., Yang, G.F.W., Eason, A. (1990) Physical therapy and rehabilitation medicine. In: *The Management of Pain*, 2nd edn. (eds J.J. Bonica, J.D. Loeser, C.R. Chapman & W.E. Fordyce), pp. 1769–88. Lea & Febiger, Philadelphia.

Lefcourt, H.M. (1982) *Locus of Control: Current Trends in Theory and Research*, 2nd edn. Erlbaum, London.

Lentz, S.S. (1995) Osteitis pubis: a review. *Obstetrical and Gynecological Survey* 50(4), 310–15.

Letsky, E. (1991) The haematological system. In: *Clinical Physiology in Obstetrics* (F.E. Hytten & G. Chamberlain), pp. 39–82. Blackwell Science, Oxford.

Levene, M. (1995) Pain relief and sedation during neonatal intensive care. *European Journal of Pediatrics* 154(8) (Suppl. 3), S22–3.

Lewin, K. (1935) *Dynamic Theory of Personality*. McGraw Hill, New York.

Lewis, C.S. (1940) *The Problem of Pain*. Century Press, London.

Lewis, J. (1990) Mothers and maternity policies in the twentieth century. In: *The Politics of Maternity Care: Services for Childbearing Women in Twentieth-Century Britain* (J. Garcia, R. Kilpatrick & M.P.M. Richards), Chapter 1. Clarendon, Oxford.

Lewis, L. (1994) Are you sitting comfortably? *Midwives Chronicle* 107(1277), 226–7.

Linton, S.J., Gotteskam, K.G. (1983) A clinical comparison of two pain scales: correlation, remembering chronic pain and a measure of compliance. *Pain* 17, 57–65.

228 *Pain in Childbearing and its Control*

Lipton, J.A., Marbach, J.J. (1984) Ethnicity and the pain experience. *Social Science and Medicine* 19(12), 1279–98.

Littlewood, J., McHugh, N. (1997) *Maternal Distress and Postnatal Depression: The Myth of Madonna.* Macmillan, London.

Livingston, J.C. (1985) The use of music and exercise to reduce the pain of pregnancy and childbirth. In: *Perspectives on Pain* (ed LA Copp). Churchill Livingstone, Edinburgh.

Llewellyn-Jones, D. (1973) *Fundamentals of Obstetrics and Gynaecology.* Faber & Faber, London.

Lloyd, G., McLauchlan, A. (1994) Nurses' attitudes towards management of pain. *Nursing Times* 90(43), 40–43.

Locsin, R.G.R.A.C. (1981) The effect of music on the pain of selected postoperative patients. *Journal of Advanced Nursing* 6(1) 19–25.

Lokey, E.A., Tran, Z.V., Wells, C.L., Myers, B.C., Tran, A.C. (1991) Effects of physical exercise on pregnancy outcomes: a meta-analytic review. *Medicine and Science in Sports and Exercise* 23(11), 1234–9.

Lothian, J.A. (1988) Relaxation: therapeutic touch. In: *Childbirth Education: Practice, Research and Theory* (F.H. Nichols & S.S. Humenick), Chapter 10. W.B. Saunders, Philadelphia.

Lowdermilk, D.L. (1993) Labor and birth at risk. In: *Maternity and Gynaecologic Care: The Nurse and the Family* 5th edn. (I.M. Bobak & M.D. Jensen), p. 1045. Mosby, St Louis.

Lowery, C.L. (1995) Sudden joint and extremity pain in pregnancy. *Obstetrics and Gynecology Clinics of North America* 22(1), 173–90.

McAllister, G., Farquhar, M. (1992) Health beliefs: a cultural division? *Journal of Advanced Nursing* 17, 1447–54.

MacArthur, A., MacArthur, C., Weeks, S. (1995) Epidural anaesthesia and low back pain after delivery: a prospective cohort study. *British Medical Journal* 311 (7016), 1336–9.

MacArthur, C., Lewis, M., Knox, E.G. (1991) *Health After Childbirth.* HMSO, London, and University of Birmingham.

McCaffery, M. (1979) *Nursing Management of the Patient with Pain.* Lippincott, Philadelphia.

McCaffery, M. (1983) *Nursing the Patient in Pain.* Adapted by B. Sofaer. Harper & Row, London.

McCaffery, M., Beebe, A. (1989) *Pain: Clinical Manual for Nursing Practice.* Mosby, St Louis.

McCandlish, R., Renfrew, M. (1993) Immersion in water during labour and birth: the need for evaluation. *Birth* 20(2), 79–85.

McConnell, A. (1995) Massage: a practical guide for health professionals. *Nursing Times Suppl.* 91(36), 3–14.

McCrea, B.H. (1996) *An Investigation of Rule-Governed Behaviours in the Control of Pain Management During the First Stage of Labour.* Unpublished D. Phil. thesis, University of Ulster.

MacDermott, R.I.J. (1994) The interpretation of midstream urine microscopy and culture results in women who present acutely in the labour ward. *British Journal of Obstetrics and Gynaecology* 101(8), 712–13.

MacDonald, R., Owen, B., Wilson, J. (1988) Patients' perceptions of obstetric anaesthetic services. *Anaesthesia* 43, 601.

MacDonald, S.J. (1991) Antenatal admission: women's perceptions of their experience. *Research and the Midwife Conference Proceedings*, 1990, University of Manchester.

MacGillivray, I. (1983) *Pre-Eclampsia: The Hypertensive Disease of Pregnancy*. W.B. Saunders, London.

McGrath, P.J. Unruh, A.M. (1994) Measurement and assessment of paediatric pain. In: *Textbook of Pain* 3rd edn. (eds P.D. Wall & R. Melzack), Chapter 16. Churchill Livingstone, Edinburgh.

Machover, I. (1995) The mobile epidural.... is it such good news? *AIMS Journal* 7(2), 10–11.

McIntosh, J. (1989) Models of childbirth and social class: a study of eighty working class primigravidae. In: *Midwives, Research and Childbirth 1* (S. Robinson & A.M. Thomson), Chapter 10. Chapman & Hall, London.

Mackey R.B. (1995) Discover the healing power of therapeutic touch. *American Journal of Nursing* 95(4), 27–32.

Macleod, J., Macintyre, C., McClure, J.H. (1995) Backache and epidural analgesia. A retrospective survey of mothers one year after childbirth. *International Journal of Obstetric Anaesthesia* 4(1), 21–5.

McLintock, A.H. (1876) *Treatise on the Theory and Practice of Midwifery 2*. New Sydenham Society, London.

McManus, T.J., Calder, A. (1978) Upright posture and the efficiency of labour. *Lancet* 1(14), 72–4.

McNab, I., McCulloch, J. (1990) *Backache*, 2nd edn. Williams Wilkins, Baltimore.

Mahomed, K., Grant, A., Ashurst, H., James, D. (1989) The Southmead perineal suture study. *British Journal of Obstetrics and Gynaecology* 96(11), 1272–80.

Maldonado, A., Barger, M. (1995) Comprehensive assessment of common musculoskeletal disorders. *Journal of Nurse-Midwifery* 20(2), 202–212.

Malkin, K. (1994) Use of massage in clinical practice. *British Journal of Nursing* 13(6), 292–4.

Mander, R. (1992a) Seeking approval for research access: the gatekeepers' role in facilitating a study of the care of the relinquishing mother. *Journal of Advanced Nursing* 17(12), 1460–64.

Mander, R. (1992b) The control of pain in labour. *Journal of Clinical Nursing* 1(1), 219–23.

Mander, R. (1993a) Who chooses the choices? *Modern Midwife* 3(1), 23–5.

Mander, R. (1993b) Epidural analgesia 1: recent history. *British Journal of Midwifery* 1(6), 259–64.

Mander, R. (1994a) Epidural analgesia 2: research basis. *British Journal of Midwifery* 2(1), 12–16.

Mander, R. (1994b) *Loss and Bereavement in Childbearing*. Blackwell Science, Oxford.

Mander, R. (1995a) Forum on maternity and the newborn: pain in labour. *Midwives* 108(1289), 180.

Mander, R. (1995b) The relevance of the Dutch system of maternity care to the UK. *Journal of Advanced Nursing* 22, 1023–26.

Mander, R. (1995c) Culture and loss in the clinical setting. *British Journal of Midwifery* 3(11), 598–9.

Mander, R. (1996) Failure to deliver: ethical issues relating to epidural analgesia in uncomplicated labour. In: *Midwifery Ethics* (L. Frith). Butterworth Heinemann, Oxford.

Mander, R. (1997a) Pethidine in childbearing. *MIDIRS Midwifery Digest,* 7(2), 202–203.

Mander, R. (1997b) An uplifting experience. *British Journal of Midwifery* (in press).

Mander, R. (1997c) The control of pain in labour. In: *Essential Midwifery* (eds C. Henderson & K. Jones), Chapter 10. Mosby, London.

Mann, F. (1983) *Scientific Aspects of Acupuncture.* Heinemann, London.

Manolitsas, T., Wein, P., Beischer, N.A., Sheedy, M.T., Ratten, V.J. (1994) Value of cardiotocography in women with antepartum haemorrhage. *Australian and New Zealand Journal of Obstetrics and Gynaecology* 34(4), 403–408.

Marcer, D. (1986) *Biofeedback and Related Therapies in Clinical Practice,* Chapter 6. Croom Helm, London.

Marchette, L., Main, R., Redlick, E. (1989) Pain reduction during neonatal circumcision. *Paediatric Nursing* 15(2), 207–210.

Marck, P.B. (1994) Unexpected pregnancy. In: *Uncertain Motherhood: Negotiating the Risks of the Childbearing Years* (P.A. Field & P.B. Marck), pp. 82–138. Sage, London.

Marrero, J.M., Goggin, P.M., de Caestecker, J.S., Pearce, J.M., Maxwell, J.D. (1992) Determinants of pregnancy heartburn. *British Journal of Obstetrics and Gynaecology* 99, 731–4.

Marris, P. (1986) *Loss and Change.* Routledge Kegan Paul, London.

Marshall, R.E., Stratton Moore, J.A., Boxerman, S.B. (1980) Circumcision 1: effects upon newborn behaviour. *Infant Behavioural Development* 3, 1–14.

Marteau, T.M. (1995) Health beliefs and attributions. In: *Health Psychology: Processes and Applications,* 2nd edn. (A. Broome & S. Llewelyn), Chapter 1. Chapman Hall, London.

Martin, E. (1989) *The Woman in the Body.* Open University Press, Milton Keynes.

Marx, G.F., Macatangay, A.S., Cohen, A.V., Schulman, H. (1969) Effect of pain relief on arterial blood gas values during labour. *New York Journal of Medicine* 69(6), 819–22.

Matthews, M.K. (1989) The relationship between maternal labour analgesia and delay in the initiation of breast feeding in healthy neonates in the early neonatal period. *Midwifery* 5(1), 3–10.

Maxwell-Hudson, C. (1990) *The Complete Book of Massage.* Dorling-Kindersley, London.

Mayer, D.J. Price, D.D. (1976) Central nervous system mechanisms of analgesia. *Pain* 2(4), 379.

Meinhart, N.T., McCaffery, M. (1983) *Pain. A Nursing Approach to Assessment and Analysis.* Appleton-Century Crofts, Norwalk, Connecticut.

Melzack, R. (1973) *The Puzzle of Pain.* Penguin, London.

Melzack, R. (1975a) The McGill Pain Questionnaire: major properties and scoring methods. *Pain* 1, 277–99.

Melzack, R. (1975b) How acupuncture can block pain. In: *Pain: Clinical and*

Experimental Perspectives (ed M. Weisenberg, pp. 251–7. Mosby, St Louis.

Melzack, R. (1983) Concepts of pain measurement. In: *Pain Measurement and Assessment* (R. Melzack), pp. 1–5. Raven Press, New York.

Melzack, R. (1984) The myth of painless childbirth. The John J. Bonica lecture. *Pain* 19(4), 321–37.

Melzack, R. (1993) Pain: past present and future. *Canadian Journal of Experimental Psychology* 47(4), 615–29.

Melzack, R., Casey K.L. (1968) Sensory, motivational and central determinants of pain. In: *The Skin Senses* (ed. D.R. Kenshalo), pp. 423–39. Charles C. Thomas, Springfield, Illinois.

Melzack, R., Katz, J. (1994) Pain measurement in persons in pain. In: *Textbook of Pain* 3rd edn. (eds P.D. Wall & R. Melzack), pp. 337–51. Churchill Livingstone, Edinburgh.

Melzack, R., Taenzer, P., Feldman, P., Kinch, R.A. (1981) Labour is still painful after prepared childbirth training. *Canadian Medical Association Journal* 125(5), 357–63.

Melzack, R., Wall, P.D. (1965) Pain mechanisms: a new theory. *Science* 150 (3699), 971–9.

Melzack, R., Wall, P.D. (1991) *The Challenge of Pain*, 2nd edn. Penguin, London.

Melzack, R., Weisz, A.Z., Sprague, L.T. (1963) Stratagems for controlling pain: contributions of auditory stimulation and suggestion. *Experimental Neurology* 8, 239–47.

Menage, J. (1993) Post traumatic stress disorder in women who have undergone obstetric and/or gynaecological procedures. A consecutive series of 30 cases. *Journal of Reproductive and Infant Psychology* 11(4), 221–8.

Mendez-Bauer, C., Arroyo, J., Garcia-Ramos, C., *et al.* (1975) Effects of standing position on spontaneous uterine contractility and other aspects of labour. *Journal of Perinatal Medicine* 3, 89–100.

Merskey, H. (1980a) Some features of the history of the idea of pain. *Pain* 6 (1), 3–8.

Merskey, H. (1980b) The meaning of pain. In: *Pain Meaning and Management* (eds W.L. Smith, H. Merskey & S.C. Gross). MTP Press, Lancaster.

Meyer, L.C., Peacock, J.L., Bland, J.M., Anderson, H.R. (1994) Symptoms and health problems in pregnancy: their association with social factors, smoking, alcohol, caffeine and attitude to pregnancy. *Paediatric and Perinatal Epidemiology* 8(2), 145–55.

Midence, K., Elander, J. (1994) *Sickle Cell Disease: A Psychosocial Approach.* Radcliffe Medical Press, Oxford.

Miller, A.W.F., Callander, R. (1989) *Obstetrics Illustrated*, 4th edn. Churchill Livingstone, Edinburgh.

Mills, G.H., Singh, D., Longman, M., O'Sullivan, J., Caunt, J.A. (1996) Nitrous oxide exposure on the labour ward. *International Journal of Obstetric Anaesthesia* 5(3), 160–164.

Minzter, B. (1993) Analgesia after caesarean delivery. In: *Postoperative Pain Management* (F.M. Ferrante & T.R. Vadeboncouer), pp. 519–30. Churchill Livingstone, Edinburgh.

Moawad, A.H. (1990) Acute appendicitis during pregnancy. In: *Surgical*

Diseases in Pregnancy (ed L.A. Cibels), pp. 105–114. Springer Verlag, New York.

Mobily, P.R., Herr, K.A., Kelley, L.S. (1993) Cognitive-behavioural techniques to reduce pain: a validation study. *International Journal of Nursing Studies* 30(6), 537–48.

Mobily, P.R., Herr, K.A., Nicholson, A.C. (1994) Validation of cutaneous stimulation interventions for pain management. *International Journal of Nursing Studies* 31(6), 533–41.

Moir, D.D. (1973) *Pain Relief in Labour: A Handbook for Midwives*. Churchill Livingstone, Edinburgh.

Molloy, B.G. Sheil, O., Duignan, N.M. (1987) Delivery after caesarean section: review of 2176 consecutive cases. *British Medical Journal* 294, 1645–7.

Monto, M. (1996) Lamaze and Bradley childbirth classes: contrasting perspectives towards the medical model of birth. *Birth* 23(4), 193–201.

Moore, J., Ball, H.G. (1974) A sequential study of intravenous analgesic treatment during labour. *British Journal of Anaesthesia* 46, 365–72.

Moore, J.L., Martin, J.N. (1992) Cancer and pregnancy. *Obstetrics and Gynecology Clinics of North America* 19(4), 815–27.

Moore, S. (1997) Physiology of pain. In: *Understanding Pain and its Relief in Labour* (ed S. Moore), Chapter 3. Churchill Livingstone, Edinburgh.

Moore, W.M.V., McLure Brown, J.C., Hill, I.D. (1965) Clinical trial of audic-analgesia in childbirth. *Journal of Obstetrics and Gynaecology of the British Commonwealth* 72, 626–9.

Morey, R.J., MacDonald, R., Fisk, N.M., Morgan, B.M. (1994) Patient control of combined spinal epidural anaesthesia. *Lancet* 344(8931), 1238.

Morgan, B.M. (1984) The consumer's attitude to obstetric care. *British Journal of Obstetrics and Gynaecology* 91, 624–8.

Morgan, B.M. (1987) Mortality and anaesthesia. In: *Foundations of Obstetric Anaesthesia* (ed B.M. Morgan). Farrand Press, London.

Morgan, B.M. (1993a) Obstetrical anaesthesia. In: *Pain and its Relief in Childbirth* (G. Chamberlain, A. Wraight & P. Steer), pp. 69–78. Churchill Livingstone, Edinburgh.

Morgan, B.M. (1993b) Mobile epidurals: combined spinal epidural analgesia in labour. *MIDIRS Midwifery Digest* 3(3), 312–13.

Morgan, B.M., Bulpitt, C.J., Clifton, P., Lewis, P.J. (1982) Analgesia and satisfaction in childbirth. *Lancet* ii, 808–810.

Morgan, B.M., Kadim, M.Y. (1994) Mobile regional analgesia in labour. *British Journal of Obstetrics and Gynaecology* 101(10), 839–41.

Morin, F. (1955) A new spinal pathway for cutaneous impulses. *American Journal of Physiology* 183(2), 245.

Morishima, H.O., Pedersen, H., Finster, M. (1980) Effects of pain on mother, labour and fetus. In *Obstetric Analgesia and Anaesthesia* (eds G.F. Marx & G.M. Bessel), pp. 197–209. Holland Biomedical Press, Amsterdam.

Morrison, C.E., Dutton, D., Howie, H., Gilmour, H. (1987) Pethidine compared with meptazinol in labour. *Anaesthesia* 42(1), 7–14.

Morrow, C.P., Curtin, J.P., Townsend, D.E. (1993) Cancer and pregnancy. In: *Synopsis of Gynaecologic Oncology*, 4th edn. (eds C.P. Morrow, J.P. Curtin & D.E. Townsend). Churchill Livingstone, Edinburgh.

Morse, J.M., Park, C. (1988) Home birth and hospital deliveries: a comparison of the perceived painfulness of parturition. *Research in Nursing and Health* 11, 175–81.

Motoyama, E.K., Rivard, G., Acheson, F. (1966) Adverse effects of maternal ventilation on the fetus. *Lancet* 1 (7432), 286–9.

Mountcastle, V.B. (1980) *Medical Physiology*, 14th edn. Mosby, St Louis.

Mueller, R.F., Young, I.D. (1995) *Emery's Elements of Medical Genetics*, 9th edn. Churchill Livingstone, Edinburgh.

Mulder, E.J.H., Visser, G.H.A. (1987) Braxton Hicks' contractions and motor behaviour in the near-term human fetus. *American Journal of Obstetrics and Gynaecology* 156(3), 543–9.

Myrnick, A. (1981) Instituting a postpartum self medication program. *Maternal and Child Health Nursing Journal* 6, 422–4.

Nathan, L., Huddleston, J.F. (1995) Acute abdominal pain in pregnancy. *Obstetrics and Gynecology Clinics of North America* 22(1), 55–67.

Nazarko, L. (1995) The therapeutic uses of cranberry juice. *Nursing Standard* 9(3), 33–5.

Newson, K. (1984) Care during labour. *British Journal of Obstetrics and Gynaecology* 91 (July), 609–610.

Newton, C. (1992) Hazards of N_2O exposure. *Nursing Times* 88(39), 54.

Newton, N., Newton, M. (1972) Childbirth in cross-cultural perspectives. In: *Modern Perspectives in Psycho-Obstetrics* (J.G. Howells). Brunner/ Mazel, New York.

Nichols, M.R. (1995) Adjustment to new parenthood: attenders versus non-attenders at prenatal education classes. *Birth* 22(1), 21–6.

Nicholls, P.A. (1988) *Homeopathy and the Medical Profession*. Croom Helm, London.

Nicholson, W. (1985) Cracked nipples in breastfeeding mothers. *Nursing Mothers of Australia Newsletter* 27, 7–10.

Niebyl, J., Bell, W., Schaaf, M., Blake, D., Dubin, N., King, T. (1979) The effect of chlorotrianisene as postpartum lactation suppression. *American Journal of Obstetrics and Gynecology* 134, 518.

Nikodem, V.C., Danziger, D., Gebka, N., Gulmezoglu, A.M., Hofmeyr, G.J. (1993) Do cabbage leaves prevent breast engorgement? A randomised, controlled study. *Birth* 20(2), 61–4.

Nimmo, W.J., Wilson, J., Prescott, L.F. (1975) Narcotic analgesics and delayed gastric emptying during labour. *Lancet* 1(7912), 890–893.

Nimmo, W.S., Wilson, J., Prescott, L.F. (1977) Further studies of gastric emptying during labour. *Anaesthesia* 32(1), 100–101.

Nissen, E., Widstrom, A.M., Lilja, G., *et al.* (1997) Effects of routinely given pethidine during labour on infants' developing breastfeeding behaviour *Acta Paediatrica* 86(2), 201–208.

Niven, C. (1985) How helpful is the presence of the husband at childbirth? *Journal of Reproductive and Infant Psychology* 3(2), 45–53.

Niven, C. (1992) *Psychological Care for Families: Before, During and After Birth*. Butterworth Heinemann, Oxford.

Niven, C. (1994) Coping with labour pain: the midwife's role. In: *Midwives, Research and Childbirth III* (S. Robinson & A.M. Thomson). Chapman & Hall, London.

234 Pain in Childbearing and its Control

Niven, C., Gijsbers, K. (1984a) A study of labour pain using the McGill Pain Questionnaire. *Social Science and Medicine* 19(12), 1347–51.

Niven, C., Gijsbers, K. (1984b) Obstetric and non-obstetric factors related to labour pain. *Journal of Reproductive and Infant Psychology* 2(2), 61–78.

Niven, C., Gijsbers, K. (1996a) Perinatal pain. In: *Conception, Pregnancy and Birth* (eds C.A. Niven & A. Walker), pp. 131–47. Butterworth Heinemann, Oxford.

Niven, C., Gijsbers, K. (1996b) Coping with labour pain. *Journal of Pain and Symptom Management* 11(2), 116–25.

Nolan, M. (1990) Normal delivery after caesarean section. *Nursing Times* 86(32), 34–8.

Nolan, M.L. (1997) Antenatal education – where next? *Journal of Advanced Nursing* 25(6), 1198–1204.

Nyatanga, B. (1993) Emotional pain in terminal illness: a dilemma for nurses. *Senior Nurse*, 13(3), 46–6.

Oakley, A. (1980) *Women Confined: Towards a Sociology of Childbearing.* Martin Robinson, Oxford.

Oakley, A. (1993) The follow-up survey. In: *Pain and its Relief in Childbirth: The Results of a National Survey Conducted by the National Birthday Trust.* (eds G. Chamberlain, A. Wraight & P. Steer), Chapter 10. Churchill Livingstone, Edinburgh.

Oakley, A., McPherson, A., Roberts, H. (1984) *Miscarriage.* Fontana, London.

Oakley, A., Richards, M.P.M. (1990) Some women's experiences of caesarean delivery. In: *The Politics of Maternity Care: Services for Childbearing Women in Twentieth Century Britain* (J. Garcia, R. Kilpatrick & M.P.M. Richards). Clarendon, Oxford.

Oberst, M.T. (1995) Our naked emperor. *Research in Nursing and Health* 18(1), 1–2.

O'Brien, P. (1986) *Birth and Our Bodies.* Pandora, London.

Odent, M. (1983) Birth under water. *Lancet* ii, 1476–7.

Odent, M. (1994) *Birth Reborn*, 2nd edn. Souvenir Press, London.

O'Driscoll, K., Meagher, D. (1986) *Active Management of Labour*, 2nd edn. Baillière Tindall, London.

Olds, S.B., London, M.L., Ladewig, P.W. (1996) *Maternal–Newborn Nursing – A Family Centred Approach*, 5th edn. Addison-Wesley, California.

Olofsson, C.H., Ekblom, A., Ekman-Ordeberg, G., Hjelm, A., Irestedt, L. (1996) Lack of analgesic effect of systematically administered morphine or pethidine on labour pain. *British Journal of Obstetrics and Gynaecology* 103 (10); 968–72.

Olsen, K.G. (1991) *The Encyclopaedia of Alternative Health Care.* Piatkus, London.

O'Neill, A. (1994) Danger and safety in medicines. *Social Science and Medicine* 38(4), 497–507.

Orner, H., Friedlander, D., Palti, Z. (1986) Hypnotic relaxation in the treatment of premature labor. *Psychosomatic Medicine* 48, 351–61.

Ostgaard, H.C., Andersson, G.B.J. (1992) Postpartum low-back pain. *Spine* 17(1), 53–5.

Oxorn, H. (1986) *Human Labor and Birth*, 5th edn. Prentice Hall, Englewood Cliffs.

Paech, M.L. (1996) Patient controlled epidural analgesia in obstetrics. *International Journal of Obstetric Anaesthesia* 5(2), 115–25.

Parazzini, F., Zanaboni, F., Liberati, A., Tognoni, G. (1989) Relief of breast symptoms in women who are not breastfeeding. In: *Effective Care in Pregnancy and Childbirth* (eds I. Chalmers, M. Enkin & M.J.N.C. Keirse), pp. 1390–1403. Oxford University Press, Oxford.

Park, G., Fulton, B., (1991) *The Management of Acute Pain.* Oxford University Press, Oxford.

Parsons, G. (1994) The benefits of relaxation in the control of pain. *Nursing Times* 90(19), 11–12.

Parsons, L, MacFarlane, A, Golding, J. (1993) Pregnancy, birth and maternity care. In: *'Race' and Health in Contemporary Britain* (W.I.V. Ahmad), Chapter 4. Open University Press, Buckingham.

Pavlik, M. (1988) Positioning: first stage of labour. In: *Childbirth Education: Practice, Research and Theory* (F.H. Nichols & S.S. Humenick), Chapter 15. W.B. Saunders, Philadelphia.

Peabody, J.L. (1979) Transcutaneous oxygen measurement to evaluate drug effect. *Clinical Perinatology* 6(1), 109–121.

Peacock, E., Furedi, A. (1996) Women. *The Guardian* 22 July p.5.

Peacock, J.L. (1986) *The Anthropological Lens: Harsh Light, Soft Focus.* Cambridge University Press, Cambridge.

Pearl, M.L., Roberts, J.M., Laros, R.K. (1993) Vaginal delivery from the persistent occipito posterior position: influence on maternal and neonatal morbidity. *Journal of Reproductive Medicine* 38(12), 955–61.

Pearson, J.F., Davies, P. (1973) The effect of continuous lumbar epidural analgesia on maternal acid–base balance and arterial lactate concentration during the second stage of labour. *Journal of Obstetric Gynaecology of the British Commonwealth* 80(3), 225–9.

Penn, R.G. (1986) Iatrogenic disease: an historical survey of adverse reactions before thalidomide. In: *Iatrogenic Diseases*, 3rd edn. (eds P.F. d'Arcy & J.P. Griffin). Oxford University Press, Oxford.

Penticuff, J.H. (1989) Infant suffering and nurse advocacy in neonatal intensive care. *Nursing Clinics of North America* 24(4), 987–96.

Perkins, E.R. (1980) *Education for Childbirth and Parenthood.* Croom Helm, London.

Perl, E.R. (1971) Is pain a specific sensation? *Journal of Psychiatric Research* 8(3/4), 273–87.

Philips, H.C. (1988) Changing chronic pain experience. *Pain* 32, 165–72.

Phillips, G.D., Cousins, M.J. (1986) Neurological mechanisms of pain and the relationship of pain, anxiety and sleep. In: *Acute Pain Management* (eds M. Cousins & G.D. Phillips), pp. 21–48. Churchill Livingstone, New York.

Phoenix, A. (1990) Black women and the maternity services. In: *The Politics of Maternity Care: Services for Childbearing Women in Twentieth-Century Britain* (J. Garcia, R. Kilpatrick & M. Richards), pp. 274–99. Clarendon, Oxford.

Pickles, C. (1987) Pregnancy induced hypertension. *Midwife, Health Visitor and Community Nurse* 23(10), 438–42.

Polvi, H.J., Pirhonen, J.P., Erkkola, R.I.J. (1996) Nitrous oxide inhalation:

effects on maternal and fetal circulations at term. *Obstetrics and Gynecology* 87(6), 1045–8.

Pomeranz, B., Wall, P.D., Weber, W.V. (1968) Cord cells responding to fine myelinated afferants from viscera, muscle and skin. *Journal of Physiology* 199(3), 511–32.

Porter, J., Jick, J. (1980) Addiction rare in patients treated with narcotics. *New England Journal of Medicine* 302, 123.

Porter, M., Macintyre, S. (1989) Psychosocial effectiveness of antenatal and postnatal care. In: *Midwives, Research and Childbirth 1* (S. Robinson & A.M. Thomson), pp. 72–94. Chapman & Hall, London.

Porter, R.W., Jiang, B. (1990) *Pregnancy and Chronic Back Pain*. International Society for the Study of the Lumbar Spine, Boston.

Prechtl, H.F.R. (1985) Ultrasound studies of human foetal behaviour. *Early Human Development* 12(2), 91–8.

Price, D.D., Dubner, R. (1977) Neurons that subserve the sensory-discriminative aspects of pain. *Pain* 3(4), 307.

Price, K., Cheek, J. (1996) Exploring the nursing role in pain management from a post-structuralist perspective. *Journal of Advanced Nursing* 24(5), 899–904.

Priest, J., Schott, J. (1991) Leading Antenatal Classes: A Practical Guide. Butterworth Heinemann, Oxford.

Pritchard, J.A., Cunningham, F.G., Pritchard, S.A., Mason, R.A. (1991) On reducing the frequency of severe abruptio placenta. *American Journal of Obstetrics and Gynecology* 165(5) Part 1, 1345–51.

Procacci, P., Massimo, Z., Naresca, M. (1994) Heart and vascular pain. In: *Textbook of Pain*, 3rd edn. (eds P.D. Wall & R. Melzack), pp. 541–54. Churchill Livingstone, Edinburgh.

Pugh, L.C., Buchko, B.L., Bishop, B.A., Cochran, J.F., Smith, L.R., Lerew, D.J. (1996) A comparison of topical agents to relieve nipple pain and enhance breastfeeding. *Birth* 23(2), 88–93.

Pulsford, D. (1992) Do we need research? *Nursing Times* 88(34), 42–3.

Pursey, M. (1994) Mobile epidural – the only analgesia without anaesthesia. *Paediatric Post* 3.

Puskar, K., Mumford, K. (1990) The healing power. *Nursing Times* 86(33), 50–52.

Quine, L., Rutter, D.R., Gowen, S. (1993) Women's satisfaction with the birth experience: a prospective study of social and psychological predictors. *Journal of Reproductive and Infant Psychology* 11(2), 107–113.

Rajan, L. (1993) Perceptions of pain and pain relief in labour: the gulf between experience and observation. *Midwifery* 9(3), 136–45.

Rajan, L. (1994) The impact of obstetric procedures and analgesia/anaesthesia during labour and delivery on breast feeding. *Midwifery* 10(2), 87–103.

Ralph, C. (1991) *Transcutaneous Nerve Stimulation*. Registrar's Letter. United Kingdom Central Council for Nursing, Midwifery and Health Visiting, London.

Ramenghi, L.A., Griffith, E.C., Wood, C.M., Levene, M.I. (1996) Effect of non sucrose sweet tasting solution on neonatal heel prick responses. *Archives of Disease in Childhood (Fetal and Neonatal Edn.)* 74(2), F129–31.

Ramin, S.M., Gambling, D.R., Lucas, M.J. (1995) Randomised trial of epidural versus intravenous analgesia during labour. *Lancet* 345, 1413–16.

Ramsay, M.M. (1993) Eclampsia: a bolt from the blue? *Current Obstetrics and Gynaecology* 3(2), 88–90.

Rankin, S. (1993) Disorders of pregnancy. In: *Myles Textbook for Midwives* (eds V.R. Bennett & L.K. Brown), pp. 320–334. Churchill Livingstone, Edinburgh.

Raphael-Leff, J. (1991) *Psychological Processes of Childbearing.* Chapman & Hall, London.

Rawlinson, P. (1996) *Human Sentience Before Birth: A Report by the Commission of Inquiry Into Fetal Sentience.* Report produced by the CARE Trust, London.

Regnard, C.F.B., Badger, C. (1987) Metabolism of narcotics. *British Medical Journal* 288, 460

Reilly, D.T., Taylor, M.A., McSharry, C., Aitchison, T. (1986) Is homeopathy a placebo response? *Lancet* 2(8512), 881–6.

Reynolds, D.V. (1969) Surgery in the rat during electrical analgesia induced by focal brain stimulation. *Science* 164(3878), 444–5.

Reynolds, F. (1989) *Epidural Analgesia in Obstetrics.* Baillière Tindall, London.

Reynolds, F. (ed) (1990) *Epidural and Spinal Blockade in Obstetrics.* Baillière Tindall, London.

Reynolds, F. (1997a) *Medicine Now.* BBC Transcript, 14 January.

Reynolds, F. (1997b) Opioids in labour – no analgesic effect. *Lancet* 349(9044), 4–5.

Roberts, H., Evans, L. (1991) *The Management of Miscarriage by General Practitioners and Trainees in the West of Scotland.* GGHB and Department of Child Health Obstetrics, University of Glasgow.

Roberts, J. (1989) Maternal Position during the first stage of labour. In: *Effective Care in Pregnancy and Childbirth*, Vol. 2 (I. Chalmers, M. Enkin & M.J.N.C. Keirse), pp. 883–92. Oxford University Press, Oxford.

Robertson, A. (1994) *Empowering Women: Teaching Active Birth in the '90s.* ACE Graphics, Camperdown, Australia.

Robinson, J. (1994) Waterbirth study. *AIMS Journal* 7(1), 16.

Robinson, J. (1995) Use of heroin in labour – AIMS' concern. *AIMS Journal* 7(2), 9–10.

Robinson, J. (1996a) Death of a mother. *British Journal of Midwifery* 4(7), 381–3.

Robinson, J. (1996b) It's only a questionnaire.... ethics in social science research. *British Journal of Midwifery* 4(1), 41–4.

Robinson, J. (1996c) A charter for ethical research in maternity care. *AIMS Journal* 7(4), 11–13.

Robinson, J. (1997). Can we measure empathy? *British Journal of Midwifery* 5(1), 44–5.

Robson, S.E.E. (1992) Variation of cervical dilatation estimation by midwives, doctors, student midwives and medical students – a small study using cervical simulation methods. In: *Research and the Midwife Conference Proceedings*, 1991, University of Manchester.

Roch, S. (1993) The use of drugs by the midwife. In: *Myles Textbook for*

Midwives (eds V.R. Bennett & L.K. Brown). Churchill Livingstone, Edinburgh.

Rodgers, B.L., Cowles, K.V. (1997) A conceptual framework for human suffering in nursing care and research. *Journal of Advanced Nursing* 25(5), 1048–53.

Rogers, D.A., Dingus, D., Standfield, J., Dipiro, J.R., May, J.R., Bowden, T.A. (1990) A prospective study of patient controlled analgesia impact on overall hospital course. *American Surgeon* 56(2), 86–8.

Rogers, M. (1980) Nursing: a science of unitary man. In: *Conceptual Models for Nursing Practice*, 2nd edn. (eds J. Riehl & C. Roy). Appleton-Century Crofts, Norwalk, Connecticut.

Rollman, G.B. (1983) Measurement of experimental pain in chronic pain patients: methodological and individual factors. In: *Pain Measurement and Assessment* (R. Melzack), pp. 251–8. Raven Press, New York.

Roman, Y., Artal, R. (1986) Physiological and endocrine adjustments to pregnancy. In: *Exercise in Pregnancy* (eds R. Artal & R.A. Wiswell). Williams Wilkins, Baltimore.

Rose, A.T., Hilbers, S.M. (1988) Relaxation: paced breathing techniques. In: *Childbirth Education: Practice, Research and Theory* (F.H. Nichols & S.S. Humenick), Chapter 14. W.B. Saunders, Philadelphia.

Rosenbaum, J.F., Biederman, J., Pollock, R.A., Hirshfeld, D.R. (1994). The etiology of social phobia. *Journal of Clinical Psychiatry* 55(Suppl.), 10–16.

Rosenbaum, R.B., Ochoa, J.L. (1993) *Carpal Tunnel Syndrome and Other Disorders of the Median Nerve*. Butterworth-Heinemann, Boston.

Royal College of Midwives (1991) *Successful Breastfeeding*, 2nd edn. Churchill Livingstone, Edinburgh.

Royal Infirmary of Edinburgh (1995) *Guidelines for the Management of Postoperative Pain*. Royal Infirmary of Edinburgh NHS Trust.

Rubin, P.C. (1987) General principles. In: Prescribing in Pregnancy (ed P.C. Rubin). *British Medical Journal*, London.

Ruiz-Irastorza, G., Lima, F., Alves, M., *et al.* (1996) Increased rate of lupus flare during pregnancy and the puerperium. *British Journal of Rheumatology* 35, 133–8.

Rush, J., Burlock, S., Lambert, K., Loosley-Millman, M., Hutchison, B., Enkin, M. (1996) The effects of whirlpool baths in labour: a randomised controlled trial. *Birth* 23(3), 136–43.

Rushforth, J.A., Levene, M.I. (1993) Behavioural response to pain in healthy neonates. *Archives of Disease in Childhood* 70(3), F174–6.

Russell, J.G.B. (1969) Moulding of the pelvic outlet. *Journal of Obstetrics and Gynaecology of the British Commonwealth* 76, 817–20.

Russell, R., Dundas, R., Reynolds, F. (1996) Long-term backache after childbirth: prospective search for causative factors. *British Medical Journal* 312, 1384–8.

Russell, R., Groves, P., Taub, N., O'Dowd, J., Reynolds, F. (1993) Assessing long term backache after childbirth. *British Medical Journal* 306 (6888), 1299–1303.

Saftlas, A.F., Olson, D.R., Atrash, H.K., Rochat, R., Rowley, D. (1991) National trends in the incidence of abruptio placentae, 1979–87. *Obstetrics and Gynaecology* 32(2), 174–6.

St James-Roberts, I., Hutchinson, C., Haran, F., Chamberlain, G. (1982) Bio-feedback as an aid to childbirth. *British Journal of Obstetrics and Gynaecology* 90, 56–60.

Salar, G., Job, I., Mingrino, S. (1981) Effect of transcutaneous electrotherapy on CSF β-endorphin content in patients without pain problems. *Pain* 10(2), 169–72.

Samarel, N. (1992) The experience of receiving therapeutic touch. *Journal of Advanced Nursing* 17(6), 651–7.

Sammons, L.N. (1984) The use of music by women during childbirth. *Journal of Nurse-Midwifery* 29(4), 266–70.

Saunders, S. (1997) Breast pain in the lactating mother. *Midwives* 110(1308), 8–9.

Savage, W. (1987) The management of obstetric pain. In: *The History and Management of Pain* (R.D. Mann), Chapter 10. Parthenon, Carnforth.

Scarry, E. (1985) *The Body in Pain: the Making and Unmaking of the World.* Oxford University Press, Oxford.

Schieve, L.A., Handler, A., Hershow, R., Persky, V., Davis, F. (1994) Urinary tract infection during pregnancy: its association with maternal morbidity and perinatal outcome. *American Journal of Public Health* 84(3), 405–410.

Schott, J., Henley, A. (1996) *Culture, Religion and Childbearing in a Multiracial Society: A Handbook for Health Professionals.* Butterworth Heinemann, London.

Schrock, P. (1988) The basis of relaxation. In: *Childbirth Education: Practice, Research and Theory* (F.H. Nichols & S.S. Humenick). W.B. Saunders, Philadelphia.

Schultz, R., Read, A.W., Straton, J.A., Stanley, F.J., Morich, P. (1991) Genitourinary tract infections in pregnancy and low birth weight: case control study in Australian Aboriginal women. *British Medical Journal* 303(6814), 1369–73.

Schuman, A.N., Marteau, T.M. (1993) Obstetricians' and midwives' contrasting perceptions of pregnancy. *Journal of Reproductive and Infant Psychology* 11(2), 115–18.

Scott, D.B., Tunstall, M.E. (1995) Serious complications associated with epidural/spinal blockade in obstetrics; a two year prospective study. *International Journal of Obstetric Anaesthesia* 4, 133–9.

Scott, G., Niven, C. (1996) Pregnancy: a biopsychosocial event. In: *Conception, Pregnancy and Birth.* (eds C.A. Niven & A. Walker pp. 41–56. Butterworth Heinemann, Oxford.

Scottish Home and Health Department (1985) *Obstetric Anaesthesia and Analgesia in Scotland.* National Medical Consultative Committee, Edinburgh Scottish Home and Health Department.

Scottish Office (1995) *Supporting Breastfeeding in Your Primary Health Care Team.* Edinburgh Scottish Office.

Sechzer, P.H. (1971) Studies in pain with an analgesic demand system. *Anaesthesia and Analgesia* 50, 1–10.

Sechzer, P.H. Wachtel, J., Keats, A.S. (1968) Circulatory lability and myocardial stress. *American Journal of Surgery* 116, 686–92.

Senden, I.P.M., van der Wettering, M.D., Eskes, A.B., Bierkens, P.B., Laube, D.W., Pitkin, M.D. (1988) Labour pain: a comparison of parturients in a

Dutch and an American teaching hospital. *Obstetrics and Gynecology* 71(4), 451–3.

Shade, P. (1992) Patient controlled analgesia: can client education improve outcomes? *Journal of Advanced Nursing* 17, 408–413.

Shapiro, A.G., Thomas, L. (1984) Efficacy of Bromocriptine versus breast binders as inhibitors of postpartum lactation. *Southern Medical Journal* 77, 719–21.

Shearer, E.M. (1995) Commentary: many factors affect the outcome of pre-natal classes. *Birth* 22(1), 27–8.

Sheikh, A.A., Jordan, C.S. (1983) Clinical uses of mental imagery. In: *Imagery: Current Theory, Research and Application* (ed A.A. Sheikh), Chapter 13. Wiley, New York.

Shepherd, J., Fry, D. (1996) Symphysis pubis pain. *Midwives* 109(1302), 199–201.

Shepherd, J.H. (1990) Cancer complicating pregnancy. In: *Clinical Gyneco-logical oncology* (eds J.H. Shepherd & J.M. Monaghan). Blackwell Science, Oxford.

Shergold, L. (1986) Epidural and spinal anaesthetics. *Nursing Times* 82(26), 44–5.

Sherwood, L. (1995) *Fundamentals of Physiology: A Human Perspective.* West Publishing, Minneapolis.

Shnider, S.M., Abboud, T.K, Artal, R., Henriksen, E.H., Stefani, S.J., Levinsen, G. (1983) Maternal catecholamine decrease during labor after lumbar epidural anesthesia. *American Journal of Obstetrics and Gynecology* 147(1), 13–15.

Shnider, S.M., Wright, R.G., Levinson, G. (1979) Uterine blood flow and plasma norepinephrine changes during maternal stress in the pregnant ewe. *Anaesthesiology* 50(6), 524–30.

Shurtz, J.D., Mayhew, R.B., Clayton, T.G. (1986) Depression recognition and control. *Dental Clinics of North America* 30(4 Suppl.), S55–65.

Sicuteri, F. (1974) Floor discussion – peripheral nerve disorders. In: *Advances in Neurology 4* (ed J.J. Bonica), p. 316. Raven Press, New York.

Simkin, P. (1989) Non-pharmacological methods of pain relief during labour. In: *Effective Care in Pregnancy and Childbirth* (I. Chalmers, M. Enkin & M.J.N.C. Keirse), Chapter 56. Oxford University Press, Oxford.

Simkin, P. (1996) Intracutaneous injection of sterile water for relief of low back pain in labour. *Birth* 23(4), 249.

Simkin, P., Enkin, M. (1989) Antenatal classes. In: *Effective Care in Preg-nancy and Childbirth* (I. Chalmers, M. Enkin & M.H.N.C. Keirse), pp. 319–34. Oxford University Press, Oxford.

Simpson, D., Smith, R. (1995a) Drugs, the law and the midwife: 1. *British Journal of Midwifery* 3(8), 320–322.

Simpson, D., Smith, R. (1995b) Drugs, the law and the midwife: 2. *British Journal of Midwifery* 3(10), 553–6.

Sindhu, F. (1996) Are non-pharmacological nursing interventions for the management of pain effective? – a meta-analysis *Journal of Advanced Nursing* 24(6), 1152–9.

Singer, S. (1985) *Human Genetics: An Introduction to the Principles of heredity*, 2nd edn. Freeman, New York.

Sjölund, B.H., Eriksson, M., Loeser, J.D. (1990) Transcutaneous and implanted electrical stimulation of peripheral nerves. In: *The Management of Pain*, 2nd edn. (eds J.J. Bonica, L.D. Loeser, C.R. Chapman & W.E. Fordyce), pp. 1852–61. Lea & Febiger, Philadelphia.

Skibsted, L., Lange, A.P. (1992) The need for pain relief in uncomplicated deliveries in an alternative birth centre compared to an obstetric delivery ward. *Pain* 48(2), 183–6.

Skovlund, E., Fyllingen, G., Landre, H., Nesheim, B.-I. (1991) Comparison of postpartum pain treatments using a sequential trial design: II Naproxen versus paracetamol. *European Journal of Clinical Pharmacology* 40(6), 539–42.

Sleep, J. (1984) The West Berkshire episiotomy trial. In: *Research and the Midwife Conference Proceedings* (eds A. Thomson & S. Robinson), 1983, University of Manchester.

Sleep, J. (1991) Postnatal perineal care. In: *Postnatal Care: A Research-Based Approach* (eds J. Alexander, V. Levy & S. Roch), pp. 1–17. Macmillan, London.

Sleep, J., Grant, A. (1987a) West Berkshire perineal management trial: three years follow-up. *British Medical Journal*, 295(6601), 749–51.

Sleep, J., Grant, A. (1987b) Pelvic floor exercises in postnatal care. *Midwifery* 3(4), 158–64.

Sleep, J., Grant, A. (1988a) Routine addition of salt or Savlon bath concentrate during bathing in the immediate postpartum period – a randomised controlled trial. *Nursing Times* 84(21), 55–7.

Sleep, J., Grant, A. (1988b) The relief of perineal pain following childbirth: a survey of midwifery practice. *Midwifery* 4(3), 118–22.

Sleep, J., Grant, A., Ashurst, H., Spencer, J.A.D. (1989) Dyspareunia associated with the use of glycerol-impregnated catgut to repair perineal trauma. *British Journal of Obstetrics and Gynaecology* 96(6), 741–3.

Slevin, M., Murphy, J. (1996) Retinopathy of prematurity screening and distress. *Society for Reproductive and Infant Psychology Conference*, September 1996, Leeds.

Sloane, E. (1993) *The Biology of Women*, 3rd edn. Delmar, New York.

Smith, F.B. (1979) *The People's Health 1830–1910*. Holmes Meier, New York.

Snell, C.C., Fothergill-Bourbonais, F., Durocher-Henriks, S. (1997) Patient controlled analgesia and intramuscular injections: a comparison of patient pain experiences and postoperative outcomes. *Journal of Advanced Nursing* 25(4), 681–90.

Snyder, R. (1977) The organisation of the dorsal root entry zone in cats and monkeys. *Journal of Comparative Neurology* 174(1), 47–70.

Sofaer, B. (1985) *The Effects of a Focused Education for Nursing Teams on Post Operative Pain of Patients*. Unpublished PhD thesis, University of Edinburgh.

Scottish Office Home and Health Department (1996) *Report on Pain Relief in Labour*. Clinical Research and Audit Group, Working Group on Maternity Services, Edinburgh.

Sosa, R., Kennell, J.H., Klaus, M.H., Unruttia, J. (1980) The effect of a supportive companion. *New England Journal of Medicine* 303, 597–600.

Spanos, N.P., Carmanico, S.J., Ellis, J.A. (1994) Hypnotic analgesia. In: *Textbook of Pain*, 3rd edn. (eds P.D. Wall & R. Melzack), pp. 1349–66. Churchill Livingstone, Edinburgh.

Sparshott, M. (1997) *Pain, Distress and the Newborn Baby*. Blackwell Science, Oxford.

Spencer, J.A.D., Grant, A., Elbourne, D., Garcia, J., Sleep, J. (1986) A randomised comparison of glycerol impregnated chromic catgut with untreated chromic catgut for the repair of perineal trauma. *British Journal of Obstetrics and Gynaecology* 93(5), 426–30.

Spross, J. (1993) Pain suffering and spiritual well-being: assessment and interventions. *Quality of Life* 3(3), 71–9.

Stalheim-Smith, A., Fitch, G.H. (1993) *Understanding Human Physiology*. West Publishing, Minneapolis.

Stamp, G.E., Williams, A.S., Crowther, C.A. (1995) Evaluation of antenatal and postnatal support. *Birth* 22(3), 138–43.

Stanway, A. (1992) *Alternative Medicine: A Guide to Natural Therapies*. Bloomsbury Books, London.

Steer, P. (1993) The methods of pain relief used. In: *Pain and its Relief in Childbirth* (G. Chamberlain, A. Wraight & P. Steer), Chapter 6. Churchill Livingstone, Edinburgh.

Steffes, S.A. (1988) Relaxation: imagery. In: *Childbirth Education: Practice, Research and Theory* (F.H. Nichols & S.S. Humenick). W.B. Saunders, Philadelphia.

Steinberg, E.S., Fishman, E.B., Santos, A.C. (1996) Local anesthetics. In: *A Practical Approach to Pain Management* (eds M. Lefkowitz & A.H. Lebovits), pp. 32–40. Little Brown & Co., Boston.

Sternbach, R.A. (1968) *Pain: A Psychophysiological Analysis*. Academic Press, New York.

Sternbach, R.A., Tursky, B. (1965) Ethnic differences among housewives in psychophysical and skin potential responses to electric shock. *Psychophysiology 1*, 241–6.

Stevens, B. (1996) Pain management in newborns: how far have we progressed in research and practice? *Birth* 23(4), 229–35.

Stewart, M., West, C. (undated) *The Birth of Your Baby at the Simpson*. Royal Infirmary of Edinburgh, Edinburgh.

Stewart, M.L. (1977) Measurement of clinical pain. *Pain: A Source Book for Nurses and Other Health Professionals* (ed A.K. Jacox), pp. 107–138. Little Brown & Co, Boston.

Stirk, F. (1991) Sickle cell in pregnancy. *Nursing Times* 87(41), 36–8.

Stroebe, W., Stroebe, M.S. (1987) *Bereavement and Health: The Psychological and Physical Consequences of Partner Loss*. Cambridge University Press, Cambridge.

Sturdy, D.E. (1990) Acute painful conditions of the perineum. In: *Pelvic Pain in Women* (ed I. Rocker), pp. 86–8. Springer-Verlag, London.

Sutton, J., Scott, P. (1994) Optimal fetal positioning: a midwifery approach to increasing the number of normal births. *MIDIRS Midwifery Digest* 4(3), 283–6.

Swanberg, E.C. (1979) Adhesiveness to urinary tract epithelial cells. *Journal of Urology* 22(2), 185 de Swiet, M. (1991) The cardiovascular system. In: *Clinical Physiology in Obstetrics* (F.E. Hytten & G. Chamberlain), pp. 3–38. Blackwell Science, Oxford.

de Swiet, M. (1995) Thromboembolism. In: *Medical Disorders in Obstetric Practice*, 3rd edn. (ed M. de Swiet), pp. 116–42. Blackwell Science, Oxford.

Symes, N. (1994) OP position a challenge for midwives. *MIDIRS Midwifery Digest* 4(2), 194.

Szasz, T. (1957) *Pain and Pleasure: A Study of Bodily Feelings.* Tavistock, London.

Taddio, A., Katz, J., Ilersich, A.L., Koren, G. (1997) Effect of neonatal circumcision on pain response during subsequent routine vaccination. *Lancet* 349(9052), 599–603.

Tarrant, J. (1993) Recent research on perineal repair. *Modern Midwife* 3(40, 24–6.

Tasharrofi, A. (1993) Midwifery care in the Netherlands. *Midwives Chronicle* 106(1267), 286–8.

Taub, A. (1974) Floor discussion: peripheral nerve disorders. In: *Advances in Neurology* 4th edn. (ed J.J. Bonica), p. 318. Raven Press, New York.

Taylor, S.E. (1983) Adjustment to threatening events: a theory of cognitive adaptation. *American Psychologist* 38, 1161.

van Teijlingen, E. (1994) *A Social or Medical Model of Childbirth? Comparing the Arguments in Grampian (Scotland) and The Netherlands.* Unpublished PhD thesis, University of Aberdeen.

Terenius, L., Wahlstrom, A. (1974) Inhibitor(s) of narcotic receptor binding in brain extracts and cerebrospinal fluid. *Acta Pharmacologica et Toxicologica* 35(Suppl.), S55.

Terman, G., Lewis, P., Leibeskind, M.J. (1984) Endogenous pain inhibitory substrates and mechanisms. In: *Advances in Pain Research and Therapy*, 7th edn. (eds C. Benedetti,. C.R. Chapman & G. Morricca), pp. 43–56. Raven Press, New York.

Tew, M. (1995) *Safer Childbirth? A Critical History of Maternity Care*, 2nd edn. Chapman & Hall, London.

Thomas, T.H., Fletcher, J.E., Hill, R.G. (1982) Influence of medication, pain and progress in labour on plasma beta-endorphin-like immunoreactivity. *British Journal of Anaesthesia* 54(4), 401–408.

Thomsen, A.C., Espersen, T., Maigaard, S. (1984) Course and treatment of milk stasis. *American Journal of Obstetrics and Cynecology* 149, 492–5.

Thomson, A.M., Hillier, V.F. (1994) A re-evaluation of the effect of pethidine on the length of labour. *Journal of Advanced Nursing* 19(3), 448–56.

Thomson, V. (1993) Psychological and physiological changes of pregnancy. In: *Myles Textbook for Midwives* (eds V.R. Bennett & L.K. Brown), pp. 94–105. Churchill Livingstone, Edinburgh.

Thornton, J.G., Lilford, R.J. (1994) Active management of labour: current knowledge and research issues. *British Medical Journal* 309(6951), 366–9.

Timm, M.M. (1989) Prenatal education evaluation. *Nursing Research* 28(6), 338–42.

To, W.W.K., Ngai, C.S.W., Ma, H.K. (1995) Pregnancies complicated by acute appendicitis. *Australian and New Zealand Journal of Surgery* 65(11), 799–803.

Trenam, G. (1994) A teaching strategy to identify the form of pain relief most suited to couples' needs. *International Journal of Childbirth Education* 9(2), 39.

Trevor, A.J., Miller, R.D. (1992) General anaesthetics. In: *Basic and Clinical Pharmacology* (B.G. Katzung). Lange, Connecticut.

Tucker, G. (1996) *National Childbirth Trust Book of Pregnancy, Birth and Parenthood.* Oxford University Press, Oxford.

Tuffnell, D.J. Bryce, F., Johnson, N., Lilford, R.J. (1989) Simulation of cervical changes in labour: reproducibility of expert assessment. *Lancet* ii, 1089–90.

Twycross, R.G. (1994) Opioids. In: *Textbook of Pain*, 3rd edn. (eds P.D. Wall & R. Melzack), pp. 943–62. Churchill Livingstone, Edinburgh.

Ueland, K., Hansen, J.M. (1969) Maternal cardiovascular dynamics: 2 Posture and uterine contractions. *American Journal of Obstetrics and Gynecology* 103(1) 1–7.

UKCC (1991a) *Midwife's Code of Practice.* UKCC, London.

UKCC (1991b) *Midwives Rules.* UKCC, London.

UKCC (1992) *Standards for the Administration of Medicines.* UKCC, London.

Ussher, J.M. (1996) Female sexuality and reproduction. In: *Reproductive Potential and Fertility Control* (C.A. Niven & A. Walker). Butterworth Heinemann, London.

Vangen, S., Stoltenberg, C., Schei, B. (1996) Ethnicity and use of obstetric analgesia. *Ethnicity and Health* 1(2), 161–7.

Vanner, R.G. (1993) Mechanisms of regurgitation and its prevention with cricoid pressure. *International Journal of Obstetric Anaesthesia* 29(4), 207–215.

Varneyburst, H. (1983) The influence of consumers in the birthing movement. *Topics in Clinical Nursing* 5, 42–54.

Velvovsky, I., Platnov, K., Ploticher, V., Shugom, E. (1960) *Painless Childbirth Through Psychoprophylaxis.* Foreign Languages Publishing House, Moscow.

Velvovsky, I.Z. (1954) *Psychoprophylactic.* Medguiz, Leningrad.

Vogler, J.H. (1993a) The first stage of labour. In: *Maternity and Gynecologic Care: The Nurse and the Family*, 5th edn. (I.M. Boback & M.D. Jensen), Chapter 17. Mosby, St Louis.

Vogler, J.H. (1993b) The second and third stages of labour. In: *Maternity and Gynecologic Care: The Nurse and the Family*, 5th edn. (I.M. Boback & M.D. Jensen), Chapter 18. Mosby, St Louis.

Vogt, J.J., Meyer-Schwarz, M.T., Foehr, R. (1973) Motor, thermal and sensory factors in heart rate variation. A methodology for indirect estimation of intermittent muscular work and environmental heat loads. *Ergonomics* 16, 45–60.

Walco, G.A., Cassidy, R.C., Schechter, N.L. (1994) Pain, hurt and harm. *New England Journal of Medicine* 331(8), 541–4.

Waldenström, U. (1988) Midwives' attitudes to pain relief during labour and delivery. *Midwifery* 4(2), 48–57.

Waldenström, U., Nilsson, C-A. (1992) Warm tub bath after spontaneous rupture of membranes. *Birth* 19(2), 57–63.

Wall, P.D. (1964) Presynaptic control of impulses at the first central synapse in the cutaneous pathway. *Progress in Brain Research* 12 (whole volume), 92–118.

Wall, P.D. (1970) The sensory and motor role of impulses travelling in the dorsal column towards cerebral cortex. *Brain* 93(3), 505.

Wall, P.D., Jones, M. (1991) *Defeating Pain: The War Against a Silent Epidemic*. Plenum, London.

Wall, P.D., Sweet, W.H. (1967) Temporary abolition of pain. *Science* 155, 108–109.

Wallace, B., Fisher, L.E. (1987) *Consciousness and Behavior*, 2nd edn. Allyn Bacon, Boston.

Wand, J.S. (1990) Carpal tunnel syndrome in pregnancy and lactation. *Journal of Hand Surgery* 15(1), 93–5.

Wang, E., Small, F. (1989) Infection in pregnancy. In: *Effective Care in Pregnancy and Childbirth* (I. Chalmers, M. Enkin & M.J.N.C. Keirse), pp. 535–64. Oxford University Press, Oxford.

Waters, J., Thomas, V. (1995) Pain from sickle cell crisis. *Nursing Times* 91(16), 29–31.

Watson, N., Mander, R. (1995) Advertising infant formula in the maternity area. *MIDIRS Midwifery Digest* 5(3), 338–41.

Way, W.L., Way, E.L. (1992) Opioid analgesics and antagonists. In: *Basic and Clinical Pharmacology*, 5th edn. (ed. B.G. Katzung). Prentice Hall, Norwalk.

Welchew, E. (1995) *Patient Controlled Analgesia*. B.M.J. Publishing Group, London.

Welford, H. (1996) Postnatal depression: focusing on a neglected issue. *Midwives* 109(1301), 165–7.

Werner, W.E.F., Schauble, P.G., Knudson, M.S. (1982) An argument for the revival of hypnosis in obstetrics. *American Journal of Clinical Hypnosis* 24, 149–71.

Wertz, R.W., Wertz, D.C. (1979) *Lying In... : A History of Childbirth in America*. Free Press, New York.

Whelton, J. (1993) Fetal medicine. In *Midwifery Practice: A Research-Based Approach* (J. Alexander, V. Levy & S. Roch), Chapter 4. Macmillan, London.

WHO (1991) *A Proposed Standard International Acupuncture Nomenclature: Report of a WHO Scientific Group*. World Health Organization, Geneva.

Wideman, M., Singer, J. (1984) The role of psychological mechanisms in preparation for childbirth. *American Psychologist* 39, 1357.

Widmer, L.K. (1978) *Peripheral Venous Disorders*. Hans Huber, Bern.

Wilkie, D.J., Savedra, M.C., Holzemer, W.L., Tesler, M.D., Paul, S.M. (1990) Use of the McGill Pain Questionnaire to measure pain: a meta-analysis. *Nursing Research* 39(1), 36–41.

Williams, M, Booth, D. (1985) *Antenatal Education: Guidelines for Teachers*, 3rd edn. Churchill Livingstone, Edinburgh.

Williams, S., Hepburn, M., McIlwaine, G. (1985) Consumer view of epidural anaesthesia. *Midwifery* 1(1), 32–6.

Willis, W.D. (1982) Control of nociceptive transmission in the spinal cord. In: *Progress in Sensory Physiology* (eds H. Autrum, D. Offoson, E. Perl & R.F. Schmidt), pp. 8–39. Springer-Verlag, New York.

Willson, H. (1992) Painful facts. *Nursing Times* 88(35), 32–3.

Wilshin, J., Wilson, P. (1991) A question of delivery. *Nursing Times* 87(43), 52–4.

Wilson, M.E. (1974) The neurological mechanisms of pain. *Anesthesia* 29(4), 407.

Wilson, P. (1990) *Antenatal Teaching*. Faber, London.

Wilson, S. (1994) Obstetric anthropology. *Student British Medical Journal* 2(4), 477.

Wolff, B.B., Langley, S. (1977) Cultural factors and the response to pain. In: *Culture Disease and Healing: Studies in Medical Anthropology* (D. Landy), Section 34, p. 313. Collier Macmillan, London.

Woods, M. (1989) Pain control and hypnosis. *Nursing Times* 85(7), 38–40.

Woolf, C.J., Thompson (1994) Stimulation-induced analgesia: transcutaneous electrical nerse stimulation (TENS) and vibration. In: *Textbook of Pain*, 3rd edn. (eds P.D. Wall & R. Melzack) Churchill Livingstone, Edinburgh.

Woolf, V. (1925) On being ill. In: (V. Woolf). *Collected Essays IV*. The Hogarth Press, London.

Woolridge, M. (1992) Dubious research on a dubious practice. *MIDIRS Midwifery Digest* 2(2), 198–9.

Woolridge, M.W. (1986) The 'anatomy' of infant sucking. *Midwifery* 2(40), 164–71.

Wraight, A. (1992) Pain in labour: the 1990 confidential enquiry into the relief of pain in labour. *Research and the Midwife Conference Proceedings*, 1990, University of Manchester.

Wraight, A. (1993) Coping with pain. In: *Pain and its Relief in Childbirth* (G. Chamberlain, A. Wraight & P. Steer), Chapter 8. Churchill Livingstone, Edinburgh.

Wright, S. (1988) Why use measurement? *Nursing Times* 84(4), 73–5.

Yang, M.M.P., Kok, S.H. (1979) Further study of the neurohumoral factor endorphin in the mechanism of acupuncture analgesia. *American Journal of Clinical Medicine* 7, 143–8.

Yang, Z., Cai, T., Wu, J. (1984) Psychological aspects of components of pain. *Journal of Psychology* 118, 135–46.

Yelland, S. (1995) Using acupuncture in midwifery care. *Modern Midwife* 5(1), 8–11.

Yudkin, P., Frumar, A.M., Anderson, A.B.M., Turnbull, A.C. (1979) A retrospective study of induction of labour. *British Journal of Obstetrics and Gynaecology* 86(4), 257–65.

Zborowski, M. (1952) Cultural components in responses to pain. *Journal of Social Issues* 8, 16–30.

Ziemer, M.M. Paone, J.P., Schupay, J., Cole, E. (1990) Methods to prevent and manage nipple pain in breastfeeding women. *Western Journal of Nursing Research* 12(6), 732–44.

Zimmerman, L., Pazehl, B., Duncan, K., Schmitz, R. (1989) Effects of music in patients who had chronic cancer pain. *Western Journal of Nursing Research* 11(3), 298–309.

Zimmerman, M. (1981) Mechanisms of pain and pain therapy. *Triangle* 20(1/2), 7–18.

Index